the serial killer letters

A Penetrating Look Inside the Minds of Murderers

By Jennifer Furio

The Charles Press, Publishers
Philadelphia

The Charles Press, Publishers
Post Office Box 15715
Philadelphia, PA 19103
(215) 496-9616 Telephone
(215) 496-9637 Telefax
mailbox@charlespresspub.com
http://www.charlespresspub.com

Library of Congress Cataloging-in-Publication Data

The serial killer letters: a penetrating look
inside the minds of murderers / Jennifer Furio.
p. cm.
ISBN 0-914783-84-X (alk. paper)
1. Serial murderers — United States — Correspondence.
2. Serial murderers — United States — Psychology — Case studies.
3. Serial murderers — United States — Biography.
I. Furio, Jennifer.
HV6529.S47 1998
364.15'23'092273 — dc21
98-21990

Printed in the United States of America

Second Printing

Contents

Acknowledgments

Putting together this book has been an incredible experience for me. Immersion in the criminal subculture and becoming involved, sometimes very closely, with these men was frightening, confusing and fascinating. Coming through it was not easy.

My goal was to produce a book that would not only have important scholarly value, but mainstream true crime appeal as well. This was not an easy task and many people helped me along the way. Besides my incredibly understanding husband and children, I had two strong sources of support and expertise. One was Lauren Meltzer, my editor at The Charles Press, Publishers — a perfectionist with a keen eye who knew exactly how to draw a balance out of me and would not let me settle for a less than top quality. I must thank Lauren for being so patient with me, a first-time author; I appreciated her willingness to take my many phone calls and to respond so thoughtfully to my repeated requests for direction. I'm grateful for having had the opportunity to work with such an accomplished professional.

I would also like to thank Ruth Stansfield, not only for her editing and her fine writing, but also for absorbing herself so thoroughly in the task of bringing the book to completion. Ruth had the rare ability to understand other people's visions — Lauren's intent and logic and my personal perspective and goals.

I would like to thank my family for standing beside me through this often difficult project. In a very real sense, my husband and two children became involved along with me in a very dark world. They endured and understood the emotional ups and downs that I went through. For the past two years we were very isolated in an odd world of our own. I can't adequately thank them for the sacrifices they made, individually and as a family.

Finally, I want to offer my sincere gratitude to all of the men who corresponded with me, both those whose letters were published and those we decided, for one reason or another, not to include. I fully appreciate how difficult it was for them to talk openly about very personal and painful subjects — their rage, anguish, shame, confusion and remorse, the loneliness of prison life and the agonizing frustration of dealing with the legal system. I thank them and commend them for their courage.

One last thing. I must stress that throughout this whole project, I always had the victims and their families in my mind and heart — and I always will. To a great extent, the depth of pain these women were forced to endure and the grief that their families are probably still experiencing made me want to create this book in the first place. I believe that until we understand what drives people to kill one another, there will always be more victims. It is my hope that with greater understanding, more awareness and grace, there will be less hate and less victimization.

J.F.

Preface

November 16, 1996

Dear Mr. Buono:

I am writing to you because I am interested in finding out what happened to you — how you ended up in prison. Right now I am corresponding with several incarcerated men who have been convicted of murder. Some of them say they're innocent. Others admit their guilt.

I know that there are innocent men in prison and guilty men. Those who are innocent are suffering for crimes they did not commit. And maybe the guilty men also suffer because they have to live with themselves. And many of them, both guilty and innocent, are facing death, living isolated on death row with no one to talk to.

What about you? Are you guilty or innocent? I don't think it's possible for anyone, no matter how tough their skin, to ignore and abandon past "transgressions," especially when they are the worst, most violent hate crimes imaginable. I know what I've read about you in books, but I realize that these "biographical" books are not always accurate. I would like to hear your side of the story. Also, please rest assured that I'm an open-minded person and that I have no interest in judging you. In my opinion, honesty is all important. It can set you free. It can help you live with yourself. That is not to imply that I'm assuming you're guilty — I just want you to tell me — honestly — how you ended up in prison.

Some of the guys who have written to me have bravely owned up to their crimes and have made generous efforts to explain what happened to them. Some have told me about their childhoods, most of which were horrible beyond belief. It's clear to me (but I don't think always to them) that many of them were victims themselves — victims of abuse and neglect. The things they've told me about their early years and especially about their mothers are so awful, it makes me cringe. Not that a bad childhood works as an excuse for killing people, but it certainly can have catastrophic effects later in life. The stories I have heard are scary and tragic, but I still want to know. Don't you agree that it's important to understand why things happen? Especially when they are as drastic as a murder conviction — or many murder convictions?

If you're guilty, can you admit it? Or maybe you already have. What drove you to commit the crimes? Do you know? Or haven't you been able to figure it out? Maybe you haven't even tried to understand. If that's the case, maybe now is a good time to start. I am not afraid to hear the truth. No matter how frightening or shocking your story is, I would be grateful if you would share it with me.

If you're innocent, isn't it important that others know? That you make an effort to make your voice heard? I'm sure you've already told the people who needed to know (lawyers, judges, jury, etc.), but will you consider sharing this information with me?

I realize I'm asking you to divulge some very personal information, so it's only fair that I tell you a little about myself. I live in Bellingham, Washington and I teach Sunday School. I am married and have two young children. I spend most of my time taking care of them. This may seem like a boring life to you, but it's not to me. In fact, my love for my children is indirectly related to why I wrote to you in the first place. I love my children and I don't want them to have to grow up into a world seething with hate and violence. Of course, I personally cannot stop either of these, but my thinking is that the more we understand how these things happen, the better equipped we'll be to approach them, deal with them and maybe even prevent them from occurring in the first place.

Even though I am frightened and sickened by these crimes, I also believe in grace. I really do. No matter how horrible the crime, I feel everyone deserves the opportunity to be forgiven.

Please write back to me. I know you don't know me and that it might be difficult to reveal this personal information to a complete stranger, but at least it will give you a chance to speak your mind. I'm here to listen to you with an open mind and an understanding heart.

Sincerely,
Jenny

The above is a letter that I sent to one of over 50 incarcerated men who have been convicted of murder and in most cases, serial murder. Most of them responded and over the past two and one-half years, we ended up developing quite an in-depth discourse — their half of which makes up a majority of this book. Not all of them were so keen on the idea of telling me anything. The following letter from a friend of Angelo Buono's, Kenneth Bianchi's partner in "The Hillside Stranglings," is a good example of someone who was very angry that I wrote in the first place:

December 18, 1996

Dear Mrs. Frio,

I have been authorized by Angelo Buono to respond to several letters you have written to him seeking correspondence with him. I am here to say: **KNOCK IT OFF!** If you cant take non-response as an answer, you've got problems and Mr. Buono does not care to be burdened with them. He's got more than enough of his own as an **INNOCENT** man, wrongfully and maliciously prosecuted, convicted and sentenced to die for CRIMES HE DID NOT COMMIT! He does not care to be used by you as your latest addition to your collection of "murderers" nor does he feel this is the way you should be spending your time as a wife, a mother, and still a young person. If the way you are spending your time and energy is to go around **DEMANDING** the attention of persons you believe to be serial killers, Honey, **YOU got problems and you need therapy!** And Mr. Buono is not a therapist. In short, Mr. Buono is NOT going to respond to your letters, and **I am telling you LAY off my man!** I trust I have made myself clear.

Signed,
P.O.

Even though Mr. Buono didn't want to have anything to do with me, his friend's letter addresses a valuable point: Why would a young mother like myself get involved with a dark project like this in the first place?

I suspect that the first thing a lot of people will think is that I am some kind of nut. Or that I have some kind of weird obsession with killers and that I am celebrating or glorifying them with this book. None of these is the case. I consider myself to be a pretty normal person and I'm interested in killers because I am afraid of them and sickened by the things they do. I believe that the more we know about people who commit these crimes, the better equipped we'll be to combat the hate and violence that is so prevalent in our world. I also suspect that a lot of people feel that subjects like this are simply too ugly to read about, that they'd rather just not know about them. I can fully appreciate this attitude, but I think it's important to educate ourselves about people who rape and murder. How else can we stop them — and, for that matter, help them?

Murder is so common these days that not a single day goes by that there isn't a news report of another tragic killing, the perpetrators of which are any race, any age, any gender. In some ways, serial killers are different. Defined in the literature as murderers who kill a succession of people (three or more) over a period of time (at least 30 days), serial killers are their own special breed of murderer, a subculture. Most are men, most kill women. Most of them are not insane. In fact, many seem completely normal, at least on the surface, meaning that they can easily live and lurk undetected in our communities, killing over and over again, never stopping until they get caught. This fact is frightening beyond words. Many of them kill complete strangers who they choose randomly, in other words, their crimes are often not personal in nature. And most of them do more than just kill; they also rape, torture and mutilate their victims. Most of the people who commit serial crimes seem to be grappling with some pretty intense "issues."

There are other reasons for my interest in murderers. Growing up, I was surrounded by murder — murder that was suspected of being the work of serial killers. When I was 11 and living in Redding, California, a man (allegedly Randall Woodfield) killed a mother and her 14-year-old stepdaughter who lived close to my house. About a year later, also in my home town, a 12-year-old girl I knew was raped and murdered. I vividly remember feeling so sorry that she would never reach adulthood and know what it was like to be married or have children, that her life was cut short at such a tragically young age. Also in the Redding area, around the same time, Cameron Hooker abducted a young woman named Colleen Stan, locked her up in a box the size of a coffin for ten years, and made her his sex slave.

In Sacramento, where I went to school, I lived in the same apartment complex where Richard Chase, the notorious "Vampire Killer," had lived a few years before. While I was in college, I knew a woman who was murdered after her car broke down late at night on Highway 99. Only blocks from my house in Sacramento, serial killer Dorothea Puente had murdered as many as 13 men and women in the late 1980s. Later, after I had gotten married, three librarians were shot and killed in our local library. Then, a woman was taken from her car at the grocery store where I shopped almost every day and was raped, killed and decapitated. And when we moved to Bellingham, Washington, I discovered this was where Kenneth Bianchi, one of the "Hillside Stranglers," had committed his last two murders.

It seemed that everywhere I went people were being killed. And I know I wasn't the only one who experienced this. This is the case all across America. Somehow when it happens to someone you know, it seems a little more real and a lot more frightening. Gradually, I wanted to know more about the men who were doing the murdering. I just couldn't fathom the kind of person who would be motivated or — even worse — find pleasure in causing an innocent person blinding fear, dizzying pain and death. Who could do something like that? And more importantly, why?

Even though research has been conducted and books have been written on serial killers and the motivations behind their crimes, much of it is inconclusive and general. For my own peace of mind and safety, for the protection of my children and the rest of the world, I wanted to know more. So, I began to write letters to convicted serial killers. I asked them quite bluntly: "If you are guilty, why did you do it, and if you're innocent, why are you in prison?" Some of them admit their guilt, others deny it. In fact, many of them deny it. This does not mean that their letters lack value in any way. To the contrary, denials of guilt are every bit as informative as admissions of guilt. You can decide for yourself who you choose to believe.

I started this project to find answers to my own questions, but it didn't take me long to realize that these letters were too important to keep to myself. I think you will agree with me that they are simply remarkable. After all, they are unedited, first-person accounts of incredible life experiences that most of us know nothing about, and situations and circumstances we cannot even imagine.

When I asked each of my correspondents for permission to publish their letters, some of them were furious, refusing because they thought I had misrepresented myself. They said they didn't know I was a writer and if they had, they wouldn't have opened up to me the way they did. (In all fairness to me, I had no intention of publishing their letters until far into the project, although I guess none of them believed this.) Others refused because they said they had written to me alone, not to the rest of the world. I have respected the wishes of those who did not want to be included in the book, but I didn't leave all of their letters out. With the two whose letters I included, I simply omitted their names and whenever necessary, I changed identifying information. The letters of those men who agreed to let me share their thoughts with others are printed exactly as I received them, word for word. Even the punctuation and emphases (underlining, etc.) have been copied with painstaking accuracy.

I cannot begin to express how very grateful I am to these men for allowing me this window into their hearts and souls. I am especially appreciative to those who made the extremely difficult effort to speak openly and intimately about experiences that are painful, embarrassing and ugly. It is my opinion that everyone of them succeeded in communicating their stories with a depth and impact never before achieved. I thank them for that.

A note on the text: I had an extremely difficult time finding information for the "biographies" that precede each set of letters. Every source I checked seemed to have different information! Birth dates, charges, sentences and crimes committed differed from source to source. In some cases, even the names of victims and family members did not agree. I have made every effort to track down the most accurate information and whenever possible I cross-checked it with court records.

Edward Spreitzer

I t makes me sad just to look at the photograph of 15-year-old Edward Spreitzer. He is wearing a new three-piece suit, shiny new shoes. His grandmother has her arm looped through his and she smiles proudly. After all, Edward is her first grandchild and this is a momentous occasion; it may have taken Edward a while (he repeated 5th grade three times), but he has finally graduated from 8th grade. Edward is smiling too, but it's a shy smile. He looks a little gawky, a little awkward.

What is so heartbreaking about this photograph and all the others that Edward's mother sent me of "Eddie" as a child, is that no one in his family — not even Eddie — could have dreamed that this sweet-smiling, redheaded boy with the toothy grin would soon end up on death row, a vicious killer convicted in the infamous "Chicago Ripper" murders. After a two-year killing spree with his alleged partners — Robin Gecht and two teenage brothers, Tommy and Andrew Kokoraleis — Spreitzer ended up turning himself in and telling authorities everything he knew about the murders — which of course seriously jeopardized the freedom of his partners. At the tender age of 21, Spreitzer had participated in killing, raping and

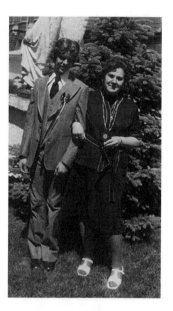

Edward Spreitzer with his grandmother on the day he graduated from 8th grade. Before long, he would end up on death row for his part in the "Chicago Ripper" murders.

mutilating dozens of women. Even though Spreitzer openly admits to his role in the murders, he says that he did them at the urging of Robin Gecht and his double-barreled shotgun. "I never ever did bad thing's alone and

I never ever will! I had gun's put in my face to force me to do the crime's. If it was not for this, I wouldn't be locked up."

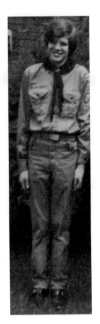

This certainly doesn't justify anything, but it does say something about the kind of guy Edward Spreitzer was at the time — weak, directionless, vulnerable, with no role models to speak of. He had problems at home with a mean stepfather who bullied and harassed him, and when his parents got fed up with him, they kicked him out. He moved from one menial job to the next and had a bad drug problem. "Sure I had a Drugs Problem. Everyone knew of that. Did Help come for that? No! I was kicked out instead. I was very vulnerable as soon as I walked out the door that day. If someone asked me to be in Porno movies, or Rob a Bank, or anything, I sure would have done it. I was not smart enough to say no, or think of it as being a bad thing. And no one would have told me it was bad."

Though he never quite admits it, Spreitzer may have looked up to Robin Gecht in the beginning. Apparently, Gecht offered him a job when he needed one and promised

At age 13½.

to teach him the carpentry trade. But nothing came of these offers. Instead,

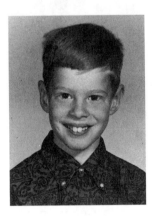

the only thing Spreitzer learned was that he was in a heap of trouble. He claims that his involvement with the murders started when Gecht threatened him: "When Robin found me, I was told he had pictures of me f - - king his wife, and that I [was the one, not Robin] who had cut her nipples off. And he would kill me. And if I went to the police, I would be locked up." Eddie believed Gecht.

Even though Spreitzer insists that he can't stand the sight of blood ("I pass out when I see blood, when the Doctor takes blood, I am on the floor. When I get a paper cut and I see blood, I am out on the floor. It don't matter how much blood, I will pass out), he was present at all of

1967, age 5.

the crimes committed by the Chicago Rippers and actually responsible for stabbing one victim and slicing off the breast of another. Spreitzer claims, in his halting style (he only recently learned to read and write from a fellow inmate): "I don't feel proud for what I did. How did it feel? I got sick and passed out. All the Blood! I didn't enjoy any of it. I guess that is why I went to the police, to once and for all to stop it. Killing was not fun for me, it never ever will be. I would have rather had me head blown off." But if this is true — that he would rather have had his head blown off — why didn't he choose that route, especially if, as he says, Robin threatened to shoot him if he didn't go along with the murders? He explains, "I was young and stupid, I didn't know better." And, pitiful as that explanation is, that is probably the truth.

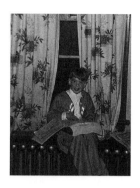

Edward Spreitzer seems so sweet and gentle in his letters that it is simply inconceivable to me that he killed and mutilated women. Perhaps the truth of the matter is that he was incapable of saying no to a man who seemed to have an iron hold on him — that is, if you believe his story about Robin Gecht. Is it possible that Spreitzer is remembering events in a way that he feels

Inscription on back, written by Eddie's mother, reads: "School play, singing & dancing on stage. St. Mary's, 1968."

exonerates him — that he would rather be seen as spineless than heartless? He seems earnest when he says, "I am not a bad person. There is no way for me to be happy. Lives were taken, in a Very Sick way. I am Sad, and feel very bad for all of this. I wish I could turn the time back, and all this never happened. But I can't. I will deal with what I done." I guess everyone "deals" with things like being a convicted killer in a different way.

Today Edward Spreitzer is on death row in Pontiac State Correctional Facility in Joliet, Illinois. His last attempt at getting a new trial was flatly denied.

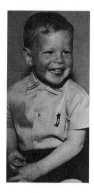

3 years old.

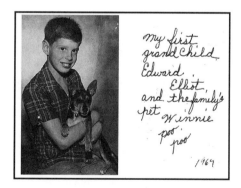

my first grand Child Edward Elliot, and the family's pet Winnie poo poo

1969

The Spreitzer Letters

June-10-11-97

Hi Jenny,

I am doing somewhat ok. I could be doing better. But we can write about that another time.

Jenny I love to write. But the problem is finding someone to write to. We are not very much liked. So we don't get much mail. But for myself alone, I do have a few pen friends. But they don't know of me being locked up. I don't feel good at all about that. But I am so lonely.

This is one reason you are hearing back from me. You say you would like to know me better. I have no problem with that. But understand only one thing. I am going to be myself. You will not have any games played, and I don't want none played on me.

Do you really host a Show about Serial Killers and write for a detective magazine?

Jenny, I am at this time still working on my appeals, this does not sound so hot with me. This could hurt me big time. You want me to be Honest. I might be able to get off Death Row, and I really want to. I don't need anything bad of me going around right now.

I don't know what you read. But if it is good that you won't judge me.

So now Jenny. as for me beinging courageous, I don't feel like this at all, I feel stupid for what I did. See there are thing's you don't know as to why I did what I did. And if I had to do this all over again, I would keep my mouth shut. Now don't get this wrong. I am not the Heartless person you read about. But no one else knows of this, because no one bothered to try and get to know the real Edward Spreitzer.

Do you want the real Edward Spreitzer?

Because like you, I myself feels horrible of how these people were killed. I feel bad for the families. But I have to deal with this every day. If I am put to Death for this, fine I will go. But there are only 2 people that do know the truth, so I am with no one to answer too.

Here is the real Edward Spreitzer. Killing was not my way of doing things,

4

that was pushed or forced onto me by a man (Robin Gecht) and a double barrel shot gun at my head. I don't feel proud for what I did.

How did it feel? I got sick and passed out. All the Blood! I didn't enjoy any of it. I guess that is why I went to the police, to once and for all to stop it. Killing was not fun for me, it never ever will be. I would have rather had me head blown off. It sure would have felt much better then what I feel now.

I have much hate for a person like myself. From what I seen, there is no Rage, it was more of a perversion. Robin was very picky on what he wanted.

That's enough for now. How about you? Besides writing with Honest Killers, What do you do? I see you are 29 with a Baby Girl.

are you married?

Me I am now 36 will be 37 Jan-5-98. I have learned to read & write when I got locked up. And have been looking for pen friends. What I am really trying to do is find the right person to have for a wife. I never had that. I want to have this even if it is for the 3 or 4 years I may have left. I never had or felt the Love of a good Women.

If there is anyone you know age 25 to 40, feel free to pass on my name & address. But if you don't, please don't feel bad of this. I will understand.

Jenny. If you are not hurt of me asking. What are you like? Besides having a Beautiful Name. Tell me of yourself. If you wish, you can send a picture of yourself. But I myself can't do the same, for last year after that Richard Speck Video Tape our prison removed all picture taking.

Well, I am sending this out now, so you will know I did get your letter, and if you write to me, I will write back to you.

Take care Jenny! And write back.

Yours Truly,
Edward Spreitzer.

P.S. Calling me Eddie is just fine. I may want to call you Beautiful or Sexy. Can I please do this?

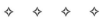

June-28-29-97

Hi Jenny,

I got your letter yesterday. I was so glad to hear back from you, and now I have the weekend to sit and spend time with you.

So Jenny sit back and relax. first you will hear of my life before Robin. to my very first time seeing him.

But first I have a few thing of your letter to talk about.

You say I seem so sad. I very much am, for I lost my case again, and there really does now look like I will be put to Death. I stopped all my letter writing. But I will keep you and one other. My heart is not into having any more. Plus it cost way too much.

You Welcomed me to write. so I will do that.

There is no way for me to be happy. Lives were taken, in a Very Sick way. I can't be happy over that. I am Sad, and feel very bad for all of this. I wish I could turn the time back, and all this never happened. But I can't. I will deal with what I done. The Families will have peace with that.

I could be looking at maybe 2 to 3 year's on my appeals, and that will be over. I will go with out a fight.

I should have known better to ask for such things, a Wife. We can't find Women to write with, let alone marry one.

It was not right of me to ask. I will stick with writing with you.

I only heard of a Little Girl. I didn't know of your other children or there ages. I am sure they are a hand full. I am also sure you're a great Mother, and you are having the time of your life with them. I understand it gets hard at time's. When they both grow up, they will understand. It will get better Jenny. Sorry to hear your Husband is away a lot. What does your Husband do that keeps him away from home?

I learned to read and write from a guy named James Free. he was put to Death 2 years ago in a first double execution in this state. James started working with me in 1990. Yes it was very hard. But I am way happy that I can. There are way more that still can't read or write, and they don't want to learn. I wanted too, and stayed on it. James wouldn't let me walk away from this.

So now you can see how I turned out. Penmanship is just me taking my time. But I would feel it is nice to read.

Jenny Thank You for writing with me. I know you & I will be good friends and with you home alone a lot, and me being lonely. We can have a good friendship, everyone needs someone to talk with. I know I do.

Sometime's I even need a shoulder to cry on. I do hope I can have that with you. and yes you have my shoulder to cry on anytime you need it. I may be a big person. I am very much gentle.

Now as for my Life before Robin [Gecht]. I had so many from one to another jobs, and that for me was hard. my longest job was bel-fast auto part's 1 1/2 years. all I did was sit in back, and when a part was needed, I would get it. I turned brake drum's, and much more. $5.00 an hour I was ok, had a car. But I was kicked out of home. my car was my home, and winter's, I went from one friend till I over did my Welcome.

Winter's was hell for me.

Then on my 20th Birthday, a party was given for me. I met Christina

Kokoraleis, and we became Girlfriend & Boyfriend. for about 15 months we were joint at the hip.

But one day she moved, that hurt. I lost my job, and went to find her.

Jenny, Christina was a nice girl, there was no sex, we just kissed and felt each other's bodies. Christina was a Virgin. And she was ever so Beautiful.

Well, Andy [Kokoraleis, Christina's brother] told me where to find her. I broke every speed limit to get to her. She babysat for Robin's kids. It was around January of 1982 when I was hunting for a job. I showed up to get Christina and she was going to help me find a job, mostly with the applications.

Well that was the first time I met Robin, and his shotgun. When I seen that door blow up, and the sound of the shotgun, I couldn't hear for a week. I went back, because Christina was still there. Andy was fired so Robin was looking for a helper. So I got the job.

Now all was cool for the first 5 monthes. One day Robin snapped, I drove his wife to the Hospital. Robin cut off her nipples. She was kept in for 5 days, I ran, and Robin came looking for me.

When he found me, I was told he had pictures of me fucking his wife, and I cut her nipples off. And he would kill me. And if I went to the police, I would be locked up.

I said no, get the fuck away.

I was ok at that time, for it was day lite, and I was walking into a food store. People everywhere. But he was everywhere. I know the truth, and he was scared. So was I.

But let me tell you of the pictures he might have had. It was around June or July 82. Rose [Robin's wife] was laying in the sun, and I was talking with her of painting around the window's. I was told how Robin didn't like tan lines. So I was putting lotion on, and she turned over, and I put lotion on her breast's. I didn't do anything else. I don't even know if this picture thing is true.

Jenny I was a big Marijuana smoker back then, But, Robin really wanted to kill me. I had this, and maybe the picture's hanging over my head.

I tried to talk with my Stepfather, he felt I was playing a game, so I was forced to do what I did.

Jenny, Please know this. I went to many people for help. And I got none. I even called the police, and had all his gun's taken. But at the time, I didn't know of all the gun's he had in the attic. And the police didn't go up there.

I was stuck, and no were else to go.

When all these murder's happened, I was sick all the time, see I pass out when I see blood, it has been like that my whole life, even in here, when the Doctor takes blood, I am on the floor. When I get a paper cut and I see blood, I am out on the floor. It don't matter how much blood, I will pass out.

So you wrote to Robin. Since I started reading. And you will see why I really wanted to learn. I wanted to read of what everyone said from the police investigation, because I was given the police reports.

I was upset to learn that Robin did have 7 pictures of me and Rose, and they are of how I told you. They are loged in with the police.

I don't care if you write to Robin. But I would be careful, he has a big family, and they might be just like him. I learned much of him, locked up 17 time's for rape High School Girl's. 400 speeding and parking ticket's. 401 gun's came out of his house on Oct-10-1982. 351 knives. (Mostly for Hunting) and much more.

I didn't know of you writing to him, I don't and will never want to see him ever again.

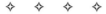

6-29-97. 11:30 AM

Yes I went to bed at 3:30 AM writing to you. No I don't have bad dream's. I like to write late at night. Everyone in bed, no one to bother me.

And as for Robin beinging an excellent liar, yes I did know of that, But after I was locked up.

As for Robin really Believes he's not involved. He should be, the courts want so bad to give him more cases. But they don't have enough on him to do that, and they are hurt by this.

I was talked to by an Elgin Police Lieutenant on June 19-97. I am waiting to hear back from him. Because he was to go see Robin.

So I will see how that went. I will write him (Police) next week.

Robin's only locked up for One murder. The Girl lived, and picked him out in a line up. I was so happy for that. All this was over. No more killings.

Now as for this fascination of Breasts. That Jenny was Robin's sick mind. Don't get me wrong, I don't [not] have a sick mind. I have and always will have a fascination for Breasts, Legs, feet, ass, and everything else on a female Body. And they will be alive.

I am not one to hurt Women, or even kill women. Jenny, I know you don't understand this. I don't myself.

All I can do is write down how I feel. Jenny I really didn't like what I was forced to do, it was the last thing on Earth I wanted to do.

My year's as a teen, and even some 6 years ago, was why I love Breasts. As a teen, I loved Girls, I loved the feel of there Bodies, I was kicked out of a grade school for having sex. I loved having sex, on Buses, in cabs, and on train's. Yes so people can watch.

And 6 year's ago, I had a 40 year old Lady who was writing, and also came to see me. Well, I am fully up on why Breasts are important to Women.

The Lady came down with a Baby she had just had. I had gotten to suck on her Breasts, and taste Breasts Milk. Jenny I enjoyed myself.

I still write to this Lady, But with her last move, it is hard for her to come see me.

Breasts are a Very Good thing. I am one to fully appreciate the Beauty of them. I like to see them, write about them, and feel them in my hands and mouth. Also the rest of the Body.

You say I can keep writing to you about yourself, and myself, and you will answer question's I was so glad to hear this Jenny.

I was scared that you would be scared, and you would not write back. But you did. I am very glad of this Jenny. Yes I do want To Know about you, and I will be glad to tell you of myself. But for me in here, there are no limits of what I can write on paper, and the same is for you.

But, are there limits of what I can write with you? Can I write and be free to write the way I feel? Yes there are things I wish to ask of about you, as also to write if myself, you & I being alone all the time. A good friendship can be what we need.

How would you feel allowing me to call? With the phone, if you allow this, there is a time limite of 35 min. But we are free to speak our mind's. This will be nice when you & I are so lonely. You can have a friend to talk with. I can only use the phone 2 times a week. Think about this, I don't want to rush you. I would love to have someone to talk with. And I sure don't want you to do anything you feel is wrong.

Don't be scared of me calling. I know you are married, I will not hurt that, you can even ask you Husband if this is ok. I don't do anything behind his back.

Now Jenny. Yes I was coersed into this. Me by myself would never hurt ever hurt a Woman, How could I? God put them on Earth, and made them look so Beautiful & Sexy. I am ever so glad of this. You are a Beautiful & Sexy Woman, and I will be hurt if you feel I am wrong. Yes I will tell you of this.

You are not wrong, under different circumstances, I could have been married with kids. And had a good life. I think of what my life would have been like, who my wife would be, and all that.

I dream of this all the time. And since my last letter, I had my cousin check on a few things.

I had him go to our old house. Now the people who lived next to us. Well the Son I really wanted to find, because he seen how I was treated by the police. Well I found him along with his 3 Sister's.

I wrote to his family. He don't live at home, so if I had a chance to get back in court, this is still cool. For if the Girls write, it will be good for David to say what he saw. And it will not be planned out, for I don't write of my case.

I have no heard from them yet. I hope I be allowed to write.

David did call and tell my Lawyer what he seen. Now my Lawyer will see if he can get something done with that.

I am sending this out now.

Take Care Jenny,

Your Friend
Edward Spreitzer.

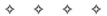

Hi Jenny,   July-16-97

I just now got your letter. And I am fast to write back.

Jenny I wish you would have written to me along time ago. Even though your letter was small, you had me in tears. I feel that I found a person who believes me, that is why I cryed. I have talked with my Lawyers for 11 years, and now as what I see, I just come out of the Seventh Circuit, and am appealing what they Decided.

I am looking at maybe 3 to 4 years till I am put to death.

Jenny, My letters are the real me 100% true. If you feel this will help me. then let's do this, I only want to keep my family out of this, for if this sets me free, I will be with my Parents, or even more there names.

I am so glad to hear you loved my letter. I put much of myself in my letters, I am just beinging myself, and that is what you wanted. I have nothing to hide. I am not a bad person Jenny, I write the way I feel, and now you see that. I truly love Women, I would never ever hurt any of them, no matter what.

You want to print my story, fine Let's do it!

and I will wait for you to write again. I still want to be allowed to call, or if you wish you can visit me face to face.

I am sending this for it is important.

Take Care.

Your Friend,
Edward Spreitzer.

July-22-23-97

Hi Beautiful.

I am doing fine, and hope the same for you and your Family.

I have been unable to sleep. Don't get this wrong, it has me thinking of You Loving my last letter. You say you will write a long letter. I am sure to keep my eyes open for that, and I will be fast to answer back on it. I have nothing else to do. I have one person to write with, and you see who that is, for my letter is in your hands. It does me good to write with you. You say I am Sweet and Human, and people need to see this.

People have seen this many time's over, the officers who work here, when they need parts' for their car's, truck's, I know of when part's are put on sales. For cars and trucks for sale. You see this paper, the trade or Buy book I get. well it covers 3 States, turn it over, you can see some of the great deals around me. I am known on this unit to help others in finding some great deals.

You say I have So much personality, and so much to give. My personality has always been the same. I have to see, hear, or read of any man that hurts a women, there is no reason for that. That goes the same for Kid's. And this is all I hear about on the news day & night.

I don't have no respect for a man who does harm to a women & kids. This Dead Beat Dads. We have a station on the radio that is nothing but this 24 hr's a day all year round. that is sad! But men are so really Stupid out in the free world.

I would love to have a family. These men have, and now they want out.

Just like now. I read of a Lady who had pleased 300 men in 10 hr's, and, another girl want's to do 400. They will have this on every talk show soon, I don't understand thing's like this. My first thought. Where did they get 300 men. I would feel some had Wifes, kids. This was all Video Taped, and is on sale World Wide. I don't see how anyone can be proud of this. The Women, or the Men. I can look in any paper and find a job even pushing a broom for $5.00 an hour. that will be fine by me. I wunder what this Women's family think's. 300 men, and one will go for 400. ouch. How can someone think of doing this?

Personally, mine is fine. I am ever so glad that you like it so much, even more that you allow me to be myself in my letter's. I have a Big Heart in me, and it is filled with nothing but Good.

So what I am 5'10" at 240 lbs. I am nothing but a Big Teddy Bear. I could carrie you in my arm's all day long. I would be ever so Gentle.

Everyone on this unit knows I don't play games, and I don't want any of that around me. I am here doing my time, I don't need friend's in here. I get by just fine. Everyone knows how I am, if I can help when it is needed, I do what I can. No one has any problems at all with me. So I am left alone. I have nothing to fear from these guy's. See all us guy's who have been on the Row for along time, we hang out together. the new ones coming in now, are so young, and Wild, more foolish if anything.

I just want away from all this. I put my heart in every letter. Because this is a Special thing for me to have. I know what you want. I have no trouble with that. But at the same time, I wanted to hear of your Sexy Self. I don't want for you to be hurt of this in any way. I guess I will hear from you on this part of my letter. I hope I did no harm by calling you Beautiful and Sexy. I do hope I can be allowed to call you Beautiful and Sexy.

I truly feel that you are a Very Beautiful and Sexy Lady. I do feel good telling you this. I do hope you smiled when hearing of this.

I wish I could send you a picture of myself. But we are no longer allowed to get them. I would Love to see who I am writing with. But it wouldn't be fair, for you couldn't get one of myself.

But Jenny, this is left up to you . I will write to my Mom, and see if she can send you one of me. I have very long Red Hair, Mom loves it so much, and she also has Red Hair.

I take after my Mom, I am cool with this. I hope you are also.

Thank You for thinking of me as beinging Sweet and Human, and most of all, for having so much personality.

You are hearing of the real Edward Spreitzer, and that is what you so much wanted.

I am sending this out.

Take care Beautiful! Write again!

> Your Friend,
> Edward Spreitzer.

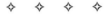

Aug-1-2-3-97

Hi Beautiful.

I am doing much better, now that I heard from you on my letter, I hope you and your Family is doing Well.

Now as for your letter, I see I have much to answer. I have all weekend, so let me get started by saying that I am most Glad to hear of you beinging so happy of reading my letter's. You would never believe just how you have me feeling at this time.

Come Monday Aug-4, I am calling my Lawyer. I have Proof that the Police lied on the stand. I will have copies made and set out to you. Because this is a major thing as to why I am locked up, and will be put to Death. I have 10 other thing's that will stop me from beinging put to Death, over the next few letter's. I am putting thing's together to show you I don't belong here at all.

The failure of having none of my Lawyer's to investigate this has hurt me so bad. They don't even care to have me DNA tested. They say it is too late. Most of my Lawyer's would have told you I didn't have a Legal leg to stand on, so they all have me dead and gone already.

Yes I as well as my Family were poor. I remember back in 1968 or 1969 we lived in a Van in the country, I was about 8 or 9.

My Mom was running from her husband, and we had no were to go, my Sister & I played in the woods around the Van, we were there the full summer and half the Winter. I know of this because I have no toe nails from the frost bite, it was a really Bad winter, sometimes we couldn't even get out, because the door's of the Van were frozen shut.

How did I do in School? Very bad, I had special classes. I did the 5th grade 3 time's. I was 15 when I graduated Grad School. I passed by the skin of my teeth, it was more with them special classes, for read & math. The teacher of them special classes was also our Babysitter. I had a big Crush on her. I didn't have it in me to want to learn, I didn't even like going to School. I was so very slow. I got my ass kicked everyday, and was made fun of. I just didn't fit in.

How did I get along with the Police? I was doing fine, I took a lie test's, don't know if I passed or not. I told the police everything I knew, and even took them out to show were the Bodies were.

All was fine till my Stepfather showed up, and told the police I was a lier, don't believe anything I say.

Well at that time, I wished I was dead, the next 5 day's was pure hell. Detective Flynn and his partner kicked my ass. I was taken out on Nov-8 at 1:30 AM it was raining. We got to a park call Shiller Wood's, over by a Big Hill, a shallow hole was dug. I was pushed into this, and covered to my neck in mud. I had Detective Flynn and partner fire there gun's in the ground next to my head. Both had reloaded 3 times. I had mud over my face, in my mouth. They finally ran out of Bullet's. I was pulled out, and was taken to one self wash car wash, and was cleaned up before I was allowed back into the car.

Now as there shift changed, 4 Detective's showed up, and the 4 ran me out to an old house in Roselle Ill. Roselle RD and Lake St. I was in this old house cuffed up, I had the ass kicking of my life. I asked them to kill me, I was hurting, Bleeding, and everytime I passed out, the 4 of them pissed on me to wake me up.

At one time they left, as was gone for over an hour. I couldn't yell for help, for they had something over my mouth, and I seen 2 Roselle Police car's.

When they got back, I was put in the car, and was going back to the station. An Assistant States Attorney Bukey & Detectives Flynn and Partner took me out. We pulled in to a picknick area across the street from St Mary Cemetery.

I was asked question's by the States Attorney, and if I didn't answer, I was hit with a Car Jack that was laying around. I was punched in the mouth by the States Attorney. The Big Ring he had on Broke my front tooth, and getting hit with the Jack, cracked 2 Ribes. I was taken to the Hospital. But there are no records of this, it was like I never went.

Was I ever pushed to answer questions? I did an 84 page Statement, on having my ass tortured to an inch of my life. I did whatever I could to get them to stop, and have them all happy.

Were I ever alone when I did bad thing's? I never ever did bad thing's alone and I never ever will! Is there ONE thing that you could think of that maybe set you over the edge, something or someone that made you do thing's, thing's you could prove you wouldn't do again?

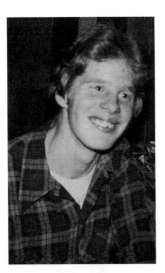

"I myself feels horrible of how these people were killed. I feel bad for the families. But I have to deal with this every day. If I am put to Death for this, fine I will go."

The only one person who had forced me into this was Robin, if it was not for him forcing me, I don't know what my life would be like. But for me having had many talkes with my Cousin's, I could live with my Brother's, and many pen friend's, I could work in a Auto Shop to driving limo's. I would love to go back to School first. My trouble's with the Law will be over. I follow every rule there is, I have stayed away from all trouble for the 15 year's I have been locked up. No one can say anything bad about me at all.

I was not set over the Edge. I had gun's put in my face to force me to do the crime's. If it was not for this, I wouldn't be locked up.

As for thing's I could prove I wouldn't do again. I can only say this, I have done everything to make myself a much better person, I can only Promise, this will never ever happen again from myself! I only hope I get the chance to show everyone I can keep my promise.

If you could even get life instead of Execution. What would that mean to my Family, my parents? I only know at this time how my Brother's would feel. They would be happy for me, I have not talked with my parent's for sometime. I would think Mom would be happy of this since I am her first Son.

Stepfather I don't know, he has been waiting for me to be put to Death, I heard this from his mouth once. I know I wouldn't be allowed to move back home, Stepfather would kill me first.

How old was I when this Started happening, at least, the planning? I was 21 year's of age when this started. There was no planning at all, it was a day by day thing. Robin would just have me to drive around. When he seen a girl he liked or disliked I would stop. Robin would have her in the back fucking her. Robin was the lead man in all of this.

When did I know this would Start? I didn't! from what I read in the Police reports, all this started on July-7-1978. I didn't know Robin at that time, I didn't even live in Illinois at that time. But I am not locked up for them crimes. I was in Kentucky the full year of 1978. My Stepfather's Brother had a Strock, I went out there to help with thing's he couldn't do. I even had to get my Driver's License's out there, so I could go to the store, post office, and drive a truck for his stain class company.

As for the Kokoraleis Brother's, I don't know much about them, I do know Robin lived next to them back from 1974 to 1979, and then Robin moved to Chicago. I first met Andy KoKoraleis on my Birthday of Jan-5-1980. After that everytime I seen Andy he was Drunk or High. I didn't know Tommy at all. No the KoKoraleis Brother's didn't force me into anything. I felt they were in the same boat I was in. But, I could be wrong. After all they did know Robin way longer then I have.

Now as for what I do in Prison, I fix T.V.s, Radio's, typewriter's, fan's, Watches, and whatever else, the Unit Coffee Pot, the Clocks, and the phones that the Inmates use. I fix thing's one at a time, so I don't have any problem's with the inmates, also I fix them in my cell, and I am only allowed so much at any one time. But that is good, I can get a T.V. fixed and only think of that, and everyone is happy.

As for learning to read & write. Well an inmate named James Free got me Reader's Digest The Large Type Edition. Here are some pages so you can see what I am talking about. I learned to read from this first. For me writing was the hard part. I had to learn how to write, as if I was writing to someone. It was like learning how to talk, to learn how to mean what I write, so the person will understand what I write. See like now, I am writing like I am talking with you, as if we were face to face, or my writing is no good, you would not understand anything. I find it most easy when I have a picture of who I am writing to, I can look and talk and write as if it was for real. It really does help.

No I am not crazy. This does help me to write.

When I was free, I was not pushed into learning. I did real bad in School, and that is if I even felt like goinging. I had no one to set me down and tell me how important an Education really is. Now I do know, and I am doing everything I can to learn what I don't know. It is hard at times. But I try my

Very Best. Yes I am trying to work on myself, and become a better person.

Do I work? No because I have a Sexual Offense, and some work is done around female Officer's, so I am not allowed to get a job. I don't have a problem with the female Officer's, I talk with them everyday & every night. James Free was put to Death 2 year's ago, and now when I have troubles I do have a few people to turn too, and one is a female Officer. I do get along with everyone. Inmates as well as Officer's Males and Females. Am I a Model prisoner? Yes I am, in here my prison record is spotless, and I will keep it that way. In here I choose to be good or bad. I choose good, because there is so much bad now, and no good. Everything around me is bad. I don't need any part of bad.

Yes you are so right this was so hard to answer. I did think of this. But I will answer from how I feel from my Heart.

I am too young to Die, and if by some chance I did wrong, I will take full responsibility for what I did, and only for what I did, I will not take responsibility for what other's do. I am still young. I can still turn out to be a good person and help other's. What would you do to keep your life? Well at this time, I will do whatever time is given me, and I am trying hard to get off Death Row. I want to keep my life. I will do anything to keep my life. And I will be Honest about keeping or trying to keep my life.

I do feel very bad for what has happened. I truly feel for the Families, my Heart and Prayer's go out for them everyday. I should be put to death. But that wouldn't bring back what I had done. I was young and Stupid, I didn't know better. If I didn't have a gun to my head, I wouldn't have had any part of this. I am not a bad person. The person who forced me to do what I did was.

No this was not hard to understand, the hard part was answering this, because people are an eye-for-an-Eye, and I really don't know if there is anything I can say or do that will make up for what I have done. But if I get the chance to prove I am a better person. I will do whatever I can. I do with all my Heart mean what I say. All I ask is for the one chance to prove this.

How will I be different? Well for the past 5 or 6 year's I have learned to read and write, and I have done everything I can to help other's. And if I can get off Death Row, the Very first thing I wish to do, is go back to School. After School, get a job where I can help other's. I can't do or say anything to prove any of what you read here. But given the chance, I will not let anyone down.

Now I will go back to you asking me through the crime scenes, as best as I can recall them.

My very first one was mostly of Robin showing me, Andy and Tom what will happen if we don't go along on this. A Black Female was picked up, Blindfolded, and Gagged. Robin shoot her point blank in the head. Put chains around her neck & legs, attached 2 Bowling Balls, and threw her in the water.

When I woke up, I was still in the Van in back of Robin's house. I understand her body was not found. And I am locked up for the crime.

Next was the drive by shooting of the 3 or 4 men standing by a pay phone. Robin had just gotten 4 new gun's and on the drive back home, I was driving. Robin loaded all 4 gun's, rolled down the window and opened fire. He just didn't care. I speeded up just to get him out of range. And when I slowed down, he open fired again. I put the gas pedal to the floor, went through 2 Red lights.

I was pulled over by Police. I got out of the Van, talked with the Police and cut up my Driver's License's right there in front of Robin, and the 2 Policemen. But we were both taken in anyway's, because the gun's were found, and were stolen. We were let go the next day.

Robin was pissed at what I had done, more for the lose of the gun's. 3 grand. I was not given a ticket for speeding. So I did get a new Driver's License's. But Robin didn't know of this. I left Robin at this point for about 2 weeks.

Next one was a Girl from Century 21. I could not drive, so I was in back drinking and getting High. And I passed out. When I woke up, I looked and seen I was at a Cemetery. I got in the driver's seat and put the lights on, and seen Robin & Andy hitting something with hammer's. When the Body fell over, I then seen it was a female, I cut the light's off, and went to the back of the Van, opened up the back door's, I puked, and popped open a Beer.

When Robin & Andy returned to the Van, they were covered from Head to Feet in blood. Robin had a 5 gallon bucket of water with Dish soap in, and him & Andy washed up. Robin dug a small hole to put the Bloody clothes in, and he & Andy had clean ones on. And we all drove home to Robin's home. I didn't go on the next two, for I got locked up for a car wreck I was in, and no one had the $300 to get me out. Yes, this was not looked into.

I wrecked up my Stepfather's 1977 Chevy Wagon, Summer of 1982 at the corner of Long Ave & Belmount Ave. I was in Jail for 3 weeks. My Driver's License's was taken from me at that time.

My next and last time out was around Sept-1982.

It was a Black Female behind a Motel in Villa Park. I was most scared of this one, Because from were we where, alote of people could see what was going on. We were next to a McDonalds parking lot, plus many other thing's and anyone could see us.

I was forced to remove one of her breasts with a wire with ring's on the end's. I would have rather taken a shot in my head. I felt the girl was dead before I removed her breasts. there was very little blood. when the wire cut in, the Breasts just fell to the ground, and I fell out also, because a car's headlights came back to where we were, Robin woke me up, and forced me to put my dick where here breasts was. I was not hard or couldn't get hard. I was sick and wanted to get away. It felt like putting it into a can of lard, wet and somewhat cold and warm, it was cold out at that time.

I do hope Jenny that this is ok, for it was most hard to write, and think back on this. But, I still do wish to help more if I can.

Your Friend.

Edward Spreitzer.

✧ ✧ ✧ ✧

Hi Beautful.   Sept-8-97

I am fine, and hope the same for you and your Family!

I hope all is well out there, for I have not heard from you for sometime, I have been trying to call, and have had no luck on that.

Yes I will worry till I hear from you, friends do that when they don't hear from them.

I miss your Beautiful sounding Voice. I hope you did get my letter, please let me know, for this place dose does at times too fail to send mail out.

In that case I would need to know, so I can findout what happened.

I am also scared that if you did get my letter, maybe I had hurt you by what I have put on paper, and you no longer wh want me for a friend. I hope this is not the case, you could just be busy with no time to write or talk on the phone.

I will try once a week to call. Plus you will know I am worried.

Jenny. I truly hope you and your Family are ok! Please Let me know of this!

Take Care!

Friends alway's.

Edward Spreitzer.

✧ ✧ ✧ ✧

Oct-7-8-9-97

Hi Jenny.

So Sorry for my delay in writing. We had some 3 shake downs, and I now have my cell back in order.

First is about your Phone. Do you know there is a Block on you Phone? I guess it was put on the last few day's or so.

I am not tripping of that. I enjoy writing so much more anyway's. But it was so nice to hear your Voice every once in a while. With me it was only the one time. Maybe I will get to talk with you again.

But for now letter's will be just fine.

My case is now done in the Seventh Circuit. I was denied again. Now my case will go to the United States Supreme Court.

I will see my Lawyer in a Week or two. I will not hold my Breath on that. Now as for your letter's.

You want to know of Rape in Prison. How Guard's turn their cheeks? Well, Rape sure does happen in every Prison around the World Every day.

I had been Raped myself back in 1984 when I first went to Stateville. I had a job working or learning to work on newer cars, for that time me and 7 guy's worked on State Police Car's, mostly on the Engine's. Well on my return to my cell I wanted to take a Shower, I was alone at first, and the Guard let 4 other men in and locked the Shower door. for 1 full hour I was raped. I knew the Guard was there, I heard him laughing. I yelled my ass off. When they found me passed out, I had 200 Stitches all around my ass, it was ripped open.

And no one ever asked what happened. I feel that everytime someone young & new goes to Prison this will happen to them. As for the Guards, they will say it is impossible to keep an eye on everyone. So nothing is ever done of a Rape in Prison.

The same is for Females in Prison. They get Rapped in Prison. By the Male Guards. We heard of this in Dwight, the Female Prison down the street from me. Females came up Pregnant. Big news on the TV and Radio last year around July & August.

Rape is a part of life in prisons. It will never stop and no one can stop it. They really can't.

Now for matter number 2.

First off Jenny. It feels ever so good to read this letter. Getting mail from anyone is always good.

Second when you Thank Me for being Honest. This is what you wanted. I feel if this don't help me it may help others to understand people like me.

Jenny it has been hard to do this. Plus having you understand.

You ask what happened to make me so Vulnerable?

I feel it was the Drug Addiction. Anyone who had Marijuana back then were who I hung out with no matter what.

The Vulnerable part. When you smoke Marijuana, there is no thinking everything around you sounds & looks good. It was my escape from all of what was happening around me. Back then anyone could have had me do anything and it was done. I would only know what happened when I came down from the High.

The only problem of all this. Had me so scared to tell the Police of this, or I would have right after the first one. I relied on what others said, because I was high, I had no judgement of wrong or right.

I remember back in 1975, 10 people were getting high by some train tracks and a train was coming. A Girl stood on the tracks, the train hit her and busted her up. Parts everywhere. We all were way to high to even get up to get her off the tracks before the train came.

The next day, I went to talk to her family. I learned that she had tried to kill herself many times. I couldn't understand why. She was so Beautiful. I still think of this every now and then.

My life Sucked back then!

You are the Very first person who has ever given me any chance of talking.

All my Lawyer's Never cared to hear of how I felt of anything. Sure I have told them what I have told you, but nothing was ever done. My whole case is filled with injustice, I was hung out to die, and I felt no one cared.

I still feel this way. No one ever really looked into my case from day one, other wise I wouldn't be on Death Row.

My Whole Family Believed the Police and what was put in the paper's. Never once has anyone come to talk to me. Sure I had a Drugs Problem. Everyone knew of that. Did Help come for that? No! I was kicked out instead.

I was very vulnerable as soon as I walked out the door that day. If someone asked me to be in Porno movies, or Rob a Bank, or anything, I sure would have done it. I was not smart enough to say no, or think or it as being a bad thing. And no one would have told me it was bad.

Injustice. First would be my Step Father, Frank and my Real Father, Edward Sr. My Real father left us back in 1970. Stepfather came in 1974. I was 13 years old. Sure he put us in a Nice House and a good School. He married my Mother in 1977, and I knew I was in trouble, for he was out for my ass first, because I was older.

My Mom think's the World of him. But when she was not around, Hell was in the House. He had this thing called cat of 9 tails. A long Broom stick handle with 9 very long stripes of leather on this. There was not any part of my body he ever missed. Every time he came home, I hide, that house was good for that many great hiding places, and I wouldn't come out till 5:00 AM when he went to work. When he came home, I hide again. I got the flash lite, and a radio with ear plugs. No one could ever find me.

My Real father was drunk all the time, he mostly threw things and made me face the wall on my knees all night long. I was pissed very much for all the abuse he did to my Mother.

Your main focus is why I am where I am? I am here for 2 reasons. 1. When my Mother & Stepfather walked into the Police Station and when Stepfather said the word I am a liar. I don't know how to tell the truth. My life was over. 2. Was Robin. I had no place to live, no job, nothing. Robin let me sleep in the basement. I first felt I was really going to learn a good trade. But that blew up in my face.

And now I set here waiting to have my ass put to death.

You are sick, or have a sick feeling about the entire case. I have been feeling the same way for 10 years and have not stopped. I am even more sick now then ever before. Why? Because from my last letter, I have found Christina, and have written to her, and have heard back from her.

Jenny. When I told you of that Dance, it was a High School dance. My point is this. When I told you of the Girl who we doubled with had taken pictures of me covered in Blood. Well Christina tells me they were paid to say that, and Christina was asked to do the same. But she wanted no part of that.

So I now see that one family was paid off to speak, and lie to get me on Death Row.

You will read this yourself, for I am getting copyes made. I have talked with my Lawyer of this. All he said was so! What do you want me to do? I feel if one was paid off, there are more!

I am pissed at what my Lawyer said, that hurt me bad. This to be in court could give me maybe a new trial. Injustice for Real!

I was so Very Happy to hear from Christina, and she feels the same. Andy wrote to her, and gave her my name & number, and she wrote to me. The Love we had is still the same. But we are just friends.

Jenny, I do know nothing can bring back the Victim's, I wish I really could. God knows I wish I could! But I can't. I can't even express to there families how bad I feel. The Courts have stopped that.

Jenny, I really do need one Really Big Miracle. I don't feel it will be from the work my Lawyer has done.

I fully enjoy my letters I can write to you. I also wish we weren't having my case to write about. But we do. Plus I am most sure we can write also as friend's. I am most glad that you wrote and wanted to know of me as myself. I Thank You So Very Much For That. Still Friends. Glad to hear this. I do miss talking with you. I hope all is well with you and your family. Yes I have been trying to call, many different times in the hopes of talking with you. I see you have been way so busy. Jenny. Please don't feel bad about not getting my calls. Don't worry about that, I can write you anytime. And Be Happy with that also.

Now as for you. No, you have not forced me to talk about the Killings, I did that on my own, at first I didn't understand that. But I sat back to think of this. I did my Very Best to answer all that you ask, and I will keep doing so.

One other thing before I send this out. I was looking for an answer on my request of a picture of you. I didn't see of how you felt of that.

Your Friend,
Edward Spreitzer.

Nov-14-15-16-97

Hello Beautiful.

Sorry, I fell behind in my writing, because of my case.

I am doing somewhat ok. Part of my case is now going in the United States Supreme Court, and part of my case is going back to Federal Court.

I would have loved to write to the families [of the victims], and let them know how bad and sad I feel of what I had done. But there is no way for me to get the information, my own lawyer think's this is not good thinking. I know you are glad to hear me speak of how I feel of the Victims.

I want you to know my feeling's are so real and true. Jenny in the eye's of God, I have been forgiven for my crimes. Because I asked to be forgiven.

It would only be more if the families knew how I felt, and hope they can forgive me. I have talked with my Lawyer's of this, and they think I am nuts.

I am Catholic and have been since age 10 when I was Baptized, I still go to church in here every tuesday's at 1:00 pm. I have one on one talkes with the father's. I am doing all I can to be a better person. I don't write this down because it may look good on paper, or have you to feel good reading this. I fully mean all I say. I am a much better person. But the courts will laugh at this for real.

Well, Beautiful, time for me to send this out. Take Care. And Smile

Your Friend Alway's
Edward Spreitzer.

March-13-14-15-98

Hello Jenny.

It was so ever good to hear from You. I have so much to write about. But first so you can see I am not dead. And I am fine, and do hope the same for You, and your family.

I have not been feeling to good, one bad cold after another. But it is gone now. They tell us the Heater is broken, so it had been way to cold. It was fixed yesterday. So we now have heat. I can feel my toe's again!

Well, Good new's. I just got off the Phone with my Mom, and I had a nice talk, something that has not been done since my arrest. Mom is coming to Visit me on March-18. I guess we will have a lot to talk about after all the year's that went by.

Jenny, Mom say's to say Hello to you, and I am asked a few question's. Jenny, Mom was hurt to hear of the Book we are doing. Please inform my Mom that it is of the truth as to save her Son's Life. Can you Please help me with this? I am Proud that you are Proud of this. I truly Thank You for allowing me to express my side of the case, and of myself.

I truly Thank You for giving me this chance. Jenny if this Book save's my Life, You know that I will truly want for you to come and Visit me, for I will have one really Big Hug for You for all of your help.

In the

United States Court of Appeals

For the Seventh Circuit

Nos. 96-1467, 96-1520

EDWARD SPREITZER,

Petitioner-Appellee/Cross-Appellant,
v.

HOWARD A. PETERS, III, Director, Illinois Department of Corrections, and RICHARD B. GRAMLEY, Warden. Pontiac Correctional Center,

Respondents-Appellants/Cross-Appellees.

Appeals from the United States District Court for the Northern District of Illinois, Eastern Division. No. 92 C 2182—David H. Coar, Judge.

On Petition for Rehearing En Banc

SUBMITTED JUNE 6, 1997—DECIDED AUGUST 11, 1997

Before POSNER, *Chief Judge,* and CUMMINGS, BAUER, COFFEY, FLAUM, EASTERBROOK, RIPPLE, MANION, KANNE, ROVNER, DIANE P. WOOD and EVANS, *Circuit Judges.*

On consideration of the petition for rehearing with suggestion for rehearing en banc filed in the above-captioned case by petitioner-appellee, all of the judges on the original panel have voted to deny and a majority of active judges has voted not to rehear en banc. Judge Ilana Diamond Rovner dissented from the denial of the petition for rehearing en banc and filed an opinion which was joined by Judge Diane P. Wood.

The petition for rehearing is DENIED.

The U.S. Court of Appeals recently denied Spreitzer's appeal for a new trial.

I was thinking of getting myself on the internet with my case. But my Problem is, that I don't know of anyone who can help me with this. Do you know of anyone who can help me with this? Please do pass on my name and address to them as I can get started.

Well Jenny at this time I am Denied in the Supreme Court of the United States. Now I am going to the Illinois Supreme Court. But, I am going back to the Federal Court's also, as to get past work finished that was not done before. My Lawyer Say's this is good. But it is hard for me to be happy of this, for if we win, the State will appeal it, and I will lose again.

I don't have no more faith in this System. I fully can't Believe they put that Women [Carla Fay Tucker] in texas to death. That hurt everyone on Death Row down here. But now everyone is not even thinking of her anymore. 2 Men were put to Death from the Unit last month, there cell's didn't even get a chance to get cold for they had new men to fill them. And they look so young. I sware one looks to be of 16 or 17, and is he small.

He came in under the New Law, so if he can't prove his case, he will be put to Death in 3 or 4 year's. Yeah under the New Law there is no way for you to take 5 or 10 year's playing around.

Jenny I have a Major new thing in my Life, and I want to share this with you. Back before my arrest I was seeing a Girl Christina, she is Andy & Tom's Sister. Well the fact is she found me, and we have been writing back and fourth to each other since Sept-28-97. We never Broke up, so we are still legal Girlfriend & Boyfriend, and we still feel the same way now as we did back then.

Jenny I am telling you this, because Christina is the first love of my life. And I want to write to her of what we are doing, as maybe she might want to add to it. I will let you know of this.

Yeah I would love to live for a long time: I don't want to die!

I have fully enjoyed writing to you. I will keep on writing, the only one who can stop me from writing is You, or if I am put to Death.

For now I am ok Jenny.

Take Care Jenny! And Smile!

Your Friend Alway's!
Edward Spreitzer.

April-24-25-26-98

Hello Beautiful

I am doing fine today, and I hope the same for you and your family.

I am to know that you have talked to my Mother and My Sister, they fully enjoyed the time talking with you.

You are hearing nothing but the truth of how my family feel's about me. I was more then glad to help anyway I could. My family are Very Nice People. And I am glad that My Mom talked with you, and also my Sister, her name is Jennifer also.

I got to see my Niece on 3-19-98. I had much fun. Now my Niece run's to the phone everytime it ring's to see if it is Uncle calling. And she cries when it isn't.

I showed her how to write her name.

I had a Very Wonderful Day. And look for another.

I am fully to know of the bad rap Illinois is getting. The Detectives and Police are all Sloppy. They can pick up anyone and lock them up, even you. It has happened, and no one can stop this. Police are the most respected people on Earth.

People will not believe there are Bad Copes. Here check this out. You are reading of the first time I was pulled over driving Robin's Van. I drove it just one time. See my Mom had a Picnic, and I picked up a few table's & chair's from the Church. Now what I learned of this Van is simple.

When you are inside, there is a Part that is between the driver, and the back, and the back door's can only be opened from the outside. So if I was doing all this, once I am in the back of this Van, there is No way for anyone to get out unless I was let out.

I learned of that, because I couldn't work them door's, even to pick up the table's and chair's.

So the police were wrong as having me to open the back door's for them as they can look inside.

Thomas Flynn is lying. John Leonard's is the truth. But as the screw driver is put in, one person is needed at each back door to lift them. If you don't have this, them door's will not open at all. Thomas Flynn is full of shit.

Sloppy is not a word I would use, for Illinois Detective's and Police are way worse then Sloppy. They are the first step of the Justice System. They feel they can do whatever they want, and they do. I have No Respect for the police at all. I seen first hand on the wrong they can do.

My Brother Danny and I were picked up in 1979 for steeling. And we had our asses kicked because they wanted to know where the stuff was, so they can keep it for themself's. When they where told it wasn't us, they kicked our asses even more harder.

Jenny I could write all day long of this. But the Bottom line is Copes in Illinois are just no good at all.

This Cook County States Attorney Richard Beuke knew of this, he was at all the places they took me too. The police tried to kill me, and Richard was watching.

Richard drove a 1979 or 1980 Chevy Monte Carlo Gray in color. License Plates that said Bad ASSS.

Jenny when he pulled in to Schiller Wood's, a Chicago Police car hit him on the Driver's Door. And I was in the police car. I have a cut over my right eye from that, when my face hit the metal cage that was between me and the police.

Yes everyone of the Lawyer's was told of this. But nothing was ever done, or even looked into. Hell I was laughed at.

I don't feel to kindly for anyone that has to do with the Justice System.

Yes I am fine, and as for beinging lonesome, Jenny I don't feel lonesome. I am most glad to have you for a friend. I was way lost because I didn't have anyone who wanted to hear my side of the cases. No one ever asked of how I felt of anything.

You gave me a fair chance to explane my side, and I am much greatful for that. I was more then glad to sit and write with you of my cases and tell you what I felt. I know it will not get me off the hook. But I only asked for a fair chance to be heard.

I don't want to die, and if the right people read my side in my letters, I only hope they can help me.

Yes I am talking about Lawyer's.

Jenny Public Defender's ain't shit, and never have been. If I had any kind of Lawyer other then a Public Defender, I would not be on Death Row. The Public Defender's I have had, have not put a second into looking into my case at all.

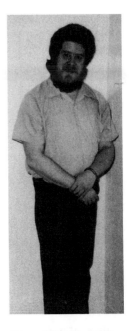

Edward Spreitzer today. "I am too young to die, and if by some chance I did wrong, I will take full responsibility for what I did, and only for what I did. I am still young. I can still turn out to be a good person and help other's. I am trying hard to get off Death Row. I want to keep my life. I will do anything to keep my life."

This is one reason I answered you back. Plus if the families read my side. They will see how sorry I fully am.

I hope that you are not Lonesome. I will try that much more to cheer you up if you are.

Your Friend Alway's.
Edward Spreitzer.

Harvy Carignan

A nger of an intensity that few people could ever imagine, frenzied anger that attacks without warning and blinds all reason — this has been Harvy Carignan's unwanted companion for most of his life — and ultimately the cause of his downfall. Reflecting on the fate that his anger had in store for a woman who had gotten too near to him, Harvy wrote: "God in all his wisdom, and me in my ignorance, had forgotten to warn her about me, to make her understand that something terrible had been happening to my brain."

Harvy Louis Carignan's life began more than 70 years ago, in Fargo, North Dakota, when he was born the illegitimate son of a local doctor and his family's housekeeper. Although his mother quickly remarried to legitimize her pregnancy, she would always blame Harvy for complicating her life. She didn't want him around and soon shipped him off to live with relatives, none of whom wanted him either. He was shuffled from one family to the next. Before he reached the tender age of 12, Harvy was put in reform school in North Dakota. After seven unhappy years he enlisted in the Army.

In the summer of 1949, while serving in Anchorage, Alaska, Private Carignan was charged with sexual assault and first degree murder of 57-year-old Laura Showalter. Even though Carignan eventually admitted his guilt, was convicted and sentenced to die, he managed to escape the hangman's noose on a legal technicality and was cleared of all charges. Not so with his next conviction — the sexual assault of Dorcas Callen — for which he was sentenced to 15 years in Alcatraz.

The prison sentence did not stop Carignan. After his release, he took up right where he left off and the assaults and murders continued...with frightening frequency. In May 1973, 15-year-old Kathy Sue Miller answered Carignan's help-wanted ad for a service attendant to work at his Seattle gas station. Miller left for the interview with Carignan and was never seen again — that is, until one month later, when her body was discovered, sexually assaulted and badly beaten.

Then, very soon after Carignan took a job as a truck driver in Minnesota, a young hitchhiker, Roxanne Wesley, was raped, beaten and left for dead. On September 13th, the very same thing happened to a 13-year-old girl. The next murder was of Laura Lesley Brock, whose battered and lifeless body was discovered in British Columbia — very close to the same time and near the same location in which Carignan had been stopped for a traffic violation. Shortly thereafter, Eileen Hunley, Carignan's live-in girlfriend at the time, was found dead. Her friend, Kathy Jane Schultz, was next.

The vicious murders and sexual attacks stopped when Carignan was finally caught. He was convicted of first degree attempted murder and first degree sexual assault of Roxanne Wesley and sentenced to 30 years. In 1976, Carignan pled guilty to second degree murder of Kathy Schultz and was found guilty of first degree murder of Eileen Hunley, his girlfriend. He was also found guilty of first degree sexual assault of Wanda Tjaden and sentenced to 30 more years. He was sentenced to life in prison at a maximum-security facility in Stillwater, Minnesota, where he remains today.

Carignan openly admits to killing Hunley and Schultz, but denies all of the other charges. He claims he is innocent of raping and trying to kill Roxanne Wesley, that they had consensual sex, and that he only hit her when she threatened to bring false rape charges against him. He says he never saw Wanda Tjaden before the day she walked into the courtroom to testify against him. Regarding Kathy Sue Miller, he says that he arranged an interview with her, but claims that they never actually met.

In many ways, Harvy Carignan is the most sensitive and articulate of the men with whom I corresponded. He is also the most difficult to

These police photographs were taken in 1964 when Harvy Carignan was arrested for burglary. He already had one death penalty under his belt — for killing a 57-year-old woman in Alaska — but a legal technicality allowed him to escape the hangman's noose.

comprehend. How could a man so well versed in the poetry of Shelley and Lovelace, so fine-tuned to feelings and emotions, have led so brutal and violent a life? Harvy himself admits that he's an enigma: "If anyone was to describe what I became they would have to use some kind of uncipherable hieroglyphics from before the Dark Ages." He believes that his problems stem in part from living most of his life in institutions, especially his younger years. "I learned nothing whatsoever about living life except from an institutional view. I lost the most important years of my life, those in which I should have learned to be an adult instead of living an institutional life and perpetuating forever childhood things and childish dreams...."

Life hasn't gotten any easier for Harvy Carignan, but now, at 72 years old, battling prostate cancer, he believes some things have changed for the better: "Finally I find myself looking forward for the first time in my life to a future for which I am prepared. I have found manhood when most men my age are slipping into their dotage. If anyone were to tell me my life was not stolen from me I would be forced to call him a liar. It was never mine, I never owned it and I am paying the price for having lived childhood long after I should have outgrown it...."

The Carignan Letters

Dear Jenny,

Happy Birthday, Jenny — and may it be your twenty-ninth and not your thirtieth. That extra year may someday prove valuable. If only I could I would give it to you for a present. As it is, I can offer no more than what you asked: a letter.

For whatever reason or reasons you wrote, thank you. I am sure it took a lot of thought and it certainly took a lot of courage. You yourself said you are not sure what your interest is. It must be a tremendous curiosity tempered by a good heart or because you are driven by a great anger. Perhaps, it was some of both. Most people write for one or the other of those reasons. I think I should have to know those reasons before I would empty my heart or bare my soul for you. You are not sure of your reasons so unless you can candidly and comfortably convey them to me, I would find it difficult to be candid and comfortable sharing myself with you. Maybe I can assist you in finding them.

You did not say much in your letter, but enough that I agree your life is sublime. Therefore, I do not believe you are looking for thrills. Subliminal minds do not allow for such. On the other hand, if you are placid, bored to the point of seeking information about old crimes, real or imagined, it might be you want to revel in the knowledge of being aware of what would be in my mind had I committed crimes you seem to believe I did, but not so you could enjoy the vicarious thrill that sometimes accompanies such knowledge. If it is not these, you may want to know for one of these two reasons: The first is for commercial purposes. The second is you want to extend a helping hand, perhaps from a heartfelt or religious standpoint. Either is valid.

Jenny, I do not find fault with your reasons, whatever they might be. You have the right to satisfy your curiosity, to enliven your sublime existence, to want to know simply because you want to know, and to offer help by extending understanding and forgiveness.

Upon more sober reflection, I suppose there could be another or many more reasons I have not touched upon. If there are, and you know them, feel free to share them with me. One of them might be the very one that would compel me to want to help you.

Please write to me. As you are by now aware I am very interested in understanding WHY you wrote, in knowing what makes you think crimes committed long ago are locked away in my head and will remain there for all eternity. That is a tremendous thought — and a scary one!

As you know by now, I do "write back," but seldom. The person and his or her reasons must interest me. I do not know your reasons, so it has to be that the way you presented your request and how you have shown your interest that interests me. I think it is because you wrote, "I have children." I read a plea for help of a kind that if I wrote and answered your questions that what I write might be of assistance to you and to them. Certainly, there is nothing the matter with aiding ones children in whatever way one can. However, for this too there must be a reason.

I write to many people. Two in Australia, two in England, one in Ireland, and one in Nova Scotia. Six months ago I corresponded with seventy different people but it became too time-consuming and I cut the list to twenty-five. Later, I limited it to twenty. You would be the twenty-first. Of course, my family is not included in this number. Some of them write often, some seldom, and some hardly ever or not at all. I leave that up to them by writing only if they write first, unless they write often. Most of the people I write to are women. Of the fifty or so I took off of my writing list, probably forty were men. The women are more loyal and deserving. I have no love interests, but some are very good friends.

Once again, Happy Birthday Jenny Whoever-You-Are. I am not averse to writing about myself. However, there must be a reason that interests me. Something that makes me feel I should and makes me want to. A first name, a number, and a request for no known reason doesn't quite seem enough. If you are sincerely interested, why don't you think about it? This might work.

Sincerely,
Harvy

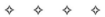

12-08-96

Jenny,

It is almost three o'clock in the morning, which reminds me of the words of a song from my youth, and I have not slept nor am I likely to. While on the present mental peregrination I thought about what I wrote yesterday and it brought much, many things, to mind, subjects and things I did not include. You wanted to know what I do in prison and what I think about. Here are some of what I do and the things I do.

I often write in the middle of the night; I sneeze into my hands although the Health Services Department asks us not to; I laugh, I grin, I grimace; I stretch, sit up when I should sleep and sleep when I should be awake; I do humorous things to feel happy, dress sloppily, shower first thing every morning, drink coffee and eat just before I go to sleep — and it doesn't bother me. I skip eating vegetables, enjoy fatty foods; I cry, sing, play the guitar — and I play it well, anything from hillbilly to the classics — and I dance with myself, jump in the air, and scream. I stretch my jaw muscles to stay awake, do my job with alacrity, do not eat in the messhall, hate cockroaches, yellow jello, plain doughnuts and thick gravy. I like candy, syrup, strawberry jam and grape jelly; I talk back to the guards, I do not smoke, and I tell bad jokes to anyone who will listen. I watch bad movies and enjoy them, like the Minnesota TWINS, watch the VIKINGS, and I am embarrassed by the Minnesota Golden Gophers — every time any of their teams win two games in a row, which isn't often, the sports announcers talk bowl bids and the teams fall flat on their collective faces the next time out — and I owned shares of the Milwaukee BREWERS when they were still the Seattle PILOTS.

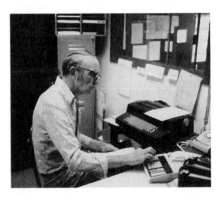

Harvy Carignan claims that he's finally learned to temper the intense anger that he says played a big part in his crimes.

I wonder about the state of the Union, worry about what is happening at home and abroad, ask why they made that stupid bitch Albright, or whatever her name is, Secretary of State, despise President Clinton as a man and I am contemptuous of him as the President, dislike politics, hate politicians, and mistrust the police. I wash my own clothes, watch a nineteen-year-old television set (Mitsubishi) and own a twenty-year-old radio (Smart. Very smart — Magnavox). I never shine my shoes, press my clothes, or use toothpicks. I do not lace my shoes all the way to the top, wear hiking boots most of the time and hang notes to myself on forbidden parts of my cell walls. I say whatever pleases me whenever it pleases me to do so to whomever it pleases me to say it to, have an extra of each of my toilet articles, buy Charmin toilet paper rather than use the state-issue, clean my cell only half often as I should, leave dishes to soak in my sink until I need to use them, use AJAX dish soap, make my bed before I do my morning ablutions, and use TIDE Soap with bleach.

I take vitamins and one aspirin a day, have property in my cell over and beyond the allowable items, seldom write cursive although I am able to write beautifully, but I seldom do because I prefer "to scratch", I love the Irish, hate the English, and abhor Asians in general except those from the once French-ruled territories. I prefer writing to women more than men except for a friend from Ohio called Mike who is an excellent letter writer. I brush my teeth irregularly, but often; refuse to wear a belt, to sew buttons, mend my shirts, or darn my socks. I keep my head shaved — when I shave — I tear my toenails, which are in-grown, instead of cutting them. I have had a prostatectomy, which is akin to being castrated, have von Hypple/Landrau Syndrome Cancer, which is in remission, and do crossword puzzles when I can check the answers. I have blue eyes, brown hair well peppered with grey, dark eyebrows in the winter and light in the summer, a beer belly but I do not drink, a ruptured navel, two stab-wound scars, seven bullet-hole scars, false teeth, and have had a broken jaw (Oh, I deserved it, did I?). I do mathematics in my head, teach my friends English grammar, speak seven languages but none fluently (Russian is the best, except English), and I am a jack-of-all-trades and am the master of most. By trade, I am an automobile mechanic but do waterproofing and cementacious work equally well, have bad eyesight, keep my fan on twenty-four hours a day, have trouble finding my plastic flatware when I need it (It is generally in the sink), and hate peanut butter. I use two pillows and two mattresses although the offical issue is one of each, cover with a sheet and blanket in hot weather and cold, wear white socks with a suit, think most policemen are scum but most prison guards are honest and trustworthy, and that people who cut off cows' tails should have their genitals removed with a roto-rooter..

I am 6' 2" tall, weight 265 pounds, wear a size twelve shoe, have a friend with the FBI, am a master liar but seldom indulge and I probably wouldn't ever lie to you. I have no reason to.

I have big hopes and small expectations, ears like a Black Lab, love Toy Poodles and shorthaired cats, am afraid of snakes and refuse to kill insects, except poisonous spiders that will not "shoo." I wash my own bedding, never turn my mattresses; I never go to church although I pray often, do not discuss the Bible even though I read it religiously, pray to God as I would talk to you — in my own idiom — and all too often tell Him what to do. I read and write poetry with a fervor, enjoy eavesdropping and put down the toilet seat before I leave the bathroom. I never attempt to kiss a girl on a first date, open doors for my dates and pull out their chairs. If they do not like it they can go home.

I was once sued for patting a cocktail waitress on the buttocks. She set her wet tray on my change and tried to walk away with it. I patted her butt to get her attention and her boss sued. I had to pay a twenty-five dollar fine and pay her one dollar after civil proceedings and she had to return my tip money ($6.00), which I promptly gave to her, which was what I was going to do if she hadn't tried to steal it. I later dated her and served time in Oak Park Heights with her son.

I tire quickly, sleep when I feel like it, do not snore (I have been accused of it but laid awake all night to listen and I did not), I own an OVATION Guitar and use cheap strings because they are all I can afford, prefer electric over acoustic guitars but we are not allowed to have them. I have one of the last word processors in the prison. We are not allowed to purchase them. Computers are anathema to the administration because they do not want us to keep records that could indict them. Poor memories by the inmates is in their favor. If we remembered names, dates, and places both the staff and administration would probably be in jail. It is pretty hard to indict them when all we remember is we were served cold potatoes on Thanksgiving.

I dislike neckties and will wear them only at weddings and funerals. I am lucky. When I die they will not make me wear a tie! The state is made up of cheap bastards and they will bury me naked with my innards in a plastic sack beside me. If I have money in my account they will take as much as is needed to cover my funeral costs. The taxpayers do not mind feeding me during my lifetime but they do not want to dress or bury me for eternity. Strange creatures, these Minnesotans. A majority of them are child abusers. It runs in families and is a way of life. Grandfathers are the worst offenders, mothers next but they are less often caught, and fathers nearly always take over where grandfathers leave off if they are caught and convicted.

More than a dozen of our legislators have been accused of felonies, others are accused of beating their wives, molesting their children, making state employees work on their campaigns, colluding to steal public funds, shoplifting, threatening their constituents, lying during their campaigns (What's new about that?) and at public hearings, and myriad other offenses against the majesty of the Law (Smile).

I am liked by most inmates, refuse to joins gangs, am a very good bridge player, hate pinochle, and dabble at poker for small stakes when I am free. I lay awake nights remembering my wives who were beautiful women, seldom think about my stepchildren, never read "girlie magazines" (They do not arouse me sexually), pray for my victims and their families and those who perjured themselves to incarcerate me. I often watch television and listen to the radio at the same time. I hate earphones, but have to use them (They cause too much wax to harden in my ears, which flakes and itches). I do not drink alcohol, smoke cigarettes or anything else, or use drugs. I quit all three on the morning of 20 June 1974. Three months later I was seeing forensic psychiatrists (Who I put on the social level with whores — they also sell themselves to the highest bidder) being made well enough to be tried in criminal court, which is a little like taking a person's appendix out so he will be well enough to hang the following day.

I hate the GREEN BAY PACKERS and the Oakland RAIDERS, feel sorry for the MARINERS because of the loss of Randy Johnson last year, think they have the best coach in the business and believe the SEAHAWKS will win with Freiz if they get rid of Meier or however his name is spelled. I admire the New York YANKEES, think Babe Ruth is the greatest baseball player ever, think players wages are too high, tickets cost too much, television is the cause of crimes and civil disobedience, and sports announcers are generally ignorant of the sport they cover.

I believe housewives with children should be paid a stipend from the federal government, so they will all be paid an equal amount, and that day care centers should be abolished. Single mothers and fathers should be paid the minimum wage, plus fifteen per cent for each child under eighteen. Child abusers should not be imprisoned but locked away for life in non-prison, but a prison-secure, setting. All offices should be elective and politicians who break their campaign promises should be prosecuted and put in jail for a term three times the length of their terms. Capital punishment should be outlawed, not because it doesn't work, but because it is brutal and sends the message that certain kinds of murder are justifiable. Retired sports figures should be placed in homes especially designed for them, governors should not be allowed to speak publicly, and lieutenant governors should not be paid because they do not work. I think the federal law that puts second-time pedaphiles in federal prison for life should be abolished, not to protect them, but because the Mexican work force the federal prison industry system was predicated upon now mostly stays in Mexico and works in American factories there. The federal prison system wants the pedaphiles because they are obeisant and will gladly work for .23¢ an hour rather than to be thrown into the general prison population. Can you imagine the Aryan Brotherhood or The Muslims being as obedient as these creeps?

I think the female guards should be kept outside the prison proper. Most of them would better serve themselves by translating the poetry of Sappho and drinking the blood of their last male sacrificial castration. Having them inside gives them too much power in the gender war. Non-lesbian females are all right but homosexuals cannot be refused jobs because of their sexual preferences. Do not misunderstand me, some few lesbians do a good job. Like with everything and everyone else, there are the few that spoil it for the many. The same goes for homosexual men. Why should they be allowed to work in what to them must seem to be the Garden of Eden (Captive apples!)?

Gangs should be broken up, but only if all gangs are eliminated. Remember, the Democratic Party is a gang that beat up people for those in Tammany Hall and made them vote the Democratic ticket. What else are fraternities and fraternal organizations except gangs. Most do not revert to violence but many have at various times during their histories.

At first blush I did not like you. Your writing was too reminiscent of someone I used to know. You were pushy and did not ask, but told me what you wanted in the grammatical voice that indicated you expected to get it. Next, I was amused by my reaction. After your second letter, I liked you and decided I could trust you. I still haven't given you what you wanted — and I may never give it to you — but you have to admit I am giving you a good foundation upon which to base your understanding.

We pay about twice as much as we should for Canteen items. We must pay the wages of four guards, which is about $38.00 an hour when everything is considered, instead of paying office clerks who have no insurance, etc. The union here is strong. I will send you a copy of what we can buy rather than go on griping about it. Food items are not taxed. Those items that are cost .0675¢ on the dollar. The reason food prices are so high is because we have a 25 per cent mark up.

I am Cellhouse Representative and the Canteen Representative. That is gratis, no pay no matter how many hours I put in. However, I do get paid on my job: $8.00 a day, seven days a week.

Well, time to go to sleep. I must watch football later today.

Sincerely,
Mr. Carignan;
Nah! It's Harvy!

19 December 1996

Dear Jenny,

Howdy Jenny from your friend Yvrah Nangirac! Let him first of all wish you and your family a very Merry Christmas and Happy New Year. It is a great time of year, the time that children remember forever and even the smallest of gifts makes them supremely happy and leaves them with memories that shape the rest of their lives. May you and your family have the best Christmas ever.

Hm-m. I am beginning to really like you, you know, for telling me about "the fascinating way in which I write." It sounds good to me! To put fascination aside, thank you. Compliments are always welcome, even those I am not sure I deserve because I do not at all see myself as a great, or even a good, writer. I simply say what is to be said about what there is to say things about and hope to be understood. If that does the trick, I am satisfied; if not, I am not satisfied. It is as simple as that.

Having read what you wrote about Ann Rule, and having had the time to ponder the predicament she put me in on the pages of her book THE WANT-AD KILLER, I think I should somewhat temper my words to better fit my feelings. I have not read the book, but my family and friends, including a very good friend with the F.B.I., told me she was fast and loose with the facts and that the truth of the book is suspect. However as much as she misused the truth and outrightly lied, I can understand her position, her desperation if you will, to build a new career as a "slicks writer." Such writers are not generally known for sticking to the facts or using them to find the truth. Sensationalism is the name of that game. Up to this point I am all right with what Ann Rule did. She did something I can understand and did for the kind of publications that most people know are sensationalized and are not always true. It is afterwards, when she drew upon "those facts" for her book, I am stymied by. I know she had just been fired from the Seattle City Police Department; actually, allowed to resign because of "failing eyesight" if you choose to believe her, and I am sure she was experiencing the pangs of silent desperation and wanted beyond reason to make good somewhere else. Well, she did. No one can deny that. She, in fact, wrote some very good books that were made into better-than-average movies. Did she get better or learn that truth is more profitable than fabrications — notice how I purposely refrain from writing the word "lies?" One must admit her fabricated book, WANT-AD KILLER went nowhere other than on the most dusty shelves of libraries, on parlor tables, and on inmates' beds. I will not go so far as to say I forgive her, although I might have, but I will say I am more kindly disposed toward her and her work because of her reasons as I understand them. Yet, before we leave this critter, please try to understand she did not only document the events of people's lives in her books; she made up events and twisted the facts to fit her version of the truth. So far as I can tell, the truth isn't in her. Nevertheless, she was trying to earn a living and one would have to be entirely callous to blame her for that. On the other hand, she hides a lot about herself. If I can believe friends who work for the Seattle Police Department she was fired from the Oregon Girl's School for sexual molestation of her charges, which allows me to give credence to the belief she might have been Ted Bundy's crime partner and later went on alone as The Green River Strangler. It is not proof, not by a damned sight, but it is deductive reasoning, the same kind of reasoning that she, as a policewoman, used to build cases against those she sent to prison without a second thought. What goes around, comes around is what I heard.

Sure, it is all right if you told others we correspond. Even if we never write another letter, the fact remains we were corresponding when you told them. May I ask who they are? I am interested in names only if they are well known or if they are writers or publishers. Will you, please, tell me? It will determine how I word what I say to you.

I can understand your having an innate compassion for victims, but why perpetrators? It is because of the third paragraph of your letter I am somewhat slow in granting you your wishes: you do not yet perfectly read what I write. The reason for this is because we have not corresponded enough and gotten used to each other's idiomata. I try hard to use perfect grammar when I should, but my idiom sneaks in nevertheless. You mistakenly understood my saying I had been accosted as I had been raped. I was assaulted with the intent to rape. This should also answer your question regarding whether or not I have been raped in prison. Not ever having been raped, the answer is obviously, "No." You are intelligent, very much so, because in spite of the mistake in understanding, you were able to discern where and why my dysfunctionalism began. In case you wonder, neither have I raped anyone in prison. I do not delve in homosexuality. To me it is a sickness I have been lucky enough not to have contacted. On the other hand, because of my compassion for homosexuals and my companionship with them I have many times been accused of being one myself. Such is life. I know better so it matters little what others think. I already told you about my founding CONS, Inc. and its purpose of protecting the old and the weak, homosexuals amongst them, from perpetrators.

...Do this for me: Remember that my past becomes a huge and pretentious shadow in the minds of those who talk about me and who let their imaginations expand as to who I am and what I did far beyond the pale of truth. One more thing: I have heard it said that when grown-ups attempt to remember their childhoods they become Aesops, more fablists than historians. I agree with that. After all, who actually can trust the mind of an adult to give credence to his childhood? The good will appear better and the bad will become worse. Of that I am sure. For instance, my mythical father was as heroic to me as the early Irish Kings and the Roman Caesars. I never doubted his courage or bravery or that he would one day appear to make me his true son. Only long afterwards did I find out who my father was and decide I could tell no one, not even my mother that I knew. For a long time, whenever I thought about him the whole of my being became an obscenity so crass and gross I refused to acknowledge him or to think about him as a human being, let alone as my father. What I was born as is no fault of mine; yet, all who knew him impute to me my father's blame and my mother's shame. Often, especially at night, I used to lay transfigured in the dim night lights of my prison cell, which I then felt was my destiny, urgent and mysterious, and I would become ineffably cry-like and, secretly, feel my soul turn inward as if to devour itself and all of me with it. It was scary. What I am letting you hear is what were my screams for help before I learned to forgive and to ask the forgiveness of others. Not being able to attain it from some people, I turned to God and sought His forgiveness. It was a long time coming. It was not because He did not want to forgive me, but because I did not know or understand how to seek and accept His grace. It is what I had called for time and time again over a great many years, ever since my youth when what was in my heart was repressed, hidden, and could be seen only after some act or another, even an act of violence. This is the mirror in which I look back and measure my diminishment. No one stepped forward to place him- or herself in the confluence of the telling currents that became my river of life. Only a long time after they reached what has become the ocean of my mistakes has anyone shown up and, then, only to point accusing fingers. Without placing the blame on anyone, it is an important fact my life is so haunted by a childhood so hideous, of such great debasement and conflict, that I have never gotten over it. It took me a long time to summon the courage to tell myself the all of it, all I could find or remember. Much of it, like the snake I fear, dread, and despise, still slithers through my memory unseen, but fearfully there. In essense, my childhood was so horrible that it did not send me marching toward my destiny, but impelled me like a jet to where and what is my life. It is what I lived each and every day of my childhood, until I grew up, found God and became he who I am today. It was "me." I was not "it" any longer because I have gotten over the fear and the shame. It made me who and what I am. It does not belong to me but to he who I was before he I am now.

I know, it sounds as if I have found a way to place the blame elsewhere, upon the shoulders of someone else. In a way, whoever thinks that might be correct. However, at the same time, he or she must admit I have changed and am not who I was. My anger, once powerful, spontaneous, and unforgivable has become manageable and managed. It does not any longer control me, but me it. To say I no longer become angry would be a mistake, a lie even, because I do, but that anger, every bit as potent and foreboding as in the past, is under new management. I control it, assuage it and channel it until it decreases in intensity and frequency and my thoughts and feelings are not controlled by it any longer. It must pass through me, my reasoning capabilities, meet at the confluence of the old me and the new so I can utilize it as I will after putting it in its proper perspective.

When I was sent to the State Training School it failed everywhere it should not have. It succeeded in making me a stranger I no longer recognized by turning me into what it wanted me to be, which wasn't anything nice. I was made to fit the needs of the institution and the perversions of the staff and the administration. If I described everything that happened I would have to use terms that could not possibly be translated as fact in the minds of most. I had to be complaisant and orthodox to the institution or I would be punished. Needless to say, I was punished beyond description. If anyone was to describe what I became they would have to use some kind of uncipherable hieroglyphics from before the Dark Ages. As a consequence, I have gone through life like an unsolveable crime that is unforgivable. People see me more for what I was made to seem to be rather than for what I became. For instance, I was in a training school so I must have been guilty of something heinous! In fact, I was guilty of nothing except being alive and even that wasn't my fault. I had nothing to do with it! Yet, people, even psychologists, will tell you that what I became was not a learned process, the effect of what was done to me. Instead, they will tell you, it is innate, subterranean, and was unbeheld until it surfaced. Only after it manifested itself in dangerous and cruel doings did my true self surface. Believe what you will. I think they are full of unadulterated bullshit; i.e., that they are liars from the core outward. Yet, the truth of the matter is I am a very intelligent being and, even at seventy years of age, I have a great aptitude and a tremendous ability. Nevertheless, my life is meaningless, one imperceptively and inevitably destroyed. How? By my own actions. Whether or not the fault is mine is of little consequence. I committed crimes, which is fact. It may not be the whole truth, but it is the facts of the matter. Never mind that never by conscious will did I perpetrate a violent crime. I never planned and carried out a personal crime in my life. The decisions were always instantaneous and carried out in the immediacy of the instance and were done before I thought rationally and stopped myself. Unmanaged anger. It is no more, but society is not forgiving. It wants its pound of flesh and as many pounds more as it can get its grubby hands on. Please, you are not a female Shylock, are you?

You are no Shylock, to be sure, but does not Shakespeare explain the declivities and verdants of my past? Someday I will fit certain crimes with these reasons. Until then just remember that such happenings and crimes are perpetrated because they do so fit.

I have a poem I want to close with. I hope you understand it as I do and love it the way I do. It is a super poem by a super person.

TO ALTHEA FROM PRISON
Richard Lovelace

When Love with unconfined wings
    Hovers within my gates.
And my divine Althea brings
    To whisper at the gates;
When I lie tangled in her hair
    And fetter'd to her eye,
The birds that wanton in the air
    Know no such liberty.

When flowing cups run swiftly round
    With no allaying Thames,
Our careless head with roses crown'd,
    Our hearts with loyal flames;
When thirsty grief in wine we steep,
    When health and draughts go free,
Fishes that tipple in the deep
    Know no such liberty.

When like committed linnets, I
    With shriller voice shall sing
The sweetness, mercy, majesty
    And glories of my King;
When shall voice aloud how good
    He is, how great should be,
Enlargèd wings that curl the flood
    Know no such liberty.

Stone walls do not a prison make,
    Nor iron bars a cage;
Minds innocent and quiet take
    That for an hermitage;
If I have freedom in my love
    And in my soul am free,
Angels alone, that soar above,
    Enjoy such liberty.

Lovelace, with Suckling, are considered the Cavalier poets. Their similarities extend to parts of their lives but, unlike Suckling, Lovelace was always in trouble and spent a great deal of time in prison. He deals with his art intricately and balances and measures his lines perfectly.

He was born rich, a gentleman, but died a pauper in a cellar in Gunpowder Alley. For months he had eaten garbage in order to survive. His pride did that to him. He had friends who would gladly have supported him.

My personal belief is he would have offended John Donne. His gallantry was facile and he treated love with lightness; Donne, on the other hand, treated it heavily, but not with more honesty. It is sometimes hard to discern the difference between his banter and cynicism. Goodness, who do you know like that?

I did not edit. It takes much too long and I do not make all that many mistakes (I hope). Please understand. I write to so many people. However, I write to only one as much or as deeply as I do you. Do not forget to help me to help you. Go for it. You can trust me anytime and anyplace. I would not tell you this if it was not true.

MERRY CHRISTMAS and a HAPPY NEW YEAR to each and all! God bless you.

Yvrah

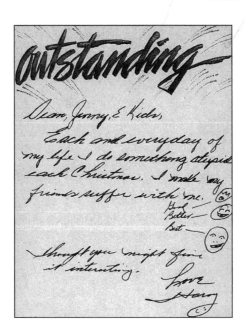

A Christmas card from Harvy.

Dear Jenny,

Hi there. For someone who has told several people we correspond and enjoys my wit and sardonics, you are remiss. It has been thirty-one days since I last wrote you — and no answer. Of course, there were the holidays and there is always a husband, children, and probably a father whose needs come before the enjoyment you derive from writing to me, if I may be so foreward as to suggest you do enjoy corresponding with me. Still, if you find the minutes to spare, please write. I have seen something special, slow-growing to be sure, but a lot more worthwhile than in most of my correspondents. I am interested in you as a writer and a very intelligent person. You seem well adjusted and to enjoy an inner peace not evident in so very many. You must live a life you enjoy. You are very much like a counselor or a policewoman. I am not asking. You will tell me when you feel the need. What I mean is you really have it together, as they say about well-adjusted people.

Dissimulation, the divergences and the lack of anyone with whom to compare myself in my youth, was the forerunner of the perfidy, the deceit and wrong doing in me. Their first appearances were the omens of a growing depravity — and, please, do not think of the word "sexual" as forming degeneracy because there was nothing worthwhile that I learned from which to degenerate — that became my future and my shame. I possessed not the power of self-control and I myself became the prey of my own inclinations. I pampered myself with continual indulgences and, as I became more and more headstrong, my passions grew mutinous. Desire, and not reason, ruled my conduct. After I learned to view myself in ways I could see my imperfections and my social ailments in a just light, and not with the jaundiced eye I had been taught to view myself through, was I able to — and surprised that I could — enjoy many good things rather than simply be discontented. And there were so many to enjoy.

This change became a method for managing my anger and dissipating my rage. You said you know my "rage but, do not feel it to such a degree." I am not sure of the degree about which you wrote, but I assume it is that which I described when I harmed others. There is a reason for your not feeling it: it no longer exists. I am not driven by desire, but by reason. One other face I should help you to understand is my victims were not strangers. Eileen Hunley was my live-in girlfriend and Kathy Schultz a friend who I was together with some seven or eight times. Roxanne Wesley was a stranger before that morning.

"What about your other victims?" you must wonder. What other victims? They are figments of the imaginations of the police and the media. People I have given rides to and argued with have been described as victims. There was one I slapped because she would not put out a "joint" in city limits is also considered a victim. In this one case, so you will think and wonder, was I not a victim and would I not have been made responsible if we had have been stopped by the police because she was smoking marijuana? I am not attempting to dispell the blame, only to make you see there is more than one side to everything. There were incidents, a few of which were crimes for which I was arrested. Nevertheless, a couple of which I stand convicted and I am now serving sentences for are amongst these. Please, do not understand this to mean that I am unjustly in prison. I am not. Some of what I am here for I am guilty of and deserved to be here. There is one I am guilty of but for which I was framed because the police had no proof. Should I be here for it? I cannot say. Neither do I really ask except to cause you to ponder the situation. I am not making an attempt to cause you to believe or disbelieve anything. I am telling you about the dissipation of my rage to the point where it no longer exists and to cause you to be aware of a few facts about people I have been in contact with during criminal and non-criminal contacts. I want you to think and ponder, to broaden the scope of your understanding about matters of all kinds and to look for and find words, phrases, and sentences with which to put your feelings into written form. After all, how little I know about the true happiness of life and how little you know about its true misery. I am only now learning about the intercourse of strangers with good offices and kind affections and you are probably only now beginning to realize they have opposites and from where they come. Therefore, let us not refuse to raise our expectations during the time we have left nor to raise our doubts to a degree we could be disappointed. The world is not as good a place as you believe and neither am I as bad as the world has been led to believe..

I do not know you in the sense of what you do other than you are a housewife. I could easily find out but I prefer to wait until you choose to tell me. That cannot be soon enough, but I am a patient man. There is something about you with which I am impressed. It is not a man/woman thing, but that which is shiny bright and squeaky clean; at the same time, you are brassy as all hell and I am fascinatingly interested with the verve and élan with which you boldly demanded that I tell you what I felt when I killed people. This tells me you are a straightforward person and I can trust you. Consequently, it is all right to like you and to let you inside my secret heart at some time in the future — all in good time — that place of inward peace called the soul where all is well with the world in spite of the sorriness of its condition.

Before you can look into my soul and comprehend what is there you must first be able to look into my mind and comprehend what is there. The riddle is: Do you want to? Do you want to spend the time to investigate allegations made by others before you accept them at face value or toss them aside as the bald-face lies that they are.

For me, art is as clean and beautiful as life is dirty and ugly. It follows sets of rules people do not. In your letters you have asked only for what are vile and ugly moments (Brassy as hell of you to ask!). My life is filled with the good and beautiful moments as well. I do not mind sharing the vile and ugly with you, but I should like to share the good and beautiful as well. I do not wish to separate them but to make a presentation and let you put them in their proper perspective. I hope to offer you a deal you cannot refuse — but not of the kind in the movie THE GODFATHER. It is not something you must accept or live to regret. My name is Carignan not Corlione.

I am not so well educated that I am an educator, but that is not my purpose. I want to apprise, not to give meaning. I want you to see the goodness in my soul as well as the badness in my heart. There are praises to be sung as well as evil to be excoriated. To say I did wrong, something the world already knows, would fall far short of your abilities and neither is it the solution, the basis upon which you should structure what you think and do. At the same time, it is not for me to convince you what the truths are, but for you to find out in your own inimical way. I will offer assistance, but I will not coerce.

Truth, like art, is as clean and beautiful as life is dirty and ugly. Truth is art. When truth is presented with that certain something that leaves no doubt about its veracity, its fidelity and ingenuousness, it is art true and simple. It is the colossus among miniatures, the skyscraper among shanties. It cannot be mistaken for anything other than what it is. It is an art form, something neither appreciated nor utilized by most of today's writers. It is what an artist discerns and puts on a canvas or the pages of a book. This brings us to the question: if you are interested, do you want to be a writer or a hack like Ann Rule and her ilk? Before you answer, you must think because her kind sells. She is the living proof of that. Money is important, but is it as important as truth?

I have turned down chances to appear on Phil Donahue, Night Line, and Oprah Winfrey, so why am I offering you what I denied them? You have one asset none of them ever aspired to: Honesty — and I admire you for it. I am giving you the opportunity to perform an art form. It will call for a lot of imagination. Can you handle it? Can you do it? I think you can. Do you want to? Think about it and let me know. Can you be comprehensive and all-inclusive? Can you create utterances of sublimity and mind-boggling profundity? Can you show I am not the lifeless background for what happened to me during my lifetime, but the living result? Can you take the material I will help you to gather and compile a factual biography about "the living result?" Can you include my psychology, criminal or otherwise? I am as far from being inside your head as you are from being inside mine — all in good time.

I will utilize both poetry and prose to show you the matrix of my mind. How and what I think will not ever become a ploy to interrupt your progress. Much of the good is fragmented and hidden amongst a plethora bad, real and assumed. You must not trust the usual sources, of which there are many. Know their origins and make every attempt to honestly understand and explain their obscurity. Can you create a running commentary that presumes to show your differences and the ways you will include your constant, permanent, and paradoxical theme? What is more, it must not be an escape from the humdrum of everyday living, but a solace and an adventure that is not only exciting and varied, but a ravishment to the point of ecstasy.

The groups I do not want you to cater to are the prurient and the psychic sick. Let them search out and create their own satisfactions. What you write must be neither a survey or an analytical appraisal of what others before you have written. In your mind, they must not exist. You must write to the point of truthful ridiculousity, but you must not appear ridiculous. Instead, you must give your readers an immediate sense of pleasure for the sheer appreciation of your art. The gap between casual reading and sublime understanding must be bridged; no, not bridged, but pulled together so a gap no longer exists. You must be rich in implication, but a closed communicator so your readers are not only absorbed, but so engrossed they will feel themselves a part of you.

A book, more than anything, is pure creation. Even in the throes of intellectual and emotional excitement the writer must achieve magic, make order out of the combined chaos of what I will tell you and what you glean elsewhere. There you must coalesce before your enchantment can exert its spell. Your book, in order to be an art of creation, must utilize many different and exact words, phrases, sentences, paragraphs, and chapters of concentrated power. You must become a miracle of controlled compilation, your combinations of absorbed creativeness a fire, a craftsmanship that glows with intensity and wreaks of an industriousness that it not only has universal appeal, but an everlasting attraction that will thwart the readers and keep them from setting it down. It must contain both an abstract beauty and your most powerful emotions. You must fill it with provoking ideas that delight in the contradictory and instruct in disagreement with those who before you treated the subject. You must awaken the imagination and excite the intellect, alert the mind and stir the soul. Each use of your personal magic, use of words, shift of picture, or abruptness of comparison must not only adorn and enrich, but enlighten and delight.

At first blush, you might proclaim, "I cannot!" but you can because I will help you find the magic to extol my virtues as well as to condemn my evil deeds. I can help you with acuteness and awareness, to persuade with careful reason, and to hypnotize your readers with a daring frenzy of words that will, like Algernon Swinburne, intoxicate them with rhythmic debauchery or like Gerard Hopkins and Hart Crane plunge them into a flood of free associations and commitive. Between us, we will turn the hallucination of already-written untruths into an unforgettable otherworld of truth that will make the nuances implicit for those able to understand and explicit for those we must convince. With redounding syllables and rousing action we will drug them with the sweet and heady delightfulness of John Keats and the witty and slightly wanton realism of Robert Herrick, that singer of the frail virtues and praiser of harmless vice. If we must, we will borrow from Percy Bysshe Shelley and utilize the superbity of his vagueness: give the readers "the joy that is almost pain" and show them "the white radiance of eternity" while hanging fixedly to "O world! O Life! O Time!"

If you can do this, you will present a combination of the imperative and the persuasiveness, bond little known facts to the already-told tale. My life has been an incredible diversity of human experience which will speak more powerfully than the rape of the truth set forth by [Ann] Rule and her ilk. I want to show worst as well as the best. I am not adverse to that. To suggest the vastness of your imagination could avoid this would be to precipitate asininity at its worst. Last of all, your extensiveness might be challenged, but as an author you would defeat your purpose if you limited the book's contents to rigid alignment. There are better and more probative ways of finding truth — the sole purpose of a manuscript of this magnitude.

The greatness of one's writing, like the beauty of one's face, is as unmistakable as it is ineffable, too overwhelming to describe, too awesome to understand. I have never seen your face and do not know its beauty, but I have read your writing and am a witness to its grandeur, its sublimity, and the possibility of its prosaic splendor. However, that is neither here nor there at the moment. That will be determined by time and circumstance, by inclination and determination. My time is short, but I have a most compelling hunch that your determination is exquisitely irrevocable. You are young and have time to spend in order to attain perfection. I am old, but your best source, so time is of the essence. I have two types of cancer, both in remission, but either could take me within two to four months if they were suddenly to reappear. My suggestion, therefore, is a test of time. I have the power of immediate recall, of perfect cognition, and a full awareness of my compulsions. I alone know what happened during every instance of my life, and why, and you have those heightened sensibilities to make people understand. I am a resource that it would be a terrible waste not to take advantage of. Call upon the complex of reason and intuition, the experience of association, and let me know your preferences and prejudices. This could work, but it is possible it would not. Therefore, let us examine the possibility. I have offered this to no one, not ever.

What do I want, expect to gain? One half of everything. If what I know is so valuable, why do I myself not write or why have I not written it myself? I lack the desire, I do not have the innate need to figure the sequences, to sort and compile the facts, and to choose such of them as will best tell the truth. We cannot possibly use everything and I am too close to it to discard the least of the relevant ones. Also, we should discuss whether it would be better for commercial reasons to say it is my "life story as told to Jenny Whatchmacallit." This is what you must think about and decide when you contemplate what I have suggested. I suppose that, most of all, it is important that I read your agenda correctly or was mistaken, that you have or do not have the desire to write the story of one intense and vast undertaking. It would include what I see when I look back on my Alcatraz experience. It is not with loathing, but it is with fond nostalgia that I revisit the surreal and devastated ruins where I wasted the decade of the 50's. My mind wanders in and out of the expunged cells, calling ghost-like to the memories of those who inhabited them, not by names, but by soubriquets willed to them by fearful time and the constant of misery.

With closed eyes I see the buildings lying ruptured, the island itself a wasteland inhabited only by the futile and wasted dreams of men who lived, died and went crazy there. The walls are wounded, bandaged with the graffiti of dementia, and the floors exhibit sores made by the footsteps that shuffled tired and wasted men to their final oblivion.

That prison, that hell on earth, that place etched in the heart of infamy, where men were interred alive and made as if dead to the world, stands stark and naked and, except for memories and ghostly murmurings of years past, the dead bereft of the gloriousness of their humanity and the exultations of their freedom, pose a presence, a vital presence, in this Castle de Sade that rests on the peak of a jagged rock jutting ominously out of San Francisco Bay. Yet, these ruins are buoyant, rife with the aura of ghastly resurrection, where, in the silence of dead dreams, screams ring out across the vastness of time, reciting eulogies to its aggrievements, anthems of ill-praise to its failure, and, at the same time, demanding a place in the annals of time while the winds sing death dirges to its extinction.

In the realm of reason, Alcatraz demands an undertaker, not a champion announcing its revival even as it grudgingly passes life and time on to those who understand its eerie emptiness and the loneliness of its suffering during its last throes of its agonizing pain.

Suddenly, as if awakening from a nightmare, everything except the walls come humpty-dumptying down and the scene fades slowly from my mind. I am as empty as the buildings, a shell deplete of everything except the hallowments made by the loneliness of forever. Together, we stand a monument to the futility that created us. Our obituary, written in untranslated runes whisper to the winds that forever change our message on the sands of time. We are seen by all and understood by none. This architectural Ozymandias lies sneering on a desert of ignorance while a world of blithe sightseers keep the horrors of the past hidden behind the joy of their happiness as they savor a vicarious vengeance themselves upon its erstwhile inhabitants, leaving the reality of this bastion of sadism to pale in comparison and, then, when they leave, they take with them their mad imaginings, and reality, like a bad dream, is forgotten and all that went on before is for nought. It is unremembered, as if it did not happen.

You have read books, heard tales and seen television documentaries about me, but do not believe them. None of them told the truth. As time has passed, each has gotten worse than the last. All of them, while based upon the premise I have committed crimes and am incarcerated, are packs of lies. I have not read or seen any of them, but I know they are filled with sick imaginings. Doesn't anyone ever bother to check out anything? If anyone would have checked they would have found that during the last fifty years most of the crimes for which I have been accused never happened and that I have not even been a suspect, investigated, or arrested for any of them except in Minnesota and a suspect for one of Washington State and cleared. The Seattle police will not admit it, but I was. It is their tenacious stupidity that makes them hang on. I had perfect alibis for the day they think the crime happened and for the day before and after. When I was not at work, I was at home without a long enough travel time in between to do anything except go back and forth.

I might be out of line. You might have decided not to write any longer. I am sorry if you have. You are one of the most interesting and intelligent people I have had the privilege of corresponding with. Thank you for what you have given me if you have no more to give.

Harvy

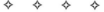

[The "petition" on the following page was written by Harvy Carignan.]

LETTER TO THOSE UNFAMILIAR
WITH THE CASES OF HARVY LOUIS CARIGNAN,
FOR WHOSE BENEFIT YOU ARE SIGNING
A PETITION FOR RELEASE

Harvy Louis Carignan was arrested by the Minneapolis Police Department on September 24th, 1974. Officers on routine patrol spotted a vehicle that resembled one described in a Memo distributed at roll call before their tour of duty, determined it was Mr. Carignan's, and arrested him.

Their Duty Captain ordered the arrestee released. The Hennepin County Sheriff's Department, without a court order or proper authority, took custody of Mr. Carignan, where Archie Sonenstahl of the Hennepin County Sheriff's Department was foisted on him as a Public Defender. The County Sheriff Deputies questioned him, read his rights under Miranda to him, told him he was under arrest, put him in a line-up consisting entirely of police officers, and at that point and time pointed out two Public Defenders, and put him in the Hennepin County Jail in solitary confinement, in the order listed herein.

Mr. Carignan was charged with kidnapping in Hennepin County. Without resolving the matter, he was taken to Carver County and kept there for more than seven months, except for short sojourns to other counties. During all his transfers, each made by the Hennepin County Sheriff's Department, Mr. Carignan was not served with court papers, except the second time he was taken from Hennepin to Carver County, and only after he arrived at Carver County where he was served by Archie Sonenstahl of the Hennepin County Sheriff's Department who had escorted him during the transfer. He was served then only because he had balked at having been taken out of Kenebac County without proper authorization, which he told authorities was kidnapping.

In Carver County, Harvy Louis Carignan was charged with Attempted Murder in the First Degree and First Degree Sexual Assault against one Roxanne Wesley. He was found guilty and sentenced to thirty years. He claims he is innocent, that the sex between them was consensual and he hit her in a rage when she made false accusations against him concerning money matters and threatened to accuse him of rape if he did not return money she purported he took from her, plus two-hundred more.

In Hennepin County he was found guilty of First Degree Sexual Assault upon Wanda Tjaden and sentenced to thirty years more. He claims never to have seen her before her first court appearance against him.

In 1976, Mr. Carignan pled guilty to Second Degree Murder in Anoka County of Kathy Jane Schultz in Isanti County. He admits his guilt.

In the same year, he was found guilty of First Degree Murder in

Sherburne County for the murder of Eileen Hunley, his girlfriend, in Hennepin County. Mr. Carignan admits killing her but denies he murdered her in the first degree.

Harvy Louis Carignan has been in prison, except for nine days in the State Hospital at Saint Peter under observation by Carver County.

Mr. Carignan has been in prison ever since. He spent more than four years at Stillwater, more than eleven years at Oak Park Heights, and the balance of his twenty-three years at Stillwater a second time. His record has been exemplary. Mr. Carignan has not had a major report in all his years in prison. Mr. Carignan has faithfully followed the work programs instead of treatment at the advice of two different Education Directors, who told him he should make use of the work program rather than make "points with the administration" because he would be past seventy if ever he was released and treatment and training would prove useless.

When Mr. Carignan was interviewed at his Fourteen-Year Parole Review, he was set off ten years although the law in his case plainly states he should have been released after twenty-five years, minus one-third off for good behavior, his other convictions to the contrary. He should have long before been paroled on them, under each of the several changing systems employed by the Department of Corrections during his time in prison.

Mr. Carignan has undergone a radical prostectomy for cancer and also has cancer that falls under the von Hypple/Landrau Syndrome, which could take his life in a matter of less than six months if it were to become malignant once again.

Mr. Carignan's remorse and rehabilitation is available in other literature and court and prison records.

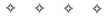

22 May 1997

Dear Jenny,

It was a tremendous learning experience to talk with you today. You see the truth much more clearly than anyone I ever talked with and, because you do, I need you badly; however, as much as I need you, your children need you more than I ever will. I am not sure how much you need or want your family, especially the extended part, to know of this, but I ask you to think about this long and hard before making a final decision. Can you exist and be happy with a life other than the one that is now yours? If it will make your life better I will walk away and let you give up on what your family deems utter foolishness. On the other hand, if you have made your choice, and intend to stick with it, I will stick by you and do everything I can to make your work the best and you a very knowledgeable and successful writer. I cannot prove everything I will tell you. Whether or not you have the means or the ability I do not know. I think it might become a full-time job and that you might need investigators to work for you because you could not possibly have enough time to do all of it by yourself.

I would like to ask if what is happening, your father's fulmination against your treatment of your children and your work, was of recent origin or has he been concerned for some time and is he only now denouncing you and the projects you have such an interest in? From where I sit I assure I am aware that your concern has nothing to do with me as an individual you are interested in or care for personally; i.e., that you are not doing this for my sake. It is evident to me that you wish to put together a study that will culminate as a help to women and that I am a source that can help you attain your goal. You have learned a thing or two about people and the public during your search, especially the criminal justice system, those who work for it, and the mindlessness by which writers make assumptions and pursue them as goals, and that you might also have come to like me as a personality you feel you can trust, but that does not mean you are blind to my faults or that you do not see me for who I am, only that you understand the wrongs I have been accused of are not always wrongs I have done, which does not mean you forgive me, only that you discern the crimes and can see and understand that I can be of service to you and your work which will, in the final analysis, be a service to mankind, and women in particular.

Now for the project: When my mother made the claim that I was a homosexual in juvenile court, she did so outside the purview of the news media and my hearing. When I arrived at the state training school and Mr. Skjod made the accusation I thought it was something he made up and I was angry with him for making such a claim against my mother. The accusation made by her and broadcasted to the boys in C Cottage by Mr. Skjod was the cause of most of my difficulties there: people believed I was a homosexual, even the superintendent. As I have told you about this, it is false. I have never in my life taken part in a homosexual act. When you write about the attacks you must make this clear. If you do not, people here will believe I was a homosexual and, although I will not be approached for homosexual acts, a certain stigma will become attached to me and it will make my life difficult and unpleasant. What is also important is that I suffered the beating and resisted the forces brought to bear: I did not succumb. This was no small success. The other thing I did not hear everything you said about was what you wrote with regards to Kathy Miller. The loudspeakers are on half the time in the cellhouse and it is very, very difficult to hear. I am so tight and try so hard to hear everything that after 15 minutes I am a nervous wreck. Regardless of whether or not you believe I ever met the girl and what you state your beliefs are, it is imperative that you include in your work the statement that I deny having ever seen or being with her on the day of her death or on any other. With all the time I have served I would have long ago made a deal with the State of Washington had I of been with her or if I was guilty. What irritates me is that the police know I am not guilty, they have evidence that proves I am not, but because this evidence is contrary to profiles they work with and do not agree with their personal beliefs they will not exonerate me. They know where I was every minute of the day Kathy Miller disappeared and the day after. One day when they were monitoring my whereabouts with a helicopter their bird broke down and, because it did and they lost track of me for some unknown length of time, they assume that I was doing something that pertains to her. What does a crippled helicopter have to do with my having committed a crime? I cannot remember for sure what day they were monitoring my whereabouts but I am sure it was days, if not weeks, after Kathy Miller was missing and, presumably, was killed. What could I possibly have been doing that pertained to her after she was dead — and according to what I remember from newspaper and television reports it seems to me she was. And what about the crimes the police committed? They colluded with my brothers-in-law when they kidnapped my wife. They lied to a judge and got him to sign an order causing my wife undue tremendous embarrassment when they took my letters to her and made them available to other police departments. The Hennepin County Sheriff's Department in Minnesota told me about them. Detective Sonenstahl told me he was afraid my wife and I were going to get back together again, which would have thwarted the case in Washington. What case? It beats me. They are so devious. Half of my problems in Minnesota, and theirs, could have been averted had they told me the truth and shown me pictures of so-called victims. I would have been able to tell them the truth, they could have researched it, and trials, even those in which I was guilty. Oh well.

Love
Harv

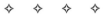

EILEEN HUNLEY

I met Eileen Hunley in 1974. She was hitchhiking and I gave her a ride. She was dirty, tired, and had no particular destination in mind, so we drove around and talked. From the beginning, I was overcome by the tremendous sense of responsibility I felt for her. Mentally, she was an innocent, a child-like creature, trusting of everyone. Being who I was and how a felt, I was left with no choice but to "adopt her", to protect her, to support her and, ultimately, to fight for her when I had to. Also, from the beginning, she frustrated me by getting into predicaments she looked to me to extricate her from. She would act without thinking. Even on the last day, when I was fighting a man she told me had just raped her, she, in child-like innocence, interfered. The fight was not a playground fight in which when one opponent gets a bloody nose he could retire. It was a deadly game, one that could not be set aside, not even when she screamed and told us to quit.

The fight itself was not because she might, or might not, have been raped, although I am sure the force and violence was precipitated by the thought. Stupid and ruthless men do stupid and ruthless things. He was stupid and I was ruthless. I think it was because of the ruthlessness I was showing, the violence I was perpetrating against my opponent, that Eileen attempted to break up the fight when she jumped on my back. Now, after it is all over, I do not believe it was to help the person I was fighting, but that it was her desire to keep me from hurting my opponent even more badly, so badly, in fact, that I might kill him. She jumped on my back twice and, the second time she herself must have been suffering excruciatingly, but she ignored her own pain and suffering because, in spite of her propensity for thinking like a child, she understood my anger, my rage, and was witness to a form of violence from which my opponent was already badly hurt and was undoubtedly going to be hurt even more badly. She, beyond all question, imputed the cause of the fight to her own actions and believed in her child-like heart that I was fighting for her honor. However, during the times she was on my back, I did not stop to think of her design, let alone her honor. What I perceived was that she was a hindrance to my ability to put an end to the fight I was in and, as a consequence, she was assisting my opponent, a person I was doing deadly combat with. Even had I perceived her actions as being designed to help me, I would have been angry with her and probably would have done the same thing: gotten her out of the fight by the most expedient and available method. Her actions had put me in jeopardy, whatever her reasons, and I was defusing that which jeopardized me. I in no way thought of hurting her for what she had done. I simply wanted her out of the action, for her not to interfere any further in my fight...

Incongruously as it seems she might have given her life to save my opponent's. He was stupid and would not give up and I was ruthless and would not quit beating him to the ground every time he got up and attacked me. If the fight had ended after the first time Eileen tried to break it up, except for my opponent's lost teeth, which after sober reflection I think might have been "pegs", Eileen's very sore, if not broken cheek bone from where it hit the manhole cover in the street, and my very sore knuckles and bruised pride, all of our lives would have been different and hers saved. However, the fight did not stop then and there. Now I think the man on the ground got up the last time, although he was himself badly hurt, in a desperate attempt to protect Eileen. He saw me slam her to the ground and imagined I was going to pummel her as I had him. Some vestige of his manhood caused him to arise to the moment and go on with the fight with no thought of winning. He could not win, but he did his best to draw me away from Eileen. He was so badly hurt when he arose the last time he could only rush me and push me across the street away from Eileen. I did not know his was a mission of mercy, but I hit him again and might have hit him again even had I known. I was in an uncontrollable rage and, after everything else he had done, I was really angry because he was interfering. To a person in my state of mind the situation had become a no-win, no-way-out proposition. The same was true for them. No matter what they might have done, my anger would have been fueled and I would have acted it out in my outrage caused I thought the two of them were against me. The only thing that could have saved them was to cease, to desist completely, the very last thing they could have done. Who can stop whatever it is he or she is doing to protect him- or her-self from a mad man, who must have seemed to them a raging beast?

After I knocked my opponent down for the last time and Eileen had jumped on my back the second time, my anger became directed toward her and what I did next was to punish her, not to kill her. During all of this the thought of killing anyone never crossed my mind. What I saw toward the end of the fight was a man my live-in girlfriend told me had raped her and while I was fighting him, she was fighting me. Was I angry? You bet I was. I was too angry to think and to be able to discern that Eileen might be attempting to help me by trying to stop the fight and that my opponent might have been making a last-ditch attempt to save Eileen after I had slammed her to the street. With this in mind, this is what happened.

On the night Eileen and I met we were riding around, she asked me if I wanted to see the collage she had worked on that day. I told her I did and we went to an apartment where her minister lived. He let us in and awakened his wife who was sleeping on the couch. They were exceptionally nice people, as were most who were connected with THE WAY sect.

Until the time Eileen invited me to see the collage I thought she was either a neophyte prostitute or a not-too-bright policewoman. Even after we left the apartment I was not convinced she was neither until we stopped outside of a house in Coon Rapids, a Minneapolis suburb. I knew someone connected with the police would not "lure" anyone outside of his or her jurisdiction. I waited in the car while Eileen went to the house. She did not enter but talked to a young man on the steps for a few minutes before she returned, and said, "Let's find a place where we can sit and talk." I suggested a restaurant. She thought it "a splendid idea." When we were seated I mentioned the person she had talked with on the steps and she said, "He didn't have much to say."

During dinner I asked her if she often accepted rides from strangers. She said she did not, but added, "I do not trust them either! The stop at my friend's house was to give him your license number!" She said it in a way that she must have known I would not be offended by. I was amused.

After supper we sat in the car in the parking lot. I thought, "She's not a policewoman. If she is a prostitute this is where she will let me know." Moments later she caught me completely off guard by when she attempted to convince me I should join THE WAY INTERNATIONAL. She talked about the founder as if she believed he was Christ at his second coming. Later, when I met the man, I found him to be a charming, well-spoken, truly charismatic man whose opinion of himself did not disagree with Eileen's! However, at the moment, in spite of Eileen's child-like thinking concerning other things, she was well versed about the church and I was quite taken with her. I wanted to go on "seeing her" and so I let her "recruit me." I cannot remember what it was she said exactly but, whatever it was, it meant she and the church was a package. Later, I learned quite a few of the girls in THE WAY felt that way, especially those being proselytized away from another sect called THE CHILDREN OF GOD. They brought with them a lifestyle that reflected badly on THE WAY INTERNATIONAL.

In time, I was happy I had joined THE WAY, as it was then called, and had become a member of this particular TWIG, which was but one of several in the Minneapolis BRANCH, which was but one of many belonging to the TREE based in Ohio. The young people, the LEAFS, in this TWIG were exceptional, some of the nicest people I ever met.

Eileen was living with a girlfriend in a lesbian relationship. She wanted her own apartment. When she learned I had furniture she asked me to move in with her, which I did on a part time basis. I was babysitting my brother's house for the summer and had to be there whenever his children were. Anyway, the relationship Eileen and I had was not based on love, but on the premise that I could put up with her, her doings, and her lifestyle without becoming jealous or angry. Eileen was faithful to nothing except the church, but neither was I and I readily accepted her lifestyle. We found ways to enjoy ourselves immensely whenever the opportunity presented itself. The only incident we ever differed about was a meeting she went to at the University that was sponsored by THE CHILDREN OF GOD. She readily admitted it was a girl she had once shared a homosexual relationship with rather than the church that drew her there. She said this girl had once attended a human sacrifice and she wanted to see for herself if it was true. I demurred. I wanted nothing to do with any sacrifices, human or otherwise. Christ had made His for me and that was enough. She went by herself and I did not get my car back for two days. That was Eileen and I had to accept her as she was or lose her altogether. By the way, the car had been driven more than 1100 miles. She had been to Wichita, Kansas.

We had some CHILDREN OF GOD converts in THE WAY and they were a breed apart. They used dope, were into unusual sexual practices, and always schemed for ways to raise money for their dope habits rather than for THE WAY. Later, I met the girl friend of Eileen's from the University and she seemed to be a very nice and sweet person, unlike the other COG's I had met. I had no way of knowing, and I really did not care, but I felt she and Eileen were still involved sexually. I know Eileen would not have kept it from me for the purpose of me not knowing. She readily performed cunilingus on Kathy Schultz when I was in the kitchen and they were in the living room of our apartment. I liked Eileen and I was willing to shut my eyes and remain ignorant to a lot of what she did. She was a tremendous sex partner and anything I would do about others would only spoil the arrangement between us.

THE WAY taught a lot about The Power of Abundant Living, meaning that God had an abundance of everything and would meet the needs of everyone faithful to Him for the asking. Of course, we were to tithe in return: ten per cent of everything we earned was to go to THE WAY. Somehow, sharing with these "brother and sisters," as they called themselves, was not at all repugnant to me and seemed very much the natural thing to do. What is more, it did seem to work. None of us ever needed or went hungry except by choice.

Victor Paul Weirville, THE WAY's founder, would later make the claim that Jesus Christ was not God but, when I first joined, Weirville was a strict Trinitarian. The Trinity is one of the prerequisites a church must teach if I am to be a member. I will not lose sight of Christ.

THE WAY held a ROCK OF AGES FESTIVAL which from five to ten thousand mostly young people attended. In 1974, it was held at the fairgrounds in Oxford, Ohio — and I attended. When I was ready to leave, Eileen was not at home, she had been gone for several days, and I would not see her again until that fateful day of the fight and she was killed. I suspected she might be with her friend from the University or with Kathy Schultz, both of whom she spent a lot of time with. I did not like her leaving without my knowing where I could contact her, but it did not anger me. She had as much right to her life as I had to mine. Anyway, so long as she was with another woman she was not with another man. I did not tell the "brothers" or "sisters" my suspicions, only that she was not home and I did not know if she was going to Ohio with us. I am not sure if I was protecting Eileen or if my ego would not allow me to. When Eileen had not returned before it was time to leave for Ohio, I went to the staging area, picked up other passengers, and went to Ohio without her.

After my return to Minneapolis I went to the apartment and let myself in. Eileen was not there. I was about to leave when I noticed the back door was open (unlocked). The elderly lady lived next door had not seen her and I was walking to my car when I heard a voice that sounded like Eileen's calling my name. There was no where she could be except in a white van parked a few feet away. I walked over to it and asked the man in the driver's seat, "Is Eileen with you?"

He answered, "Beat it, Punk!"

Before he could get his lips together I had jerked him out the window, hit him, and he was laying on the ground. He was out. I walked to the back of the van, opened the door, and Eileen and a young black man were sitting on a rug on the floor. He was fully dressed but she was wearing only a tee shirt and a pair of Argyle socks. Over her left arm were her cut-offs, a reddish-brown jacket and a pair of pinkish-white panties. In her hand were her shoes.

Eileen said, "Harvy, these guys raped me!"

She was lying. I remembered her telling, "I could never be raped. I'd just lay there and enjoy it!" She had said it facetiously, but I believed her. I knew her well enough to know her way: she always took the easy way out.

"Put your pants on and go to the house," I told her. The person I had "knocked out" was pulling on my leg and, when I tried to push him away, he bit me. I kicked him in the face so hard he flipped all the way over and landed on his back. His teeth were spewing out of his mouth like popcorn out of a popcorn machine at a movie theater. It was then Eileen jumped on my back the first time and tried to hold my arms while she screamed, "Leave 'im alone! You're going to kill him!"

I reached back, got a hold of Eileen's hair, pulled her over my shoulder, and slammed her on the street so hard that the diamond-shaped indentations on her cheek were from a manhole cover.

The man I had just kicked got up and attacked me again. It was without force or strength and, when I tried to push him away, Eileen jumped on my back a second time and their combined momentum pushed me to the side of the road. I remember saying, "You fuckin' slut!" as I pulled her over my shoulder a second time. I hung on to her hair at the nape of her neck and pushed her face into the grass until I felt something warm on my arm: it was blood. I had pushed her face into an L-shaped iron bar sticking out of the ground next to a telephone booth.

The man got up and ran. The other man had driven away after Eileen got out of the van. I remember the man on the street hollering, "Billy! Don't leave me!" But Billy had left him and now he was running up the street in the direction the van had gone.

I learned later that a hospital was within spitting distance from where we had been fighting. I thought the building was an old-folks home because I saw a lot of older people going in and coming out. There were no markings to indicate it was a hospital.

I placed Eileen's clothing on the seat of my car, and placed her in a sitting position on the passenger side of the front seat. I got in and begin to drive to North Memorial Hospital. It was the only hospital I knew the address of. On the way, Eileen died. She urinated and deficated on her clothing. I was not a doctor and had seen death only twice before in my life, but I knew she was gone.

It might seem now that I was calm and in control of my facilities, but I assure you I was not. I was excited and mixed up, thoroughly confused and unable to make sound decisions. Instead of going on to North Memorial Hospital I stopped on Hennepin Avenue, lifted Eileen out of the car, and laid her in the trunk on a U-Haul blanket.

I drove to the airport. I felt I had to get away, to escape the thing I had done. I wanted to go anywhere but I could not decide where to go or what to do. On the one hand, I knew I had to escape; on the other, I could not accept Eileen was dead and I could not leave if she needed me. I thought about going to Dallas. One of the girls I had taken to Ohio had gone to Texas to be an Ambassador for Christ in THE WAY Ministry. I had the foresight to know that if she helped me I would be putting her in jeopardy and decided against going there. The stupid thought, "How will I get Eileen on the plane?" kept running through my mind. Next, I considered Seattle, but I had left there with a cloud of suspicion over my head more than a year earlier. I knew I would be putting my family and friends in jeopardy, so I decided against that too. I remained at the airport for about five hours before I remembered I had promised a friend I would take two of her friends to Duluth with me that night. It was not only a solution, but the only solution: I had to get Eileen "out of town." I knew that whatever I did, I was in "deep shit." The thought that I would "beat the rap" never crossed my mind. It was not a matter of not getting caught, but of prolonging the eventuality as long as possible. I knew Eileen was dead. I put her in the trunk because I knew my story would be unpalatable. I had left Seattle under the cloud of suspicion that I might have committed a murder there and any explanations I could give about Eileen would be treated with the deepest of suspicion.

I was frustrated, upset because of what I had done, afraid because I did not know what to do. After five hours in the parking lot near the airport I had pulled myself together somewhat and I decided to go on living my life as if nothing had happened. I picked up the two young women who had been to THE ROCK OF AGES FESTIVAL and headed for Duluth.

After wrestling with my conscience for five hours at the airport I was tired and asked one of the women to drive. I crawled into the back seat and passed out until we got to Duluth.

I went to my brother Clinton's house, but my sister had just arrived with her family so I decided to go to sleep at Clinton's wife's parents. It was late and I went to the room they had open for me. I got up early and left immediately. When I got in my car there was a terrible stench. Eileen was in the trunk. I had consciously dismissed her from my mind but my subconscious had been working overtime. I was inwardly being torn to pieces.

I know the perfunctorial way in which I tell this makes it seem I am cold-hearted and uncaring. Nothing could be farther from the truth. The fear I felt was as much for Eileen as for myself. I had no idea about her future, where her soul was or where it was going to end up. She had professed Christ but, like me, she had not lived the kind of life a true Christian would pursue. Neither was the apprehension I felt for myself all physical. I doubted my mental abilities and spiritual qualities. Prior to this I had been "losing it." I was recovering the trauma of having quit dope, alcohol, and cigarettes all at one time on June 20th., my sister's birthday. I would become angry beyond commensuration over the tiniest of things and at a loss about what to do about it. I knew that if I approached anyone with the truth at this time in my life, including doctors, that I was "a dead duck." I attempted therefore to fumble my way through whatever arose — and, from that moment forward, no more would I fumble my way out of one situation than would I be in another. Life was absurd and I was stupid. What I did afterwards is proof of that.

I left Duluth with Eileen still in the trunk. I drove with abandon and with no destination in mind. I had no idea where I was going and neither did I care. I just knew I was supposed to drive until I got to wherever it was I was meant to go. I thought I found that when I spied a pigpen with myriad kinds of bones in it. In that instant, I thought something told me that would be her resting place.

I got out, wrapped her more tightly in the U-Haul blanket she was in and put her over the fence into the pigsty; then, I drove away.

The farther away I got, the more I knew I had chosen the wrong place. I could not leave her there. I decided that even if it meant my getting caught I had to go back and rescue Eileen from such a place. I returned. When I got there a man was putting Eileen into the back of a reddish-brown Ford pick-up.

I followed it for more than fifty miles before the driver turned off of the main highway and dumped Eileen's body over a fence and into a wood. After he drove away I was going to go to pick her up, but what looked like a Highway Patrol car was parked on the main highway. While I sat and waited for the police car to leave an elderly man came out of the wood carrying Eileen and took her a few feet into a cornfield. There he unwrapped her, examined her bodily closely — not pruriently — checked her clothing, folded the blanket, and took it with him, into the woods from where he had come. A while after he left the patrol also left. I waited a little while and, just when I was ready to go to get Eileen, the patrol car returned and parked in the same place. I waited a while longer and decided Eileen's body was just that, an earthen vessel in which her soul, now gone, had lived and I convinced myself it did not matter where the body lay. The soul had departed. I think now that my conscious mind decided it was too risky to be hanging around and I drove away. That Eileen had been touched by others was a catharsis of sorts: I could say, "If others had not touched her I would have. . . . " It was as if what I did had been done by committee and I was no longer totally to blame. I returned to Minneapolis, my guilt allayed, but not dissolved.

Life thereafter became a living hell, extremely difficult, especially when anyone would ask if I had seen Eileen. I wanted so badly to tell the people from the church, those who I felt loved her and truly cared for her what had happened, but I could not: it would not do her any good and it would hurt me immeasurably. Even if I was arrested and sent to prison it would not give Eileen her life back. That my state of mind concerning it would cause me to take Kathy Schultz's life a few days later and to fiendishly assault Roxanne Wesley was something I did not know and could not envision. I had no way of seeing the future. During the time I spent at the airport I concluded that nothing I could do, including being caught and sent to prison, would help Eileen. All the time I spent waiting to regain possession of her body served only to reinforce that belief. Later events proved it would have been better if I had turned myself in or if I had been caught, but turning oneself in, especially for murder, is not something that is easy to do. Even as I feel now the thought seems so ludicrous that I would try to live with life as it was. Only if turning oneself in would help another would it be the thing to do. It would not have helped Eileen, given her even a moment of her life back. If only society was not so bloodthirsty in its demand people who commit crimes, even those as heinous as this, might turn them themselves in for the help they could get. Why should they for a life sentence or a date with the executioner? It would be stupid of them.

I have never gotten over what I did. I have forgiven myself but even that took until I found out God had forgiven me. Society would not and I had to find it somewhere. Yet, I know in my deepest heart that what I did should not have happened, that I was wrong, and there is about me aura of guilt from which I will never feel free.

For the longest time I blamed it on my state of mind and lack of physical well-being because I had quit using dope, smoking, and drinking. The idea is ludicrous because I quit all three by choice and quitting them was the undoing of what had begun when I decided to smoke, drink, and to use drugs. I cannot remember having been conscientious, keen, ambitious, intelligent, smart, and correct all at the one and the same time and, if you think I felt stupid then, you should know how I feel now even after more than twenty-three years in prison — and each new day just adds to stupidity!

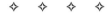

Dear Jenny,

As in the biblical beginning, it began with the "word": we wrote; next, there was "the voice" when we talked over the telephone; and, now, there is "the likeness." We had faces to place alongside everything else so we could see each other in a reality and a completeness. The total everything we had to create who we are in each other's minds.

At first, we were awkward and our getting acquainted was not unlike a tilting match or a sword fight with a series of verbal thrusts and parries by which we became acquainted and that familiarity became a friendship which grew in spite of such cataclysmic waves that rippled back and forth between us. Nevertheless, what developed was what we stood up for in the face of everything everyone threw into the arena so we might fail. We were patient souls who created a normalcy where none should ever have existed. Once we accepted there could be a normalcy, we became friends. The groundwork was laid in the beginning and became what was essentially an abnormality. As soon as we realized and understood we need not relate about what had taken place in the beginning we created moments of such normalcy the abnormalcy was gone, became extinct as the dinosaurs, and was replaced with what developed out of common sense and understanding.

Our silences became a quietness, moments of rest and relief in which we readied other words and phrases that developed into the present situation. It was during the saliency of these moments that I realized I had come in contact with the one person who was truthful enough to save what was left of a quest in which the facts and the truth would be told; that you who could, if you would, present them with such forcefulness and with such a sense of poignancy that what had already been said and written would not matter: your presentation would be brilliant and it would serve to unloose the truth that had for so long eluded a baffled public.

Jenny, truth is power, one that does not corrupt, the reason God is incorruptible and you almost are. You are exuberant and childlike, too much the enthusiast to let yourself be corrupted, unless you are blindsided. Some will tell

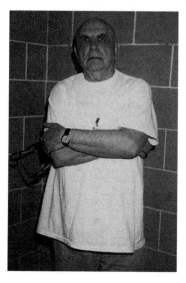

you that is what I have done, and you yourself must sometimes wonder about the truth of it, but you are too wise and much too intelligent to be taken in by the falsity of such an accusation. They have their proofs and I have mine. Please do not think I felt compelled to write this out of a false sense of gratitude. To see you as anyone other than who you are would be unthinkable. Also, to thank you would be an arrogance that would return us to the abnormalcy of our beginning. That I am thankful is understood, it is an intuition. I respect your honesty and am filled with gratitude because of your understanding, I dare not put these things into words. In fact, words would denigrate such feelings, make them less than the limitations on them. I need not say this any

Harvy Carignan today.

more than you need to convince me of integrity, your need to write about what is truth. That is a given.

Jenny, you are so uncritical of what I write I sometimes wonder if you do not sit and make silent fun of my efforts. Remember, in almost everything I sent I did not as much as edit. I wrote what came to mind as it came to mind and left mistakes and all. If you want me to be a little more careful and to put more effort into what I do, please, let me know. I can do better, not as good as you, but better than most.

I think some people commit their crimes because of guilt. They feel they are not as good as others on the one hand and better on the other and that they are being held back. I think I recognized this in some of my criminality. It caused a flux that could only be resolved by the theft of what I thought ought to be mine, that or something of an equivalent value. That, of course, was in the past. The thought somehow disappeared from my working mind after I learned to manage my anger, to be in control of my thoughts instead of allowing them to be in control of me.

Harv

In the realm of reason, Alcatraz demands an undertaker, not a champion announcing its revival even as it grudgingly passes life and time on to those who understand its eerie emptiness and the loneliness of its suffering during its last throes of its agonizing pain.

Suddenly, as if awakening from a nightmare, everything except the walls come humpty-dumptying down and the scene fades slowly from my mind. I am as empty as the buildings, a shell deplete of everything except the hollowments made by the loneliness of forever. Together, we stand a monument to the futility that created us. Our obituary, written in untranslated runes whisper to the winds that forever change our message on the sands of time. We are seen by all and understood by none. This architectural Ozymandias lies sneering on a desert of ignorance while a world of blithe sightseers keep the horrors of the past hidden behind the joy of their happiness as they savor a vicarious vengeance themselves upon its erstwhile inhabitants, leaving the reality of this bastion of sadism to pale in comparison and, then, when they leave, they take with them their mad imaginings, and reality, like a bad dream, is forgotten and all that went on before is for nought. It is unremembered, as if it did not happen.

You have read books, heard tales, and seen televison documentaries about me, but do not believe them. None of them told the truth. As time has passed, each has gotten worse than the last. All of them, while based upon the premise I have committed crimes and am incarcerated, are packs of lies. I have not read or seen any of them, but I know they are filled with sick imaginings. What I have heard what others so. Doesn't anyone ever bother to check out anything? If anyone would have checked they would have found that during the last fifty years most of the crimes for which I have been accused never happened and that I have not even been a suspect, investigated, or arrestged for any of them except in Minnesota and a suspect for one in Washington State and cleared. The Seattle police will not admit it, but I was. It is their tenacious stupidity that makes them hang on. I had perfect alibis for the day they think the crime happened and for the day before and after. When I was not at work, I was at home without a long enough travel time in between to do anything except go back and forth.

I might be out of line. You might have decided not to write any longer. I am sorry if you have. You are one of the most interesting and intelligent people I have had the privilege of corresponding with. Thank you for what you h ave given me if you have no more to give.

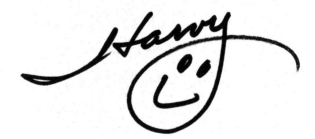

A page from one of Harvy Carignan's letters.

Roy Norris

R oy Norris cannot bear to have anyone look him in the eye. "It gives me a sickly feeling in my guts. I seldom make eye contact with anyone. I don't like leaving my cell. If I had a shower in here, they could weld my door shut for all I care." Norris says his life ended on November 20, 1979, the day he was arrested, with Lawrence Bittaker, for the brutal torture and murder of five teenaged girls.

Norris began having "problems" while he was in the Navy. A sexual assault conviction sent him to Atascadero State Hospital where he was diagnosed as a Mentally Disordered Sex Offender — even though he claims that he couldn't have raped the woman because he was still a virgin at the time. In 1975, Norris was again charged with sexual assault (which he also denies), but this time he was sent to prison where he eventually met Lawrence Bittaker, a meeting that would soon change his life forever.

On June 24, 1979, just six months after his release from prison, Norris, along with Bittaker, committed his first murder. Over the next five months, the two paroled convicts drove around in Bittaker's van, the "Murder Mac," trolling for young girls to kill. Norris reports that they had no trouble finding victims: "No bodies were being discovered and young women weren't leery in the least!" They managed to kill five girls before being caught.

Even though Norris admits his guilt in the murders — or at least his participation — he has a knack for sidestepping actual responsibility. He says the first murder occurred because they were high on the drug Angel Dust ("I came to my senses with a dead girl at my feet"). He also points an accusing finger at Bittaker. Norris says that he participated in the killings only because he thought that if he didn't, Bittaker would lay his killing hands on him. Furthermore, Norris says that it was Bittaker who twisted strangling wire around the girls' necks with pliers, who crushed their skulls with driving sledgehammer blows, who penetrated their brains with an icepick. Norris does admit that he killed Shirley Lynette Ledford, their last victim, with a coat hanger wire and vise-grips, but only because he didn't have the guts to say no to Bittaker's demand. Finally, Norris claims, unconvincingly, that the only reason he made the now infamous tape recording of Shirley Ledford's murder, complete with her chilling screams and terrified pleas for mercy, was to placate Bittaker — not for his future enjoyment, as most accounts report.

"If I had truly enjoyed raping and murdering kids," Norris writes, "we could easily have done so to 50 or 60 in the same time period." He says his obsession was to possess women and to hold them captive, but not to murder them. "I would've been keen on abducting a really hot sexy beauty for a month or so and then releasing her — but only those young women that were haughty bitches!" Even if Norris claims that his real turn-on was the abduction aspect, I find it hard to believe that anyone would be involved in murders, especially ones as gruesome and sadistic as these, unless they derived some sort of pleasure from them. No guts? I doubt it. Afraid of Bittaker? Unlikely.

Now 50 years old, Roy L. Norris lives alone in a two-man cell in Pelican Bay Prison, a maximum security facility in northern California. He will remain there for the rest of his life. He has considered suicide but he says there are some things that prevent him from going through with it: "Bittaker is one of them. I wish to be sure of his fate...death or otherwise."

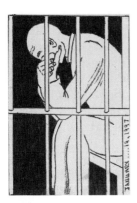 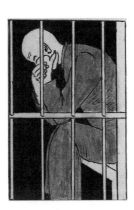 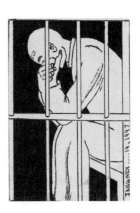

These drawings (and all the other artwork in this chapter) were done by Roy Norris. The above, drawn with a ballpoint pen, were on the outside of two different envelopes.

The Norris Letters

Dear Jenny,

On the reverse side, is a list of items that I <u>cannot</u> receive through the mail.....and a smaller list of items I <u>can</u> receive (and their respective quantities.) I will answer your questions, as truthfully and candidly as my inhibitions will allow. Further, I am here in prison because I am guilty. I testified against my co-defendant.....Lawrence S. Bittaker....currently on San Quentin's Death Row. I feel a social responsibility to answer questions that I <u>can</u> answer — for anyone who seeks answers. I will usually respond within two or three days — after receiving a letter. I am enclosing a part of your envelope...because I wish you to see for yourself....that this prison delays the delivery of our mail. In this instance, your letter arrived at the prison on January 6th, but I didn't get it until late this evening (the 16th). Ten days! I just recently received one that was delayed 16 days! The record so far. PLEASE.....PLEASE.....feel free to complain vigorously to your postal authorities! PLEASE!!

I use parentheses too much and usually in the wrong places in my sentences. And I tend to be prolific when the mood strikes me. I normally stay up all night and sleep in the day. I have a TV and we get just the basic network programming (<u>ABC</u>, <u>CBS</u>, <u>NBC</u>, <u>PBS</u>, <u>FOX</u>, <u>UNIVISION</u>, <u>BET</u>, <u>ESPN1</u> and a local radio station on channel 8 — Hits of the 70's 80's and 90's.) I don't normally watch TV soaps or Univision (I don't understand spanish) or BET (it's <u>too</u> Black) or ESPN. (I'm not a sports enthusiast). Nine times out of ten, I'm tuned to PBS for a "<u>HOW TO</u>" program or <u>most anything else</u> except OPERA.

Pelican Bay Prison — S.H.U. (Security Housing Unit) Facility ("C" and "D" facilities) is a maximum security facility...equal to a prison within a prison. I am currently housed by myself in a two man cell. There are no windows in our cells. It's a new prison that's had many problems so far. I am in my cell for twenty-four hours a day — every day. I could go to a "yard" for 90 minutes each day — but frankly, it's even more depressing than our cells. Essentially, it's a two-story concrete box — 12ft x 28ft.....with a plexiglass cover over half of it (protection from rain). Oh!, and you're on closed-circuit TV, on the yard. Except for three 10 minute showers per week, I'm in the cell all day — everyday.

Currently, I'm corresponding with fourteen people — other than my immediate family. I also write "fan-mail" — seeking autographs of celebrities and young women who appear in Playboy Magazine. One of my pen-pal friends is an Autograph Hound and I send him any autographs I get as gifts....for Christmas, his birthday and after each Special Olympics program he participates in. Though — my response rate has dropped from 1/3 (30%) to less than 1/20 (5%) since 1989. Celebrities are just overwhelmed with requests and some now sell their autographs, which stops my small hobby — cold!

1/19/97

I am involved in a Bible Correspondence Course. I've been involved with about eight different courses (denominal differences), in about as many past years. And though I say prayers every day, I say none for myself & I've not sought forgiveness....yet. I just haven't found the FAITH yet. My educational interests are all firmly based on verifiable science — which conflicts with all religions — to some degree. It's obvious to some people, that the Earth is <u>VERY OLD</u>. The idea that the Earth was created at 9:00 a.m. on October 26, 4004 B.C. - - - - is absolutely ridiculous!! Yet...the end of the world as we know it (the second coming!)...may be about to occur near the millennium. (?) Things do seem to be rather odd or crazy these days. Even I am shocked by some of the crimes that the media so diligently report until every hermit knows all the gory details. (Don't get me started!) (I tend to ramble and shift subjects, too!)

Pardon me, but who is Ann Rule?

I'm forty-eight (49 in Feb.), Caucasian, 6ft., Hazel eyes, brown hair gone white, and I weigh about 215 lbs*... (*A guess, only)

Not a single day has passed, since the first murder, that I haven't wished I'd not been involved.

Sincerely yours,
Roy Norris

MAIL

THESE CONTRABAND ITEMS WILL RESULT IN YOUR MAIL TO ME, BEING RETURNED TO YOU:

ART PAPER
CARD BOARD
CASH MONEY
CLOTH
CONTEST ENTRIES
FOREIGN CURRENCY
GLITTER
GLUED ITEMS
HOLOGRAMS
HOMEMADE ITEMS
JEWELRY
LAMINATED ITEMS
LOTTERY TICKETS
MUSICAL OR VOICE GREETING CARDS
PENCILS OR PENS
PHOTOGRAPH FRAMES
PHOTOGRAPHS LARGER THAN 8"X10"
PLASTIC
POLAROID PHOTOGRAPHS
PORNOGRAPHY (DEPICTING, DISPLAYING OR DESCRIBING PENETRATION OF THE VAGINA OR AN-
    US OR CONTACT BETWEEN THE MOUTH AND THE GENITALIA, OR OTHER PERVASIVE THEMES)
POSTERS
STAMPS OR STICKER TYPE POSTAGE (SHU PRISONERS ONLY)
STICKERS (RETURN ADDRESS LABELS AND CANCELLED STAMPS ARE TORN OFF OF SHU MAIL)
TRADING OR GAMING CARDS
UNKNOWN SUBSTANCES
USED BOOKS
other : _____

PROPERTY ALLOWED IN MAIL:

1 - CALENDAR (8"X10" OR SMALLER)
5 - GREETING CARDS
5 - MANILA ENVELOPES
12 - PHOTOGRAPHS
40 - PRINTED OR EMBOSSED POSTAGE ENVELOPES (SHU PRISONERS)
3 - WRITING TABLETS
40 - POST CARDS (OR THE ENVELOPES.. OR ANY COMBINATION UP TO 40 TOTAL PER MAILING)

SPECIAL NOTICE:

NO ITEMS DEPICTING GANGS OR GANG COLORS AND HAND SIGNS, WEAPONS, DRUGS,
FIGHTING TECHNIQUES, UNLAWFUL ACTIVITIES OR UNCLOTHED MINORS.

NO ITEMS THAT CANNOT BE SEARCHED WITHOUT BEING DESTROYED

NO NEWSPAPERS, NEW BOOKS, MAGAZINES DIRECTLY FROM PRIVATE CITIZENS.
(THESE ITEMS ARE ACCEPTABLE — ONLY FROM THE PUBLISHERS OR LICENSED VENDORS)

NO THIRD PARTY MAIL

CORRESPONDANCE FROM ANOTHER INCARCERATED PERSON, PAROLEE, PROBATIONER,
ETC. — MUST HAVE PRIOR APPROVAL

other : _____

This is the list of items Roy Norris says he cannot receive in prison, mentioned in the beginning of the letter dated January 16, 1997.

February 21, 1997

Dear Jenny,

Your February 7th letter was delivered...Thursday evening (yesterday) delayed by the prison for ten days after arrival at the prison on the tenth. (* lb. ¢ @ # $ *!!) I assume you sent the blank page along, for my reply. Don't bother, as I have more than enough paper. Besides, I prefer to use photocopy backs for my letters. They add 'interest' to my letters. I keep track of what I write on, so I don't send duplicates to anyone. The same goes for my envelope drawings.

I have some basic rules that I like to get out of the way, initially. I will follow them myself. I dislike <u>repeating myself</u>. I keep a pen-friends' letter...only until I answer all the questions, then I tear it to bits. I also code return addresses, as I've had cell-mates attempt to contact my correspondents. While I am currently...single-celled, I continue the coding of what I judge as critical information. There are many questions that you will ask — that I simply can't answer in a single letter...plain and simple! But I've been practicing since 1983...or thereabouts. If I don't answer something, I'll transfer the question to a note-page I keep handy just for that purpose...and I usually acknowledge the failure. I also answer letters within two or three days. The only reasons that I'll stop writing, are: <u>if I get the feeling you're not paying attention</u> (asking the same questions over, ignoring my questions, etc.); if you make a habit of not including the embossed envelope for my response; and if you stop responding to me. (Who is Ann Rule? Send me your birthdate, as I like to acknowledge them. Plus, I wish to know your age.)

Since you're not a "one-timer" seeking only my autograph or artwork...I'll begin with some basics. I just turned 49 on the 5th (2/5/48). I was born and raised in Greeley, Colorado. Though I don't have my High School Diploma, I do have a GED Equivelency — that would've gotten me into a college — if I'd cared to go. (Along with a good SAT score, obviously) Instead, I joined the Navy...as my grandfather and father had...and I did <u>get to see</u> a part of "the WORLD," including Vietnam. I began having 'problems' while in the Navy and after my discharge (Honorable)...

I was incarcerated at Atascadero State Hospital. After that experience, my next incarceration was at California Men's Colony in San Luis Obispo — where after nearly 2 1/2 years...I met [Lawrence Bittaker] a few months before our respective paroles. I had no idea upon my release, that we would eventually get together' again...and I didn't even have his address. He wasn't my first, second or even third choice in the kinds of people I would choose to befriend in free society. I paroled on January 15th 1979. The first murder occurred on June 24th and the last one on Halloween night. And my life ended on my arrest November 20th, 1979 (I just haven't died yet.)

If you consider my rearing in Colorado — as basically institutional (being told what to do) and the Navy, as well - - - - then my total life experience - - - <u>not</u> institutionalized — only totals about a single year, in <u>over</u> a decade. That's rather "telling"...I'd say.

I've been up all night and it's nearly 7 a.m. (breakfast). Oh!, I sleep daytimes — because I have intense nightmarish dreams at night. However, not during the daytime; yet. Plus, I am not interested in any daytime TV programming (except for PBS — "<u>HOW TO</u>" shows). A number of prisoners and staff have told me that I talk and sometimes 'rave' in my night-time sleep....so I avoid night-time sleep as much as possible. Especially so, between June 24th and November 1st of each year — when the dreams intensify more. Guilty conscience, I think!

I'll close for now and get ready for breakfast and bedtime.

———————————

2/22/97

It's a few minutes after midnight (Sat. a.m.). I'm tuned to "Politically Incorrect" with Bill Mahr. If you stay up this late, which do you prefer....Jay Leno or David Letterman? I used to watch Johnny Carson — then David Letterman. But since Letterman and Leno are at the same time now...I prefer Leno's comedy. Especially the dancing "Ito's" during the Simpson's trial. And since I've broached the subject...I think Simpson is probably guilty, but I did not get convinced in the TV Criminal Trial. (Which wasn't like any real-life trial! Money talks and makes the laws!) I don't accept the Civil Trial's Verdict, because the U.S. Constitutional guarantees against double-jeopardy. It was a sham of a trial...with an obviously prejudiced judge that allowed in evidence that meant absolutely nothing and denied Simpson's attorney's the opportunity to offer any defense. It was entirely a political revenge affair and if I were Simpson, I'd have moved any money's to off shore ac-

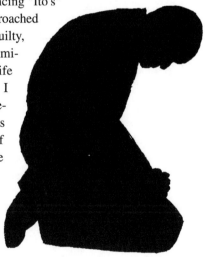

counts and the moment the court returned the children, I'd have left the United States for good. A hundred thousand dollars in some countries, is the equivalent of a million dollars here! I **WAS** just as stunned as Marcia Clark, though! I fully expected he'd be sent to this prison, for his own safety.

Do I think about the crimes? I definitely try not to. But not a single day has passed since the first murder — that I haven't wished <u>that first one</u> hadn't occurred. The "sensationalized story" states that Larry and I planned the murders while in prison. That's pure bullshit!! Stephen Kay, the District Attorney, said it to media reporters before the preliminary hearing. (He was Bugliosi's co-prosecutor against the Manson Family — but Bugliosi gave him no credit in the book. Kay has political ambitions and he craves the media attention! I've heard him talk about it.) At the same time that our case was in the courts...so was Bonno/ Bianci (The Hillside Strangler) and Bonin/Munro (The Freeway Strangler)...and the Rodney Alcala (?) murder trial in Orange County. It was reporter's "field of dreams" and Kay's personal media nightmare! So...our case became <u>more provocative</u> to meet <u>his</u> agenda.

I'm not saying our five murders weren't heinous and cold-blooded. They were...and if there had been more — the victims would really have suffered at Larry's hands! I suspect also, I would have been <u>one of them too</u>. (I'll get to that later) Also....the police in all of L.A. didn't even know we existed*. (*THE MURDERS, THAT IS) Had no idea! Until a fellow I approached (another parolee/ friend (?)) — and asked to keep his eyes + ears open for '<u>a handgun for sale</u>,' went to his attorney with the most basic idea of what was occuring. I confided in him, that I wanted a gun....probably for killing Larry, myself. His attorney tried to sell the case to L.A.P.D. (who refused for lack of evidence), the L.A.C.S.D. (refused), the Torrance P.D. (refused — for jurisdictional problems), and finally the Beach Community P.S.s (Redondo Bch, Manhattan Bch, Hermosa Bch, etc.) that "took it" as a group.

L.A.'s County Sheriff took credit, when he broke the story to reporters, only to get the media off of the Sheriff's dept. for the killing of a deranged black female surrounded by eight Sheriff's. She was threatening them with a paring knife and they pumped six rounds into her — rather than subdue her. Had I known how much pain and anguish my confessions details would create for the families of the victims...and my own family and friends, I may not have confessed. At least, not in so much detail. I should have just driven the van off one of L.A.'s elevated freeways — Halloween night. But, the families of the first four victims would still be looking for their daughters. About the only thing I can feel good about...are the lives I saved, by making them wary about climbing into the van. I received three letters from girls that remembered my doing <u>just</u> <u>that</u> — thanking me for their lives. But of course, none of this info reached the media's ears — or they weren't interested.

The first murder was a product of our experimenting with PCP (Sherman, Angel Dust, etc.). When I came back to reality, Cindy was already dead. My story, is what Larry told me had happened. I do remember some flashes of what he related — but it's all jumbled up and out of sync. I let him talk me into dumping her body and pretending all was well. The Death Penalty had been re-instated, so

I had grave concerns — obviously. But while driving — or working at Lloyd's Electronics — I often began crying ———— for what seemed little reason to me. I also toyed with the idea of turning myself in, while sitting in the Carson Sheriff's Parking Lot and the Torrance P.D. Parking Lot. I didn't, but I felt like it — very often. FEAR, kept me quiet.

2/23/97

I have problems with Christianity, because I'm a believer of EVOLUTION. While I didn't attend college, I have (had) a Vocational Electronics certificate and I'm self-taught/well read in the sciences. I'm good in math — up to quadratic equations in Algebra and I still fight with understanding Calculus. I've just recently requested a Trigonometry Text from our reading library.

I've scan-studied most religions, world-wide, for personal reasons I may get into later. The Bible's 'MESSAGE AND TENENTS' come closest to what I think is REALLY going on. The wisdom is the sharpest (possibly wrong adjective, but close). Forced to choose...I'll take Christianity. (Protestant)

Where did you obtain my address...and have you written to Bittaker? Who else writes to you...consistently?

Didn't women respect me in my life — or what pissed me off so much? This is one of those questions that will take some lengthy answering. No easy answers. I wish I could be definitive and exact about specific incidents that led me to my fate...but there's just too many things (small, medium, and large) that affected me. For a long time, I thought I may have been slightly retarded...but now I believe I didn't have a grasp of the world — like some kids did. I recall, reacting to people — rather than interacting <u>with</u> people. A social cripple...(?)

This is enough for my second response, eh?!

Sincerely yours,
Roy L. Norris

P.S. — No, I've never met Lawrence Singleton.

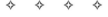

March 12, 1997

Dear Jenny,

Except for the occassional cartoon that I traced onto a page or envelope, I wasn't the least bit interested in drawing...until pressured by correspondants for some "criminal art." But I'm a bit of a perfectionist personality [drawing of a key] and I <u>had</u> to draw something that was recognizable for what it was — and easily. So I had to learn how to draw some <u>specific</u> <u>things</u> — <u>at the very least</u>. I mastered the head of a cougar or mountain lion and a small shore scene — before getting into flowers. I'm a slow learner and only recently — have I attempted to "loosen-up" a bit. Your "sketch" is better than any of mine. (sketches)

I was born, February 5th, 1948, at nearly midnight (or almost the 6th of February — which my father's father wanted, as it was his birthdate).

My father's family...all lived within a block of us (except his sister), as my grandfather had invested World War II profits into real estate. He derived his profits from an Auto Parts/Salvage Yard. All of his family considered my mom to be a 'gold-digger'....especially my grandmother — who openly criticized my mom to everyone except my mom. Her son, Bill, begat a son* and daughter — first....and grandmother doted on them. I'm a year behind cousin Shirley and my sister is three years younger than myself. Sis and I, were the 'black sheep' of the clan....and the obvious favoritism* was evident in every aspect of our lives. From the house my father had to pay rent for — while working for his dad (the only son to do so)...to the value of the Christmas gifts at Christmas.

I remember a coal burning stove in the kitchen and waiting twice a week for the ice delivery man to put block ice in our ICE BOX on the porch. (The only house my grandparents owned — that didn't have gas stoves and heaters...and electricity. In a city — no less!) Mom used a wash board for our clothes, until I was about 3½ years old. I remember the day when electricity was installed and gas piping came in. Everything was used, of course, (from grandma's house) but mom cherished the refrigerator, gas stove, washer and wringer (that used hot water from the stove, still!). We didn't have running hot water for a few more years.

I should add to the previous segment...that my grandmother blamed me for many things I was led into — or talked into — by both of my older cousins. This occurred so often, that I got to the point of not even bothering to defend myself. I simply accepted the blame and punishment. (Note: [Drawing of a key] As you might guess, this was likely the beginning of many supressed and angry feelings in regards to two female personality types.)

Mood controls much of my life now. In the past, I avoided being a moody person — by suppressing nearly all of my feelings. [Drawing of a key]

Today is my sister's forty-sixth birthday. That sounds so strange to my ears! Because...[drawing of a key] I never really expected to live beyond forty years of age. To explain, I must go back to the summer of my sixteenth year.......while 'hanging out' with a friend who worked at a gas station downtown (clean-up work mostly and pumping gas), I overheard some crude language about what a guy would do — if he ever got the chance with a certain woman that <u>walked past the station every evening</u> — in route to her parked car in the lot across the street. The fellow sounded quite serious to me and about an hour later, she walked past. This guy tapped on the window and when she turned — she saw me and waved. It was my Aunt Margie! The guy was surprized, as she'd never acknowledged <u>him</u> before.

Margie lived across the street from us for a while — then she and my Uncle moved about a mile away (but still in town). Margie was a bit brazen. She was the first woman in our town to dare wear a bikini swimsuit. Normally, she wore tight clothing...mostly dresses, about an inch higher than the current trend and high-heeled shoes. Until I heard about Amelda Marcos's shoe collection, I thought Margie was eccentric with her collection. I liked her legs (great!)...but I didn't care for the rest of her much. A bit too busty for my tastes and she had a mole just below the left corner of her mouth. (Why do women...and some men...like that? It's a nasty imperfection that makes me cringe. Many times, I've been in awe of a gal's face, until she turned fully towards me and I saw a mole. Instantly, she became invisible to me! I [drawing of a key] adore beautiful women!)

My Uncle Lee, was a semi-truck owner and driver, out of town a lot. He's the oldest of my father's brothers and he talked badly about Margie, in my early years. He felt she was running around on him — while he was on the road. I'm sure, his mom (grandma) was (again) responsible for his attitude. Because Margie and my mom often felt bruised by family gossip, they were friends.

Okay...now back to events. I considered telling my Uncle about the overheard conversation...but considering his tendancy to be a hot head and that he would likely use it against Margie (and provide grandma with more fodder for gossip), I chose not to. I also considered telling my father, but I saw that as just a postponement of the same results. I never even considered telling mom...and now, I wonder why!? Regardless...one morning (about 10 a.m.) in...(?)...late June, my father told me to go up to Aunt Margie's and get a 'urine sample' to deliver to her doctor. She was at home — sick.

Well...after doing the errand...I returned to Margie's and told <u>her</u> about the overheard conversation. Her reaction wasn't even slightly concerned, <u>enough</u> — as far as I was concerned, and I re-emphasized what I felt he had implied. And again, she seemed unconcerned. Frankly, I was stymied or more precisely ... wholly confused! (Now comes the crux.) Being totally in-experienced in speaking of such things — (and likely suffering from a degree of social-retardation)...I attempted to imply that I could understand...why the guy might be thinking such thoughts...and I criticized her choice of clothing style and possibly provocative mannerisms.

To be honest, I don't remember — for sure — what came out of my mouth. My motivation, however, was of concern for her.

Her reaction, was immediate and very angry. So angry, I knew I couldn't explain myself — so I left. I returned to the Salvage Yard and the tasks I had been at before the errand. Maybe — Half an hour later my father appeared...VERY ANGRY (RED FACE ANGRY)...and told me that Margie had called. He said he had to go down town, but when he got back he'd give me a beating I'd remember until I died.

Well...!! I decided not to wait for that beating — which I didn't deserve — and obviously couldn't explain my way out of...so I closed up the business, took my weekly earnings for the week, grabbed some clothes...and ran away from home...in the car my father had given me (A 1952 Cadillac Coupe DeVille. A luxury car in 1952, twelve years earlier. Powered everything!) Using a false ID I'd gotten from <u>my cousin BOB</u> (Shirley's older brother), I bought a case of COOR's beer and headed for the hills, literally. The Rockies...and a place I'd discovered while up Deer Hunting the year before. A small valley with a tiny brook flowing over worn smooth rocks. (I'd left a note in a drawer — about Margie misunderstanding me — and what I intended to do.) I sat in the car and drank about a 6 pack of the 3.2% beer that was legal to 18 year olds — then. I felt like the Japanese — when they've LOST FACE. When drunk enough, I used a diabetic syringe to squeeze about a cc of air into my left arm vein and smiled as I watched it go up my arm. I should not have awakened — after passing out. The cc was more than enough air to have stopped my heart. At least, every doctor I've spoken to so far...agrees! (With what I know now...I'd use the whole syringe if I could go back to that moment.) It was and is...sad news that my attempt failed.

Well, when I did awaken....it was about the same time of day as where I'd remembered blacking out. In fact, I got out of the car — hoping I was actually dead — but just not grasping it correctly. I realized though, that I had failed. I was also <u>stone cold sober</u> and <u>very hungry</u>. And I'd lost the intense mood — necessary to attempt such a thing.

So, at a cafe a few miles away — I discovered that I'd been "OUT" for two full days. From there, I drove to Estes Park, CO. A fellow I know, was working at the Darkhorse Theatre (acting) for the summer. I don't remember now — how many days I was there — before I was apprehended as a runaway, but I had put in a couple days work on a Dude Ranch...saddling horses and cleaning out the stalls and unsaddling the horses...hours later. At $5.00 an hour — it was nearly double what my father drew as a salary from the family business (ran <u>financially</u> by my grandmother, then). I sat in the city jail — about six hours — waiting for my father (only about 50 miles away and I was apprehended about 5 p.m.).

Dear ole dad had brought a friend to drive my car home and dad didn't say a word — until we pulled in the driveway. And then, only that mom wanted to talk to me inside.

Well, it was then that I learned that my father had been forced...into marrying mom.....and that mom had been pregnant about four months before they married (with the understanding they'd get a divorce when I was old enough to understand the situation). Mom says that he and his friends tried to induce a miscarriage by tripping her at the skating rink...and rough rides on dad's motorcycles. Mom stressed that I was to avoid sex until after I was married — but didn't say a word about Margie.

Honestly, I felt even stranger than DEATH.....afterwards. But I didn't have the necessary MOOD and FALSE courage that the alcohol induced — to try again. Instead.....alone in my room upstairs, I promised myself that if my life wasn't substantially better by the time I was forty, I'd stop trying and do the job right. I also agreed to remain virginal until after marriage... so my children wouldn't possibly <u>have reason</u> to feel as I did. (I had no idea how difficult that decision would be — but I remained chaste   TECHNICALLY   until 1975...[drawing of a key])

Hence......'because my life hasn't been substantially better'..........I've not seriously considered life beyond forty....much. I've postponed that limit, for several reasons. Bittaker, is one of them. I wish to be sure of his fate....death or otherwise.

3/16/97

The first murder...is the result of Bittaker's and my personalities — on P.C.P. (the drug: Angel Dust). It wasn't planned — at least not by myself. We'd been with some teens that hung-out near the motel that Larry lived in, while they were under the influence of the drug...and we saw nothing unusual. So...one Sunday morning about 10am, we smoked half of a Sharman Cigarello that had been dipped into a jar of PCP. We'd smoked a lot of marijuana in the past months and didn't expect anything much different. And the teens had smoked the first half.

Around midnight — that night — <u>I came back to my senses</u>...with a dead girl at my feet!! I have some memories of the day, but they are only glimpses of events that seem like snippits of a movie — spliced together out of sequence. The 'story' I related to the Homicide Investigators.....was the story that Larry told — me had happened. There's just enough info in my own personal memory — that "jives" with his rendition, that I've accepted the version as fact. The last cognizant memories I have, are the smoking of the cigarello.....until about midnight.

It wasn't an easy experience to handle — and I found myself unexpectedly in tears.....at work and in my car. Twice, that I remember specifically.....I sat in my car — in the parking lots of the Torrance Police Dept and the Carson Sheriff's Dept. — Trying to screw-up the courage to turn myself in. I didn't, obviously; but if I'd done it solely myself — I may have. California had just re-instated the death penalty.

The murders continued (three more occasions), because I didn't have the guts to say NO........until the last victim, whom I was told to kill (personally ... hands on...so to speak) by Bittaker.....because he'd finished with her. He was driving and he'd personally killed (hands on) the others. After doing it....I told Larry I couldn't do it anymore.

I did <u>avoid quite a few potential victims</u> — between the actual murders; <u>very purposely</u>. I even got three letters at mom's place — from three girls <u>that remember</u> my <u>PURPOSELY</u> making them <u>WARY</u> enough to refuse the proffered rides that they had their thumbs out for; thanking me for saving their lives. I....."<u>put off</u>" or "<u>made wary</u>" many, many young women. Only the ones I couldn't "put off" or "unsettle" — became victims. ((Note: I'm not trying to make them responsible for their own lives. I just want you to understand ....that if I had truly enjoyed raping and murdering kids, we could easily <u>have done so</u> to fifty or sixty in the same time period (at the <u>very least</u> — thirty with no problems!) No bodies were being discovered and young women weren't leery in the least!))
3/19/97

<u>About visiting me</u>.....I am <u>able</u> to be 'forthcoming' and 'candid' in my responses.....because I don't have to face you, eye to eye. I seldom meet another person's gaze, because I am embarrassed and humiliated by <u>my involvement</u> in the crimes! They (the crimes) did not make me feel good! In fact, the opposite is the case...and I detest my own fear and hesitation to confront Larry <u>immediately</u>! While I would, eventually like to see who I'm writing...in picture form...I don't wish to feel <u>your own gaze</u> upon me. Or anyone else's for that matter. In the past sixteen years, I've only had one family visit (my father from Colorado and my then, recent, step mom)...or rather...one visit, from the family. I've refused all interview requests and TV sensationalism opportunities. I have caused my family too much pain and humiliation already, not to mention the families of the victims. It's not always easy...to 'connect' with another person — via the mail — and yet remain clinically detached. I do try to maintain detachment...because I'd prefer not to become emotionally involved with my correspondents. (Except my immediate family of course)

If I thought you might want to actually visit me — face to face — I'd very likely begin toning down my responses. In all honesty, I'm not seeking an emotional involvement and or commitment with anyone. I don't write romantic or sexually thrilling fantasy letters! My <u>time</u> is difficult enough.

As you say, that you have two youngsters to care for — you'd be better off — meeting someone with a future, and not wasting precious resources on travel expenses to visit someone like me.

Well...I've used up all my space for this letter. When I get my hands on an embossed envelope — I'll mail this out.

Roy L. Norris

✧   ✧   ✧   ✧

March 30th....Easter Sunday....1997

Dear Jenny,

I've received your March 15th letter. Apparently, you think you missed a response to me. I think you just forgot the letter that prompted my last letter which I was delayed in sending, for lack of an envelope. I have no access to a telephone! I haven't spoken on one — to anyone — in more than <u>fourteen</u> years.

Where have you gotten the idea....that I hate Oprah? That's not true. She is one of the few BLACK People....that are being responsible citizens. And I was very impressed with her role in "The Color Purple" with another of my favorites....'Whoopi Goldberg.' I'll admit, that for a period of time, Oprah was bashing men pretty heavily....and I considered writing some critically-harsh responses! But my fear of getting media attention for such a letter to a talk-show personality — or — newscaster, keeps me from writing such letters. [Drawing of a key]

For example....last Friday night on ABC's 20/20, there was a report by John Stossle — about a fellow attending Brown University — accused of rape. Not a violent rape. More like a date-rape. The University, more than five weeks after the fact, (the girl waited four weeks to bring it up — to Administration) found him guilty of sexual miscontact. The Campus newspaper then ran a special page one story — even printing his name and photo! The girl even admits being drunk and....provacative — possibly. Stossle is a good reporter that goes the extra mile to allow people to speak their minds. The girl's name has never been printed and wasn't used by 20/20 — eventhough she refused to be interviewed and has been named in a slander-suit by the fellow (after being forced by peer pressure to end his studies at Brown). Yet, the girl is shown — voicing her opinions in opposition to 20/20's campus presence. My reaction. On a scale of one to ten — the girl rates a four — maybe. In my own life, I wouldn't even notice her existence. In a glance, she'd become invisible. But that's me and I already admitted being an adorer of beauty. (Why is it, or <u>is it just me</u>, that the women usually yelling "RAPE!"....are women that I wouldn't waste a second look at? Seriously — I can't remember a beautiful gal, ON TV ANYWAY, claiming she'd been raped. A number have been killed after being raped — though. When I see a gal like the one tonight, making such claims....I think...."Doesn't the guy have more class than to be involved with someone that looks like that!' Yea, I admit it's a shallow — coarse — uncompassionate and insensitive view.) I think the girl got drunk and 'out of control' on her own — and because she lacks experience (because of her looks) — she became a bit aggressive and flirtatious with a guy that didn't reject her.....and one thing led to another. I believe she was wrong to claim RAPE — four weeks after the fact — and I believe the politics of campus sexual involvement (and a strong WOMEN'S RIGHTS ADVOCACY GROUP on campus) exaggerated the situation well beyond the right and wrong of experience. I feel sorry for the guy, obviously; because it's happened to me....too many times. Specifically and allegorically. (The rape that sent me to prison in 1975, to eventually meet Bittaker, was **sex** by mutual consent!) I'm tempted to write a critical response to the Campus Paper or the University — or a — 'WELL DONE' to "20/20"....but because of WHO I AM, my response could easily be construed with creative license, to be something completely different. I've already humiliated and embarrassed my family and friends — beyond normal human limits. So I bite my tongue — so to speak....except in my mail to people who really want to understand me.

As for those "FOOLS" that suicided in southern CALIF. this past week....I just feel pity, that their lives were so empty — that they could become so involved with such an obvious CULT. No matter what, there are some people in this world, that can be lured "religiously" into acts contrary to the wisdom of the Bible and life in general. (I think about death a lot. Every single day, in fact. And I figure a day will come when I decide — there's just not enough reason to keep waking up — day after day. If it ever arrives, I won't try to take anyone else with me. Whatever awaits me on the other side of the veil, isn't for sharing with others.

Now look at the Goldman's and Brown's families — fighting over who gets what of O.J.'s property! Goldman's noble claim is tarnished by HIS BOOK and GREED! The media attention is EVIL!! It turns people into ASSHOLES!! I know — from experience!! For a time, as a 'State's Witness', I felt a false sense of importance. It's very seductive — fame! But a hollow seductress — is vanity (pun).

3/31/97

I've had my own problems with alcohol, so I know how tempting it is. I stopped drinking alcohol....in favor of marijuana, in 1968 — and haven't been drunk or even tipsy since the 4th of July of that year. But my mother became an alcoholic (a family genetic tendency) and as frustrated as I get in this environment....I won't allow myself to drink. I like being in control! [Drawing of a key] The same need to control my emotions, desires to be "in charge" of the immediate situation around me. I also avoided a HEROIN habit, because I'd have given the drug — power over my life. No matter how stoned I get on grass, I can still think well enough to know when I'm not capable of — interacting. Alcohol brings out the "creature" in all of us and grants us the right to antagonize others. After tobacco falls....alcohol will be next. It's 3 a.m. and I'm falling asleep as I'm writing this. Time to take a nap.

April 1, 97

When I was about four or five years old, my cousin Shirley (a year older) had seen her parents...."doing it." She asked if I'd ever seen my parents "doing it", but since neither of us knew what "IT" was....I couldn't answer. Well, on a Saturday morning, soon after her discovery, she talked me into experimenting (?) like her folks had done, to see why they liked...."doing it." Saturday morning was 'shopping day' for the weekly groceries, and both our moms would be gone. So on her back porch....we undress and laid down together under a blanket, and she told me to do this and do that and....nothing! Except, her mom caught us and went ballistic! Of course, I was the one blamed — and I was punished a week longer than she was.

It's a common experience for kids that age, I know now. But the 'being punished' for it, emphasized that whatever 'IT' was, 'IT' was adult activity — not for kids. As far as I remember, I didn't experience anything sexual.

However.........later on (between 1956 and 1959?) I experienced very pleasing feelings when wrestling with cousin Shirley (though no erections) and....(this is a bit embarrassing) the beginning of a shoe-fetish because of her (though I don't understand why). The fetish [drawing of a key], shifted from the original "saddle shoe" to the round toed canvas tennis shoes (like boat deck shoes.... Before the modern Adidas style athletic shoes became popular). The cheer-leaders wore them, and because of the shoe fetish (I suspect?)....I prefer a shapely pair of legs more than large breasts. In a crowd, I notice hair first (long as possible and blonde or light brown)... then the face. Then, if she's at least a six.. on a ten scale (looks), I check legs, if possible. If good legs, I can drop to a five (face). IF SHE'S WEARING THE TENNIS SHOES (AND THEY FIT WELL), I CAN EVEN DROP TO A FOUR.

An eight or better with long blonde hair — great legs and tennis shoes — would almost be irresistible for me. When I was making jewelry — I made custom items at and below cost — for young women that met those requirements....just so I could have reason to be around them. (used to buy gem grade opal in the rough — then cut — grind — and polish calibrated and baroque stones to sell to Zales, Slavick's, and other jewelry stores. Once I had my investment back, I saved the rest of the ounce to show at "Opal Parties". It's a psych-game....really, and I'll explain it later, when you know more about my past.) I should be more specific about this tennis shoe fetish.....as it's quite <u>compelling</u> if the right girl is wearing them. A better word is COMPULSION. The better the gal rates — the greater is the compulsion and obviously — the greater the risks I'll accept. I have, on occasion, followed such young women — MILES, in hopes of a possible chance meeting....in which — I can make known — that I am able to make custom jewelry and fix electronic equipment. An hour on the freeway on a cold night — on my old motorcycle — wouldn't be out of the ordinary for me — if she was an 8 1/2 to a 10. (A 10 would be Heather Locklear, about ten years ago.)

I've just reread your hand-written letter....and in regards to what Larry says about the girl in the tape recording — having been a participant. We've all heard women scream in horror movies. Directors of these movies want the best screams possible and they listen to many — many young women screaming — day after day. <u>Still</u>, we (the viewers) know that no-one is REALLY being stabbed or hacked-up or even raped. Why? Simply because an actress can't produce **some sounds** that can convince us that something vile and heinous is happening. If you ever heard that tape, there is just no possible way that you'd not begin crying and trembling. I doubt you could listen to more than a full sixty seconds of it. I heard her — when it was happening — and it sent chills down my spine. I was chain smoking marijuana — like it was tobacco — and I would've taken almost any other drug I could get my hands on at the time. Since that night, I've been forced to listen to the whole tape — <u>just once</u> (**Before** I signed the "AGREEMENT" with the D.A.). I NEVER WANT TO HEAR IT AGAIN! (Though, <u>I do</u>, in several of my nightmares!) If you could hear part of it — you would understand exactly why I don't like people's eyes on me. You'd know why I don't want to participate in the media spectacles.... and I honestly doubt you'd want to hear from me again. Just as this much attention on it — to write this little bit — gives me pause to think self-destructively. (Another reason I don't want to be emotionally envolved with anyone…is because I can't —won't — guarantee what I'll do after Larry's execution.) Larry can say or write such drivel (sp?) because you can't get a copy of the tape. Some of the Crime Collectors that write to me — have tried! You'd recognize the voice — <u>easily</u>. And <u>you'd know</u> <u>instinctively</u>!!

Sincere-ly,
Roy L. Norris

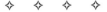

April 19, 1997

Dear Jenny,

If I haven't already informed you...my mail is inspected by 1st watch staff, then is forwarded the following day to the C-Facility Correctional Counselor Supervisor for her personal review...before it's sent on to the mailroom. Last year......ah.....January of '96, mom returned home and was confronted with numerous bills that had piled-up during her month in the hospital (surgery). A fellow I was involved with (he was/is selling small drawings of mine and 'things' — to crime buffs), had a balance of $7500 owed to me. So I wrote to him — explaining mom's situation and directed him to send the balance to her. Nothing! Each month, approximately, I sent similar letters along with queries about why he wasn't responding. He'd told me once, he was passing on the mantle of "control or management" — to others...and I assumed he wasn't receiving my letters. So I wrote to a fellow that we both know and explained my problems in getting a response and asked him to tell the other in his telephone conversation. Months had passed and I'd sent plea after plea.

In August of '96, I received an "Informative Chrono" from the above Counselor, reading...."On this date (8/2/96) I received a telephone call regarding Inmate Norris. The call was from a Mr. Craig Sanders of Danville, Illinois. Mr. Sanders had called approximately two weeks ago and stated he was having problems with Inmate Norris, do to the fact that his business had refused to do business with Norris. Norris in turn, was writing slanderous things about Mr. Sanders and his business. Mr. Sanders is now going to fax a copy of a letter that Norris has written to one of Sanders' customers — where Norris makes very derrogatory remarks and threatening statements about Sanders. Mr. Sanders has requested that Norris be stopped from making these types of threatening statements about him to others. Mr. Sanders was advised that we would start monitoring Norris's outgoing mail. When the fax is received, it will be reviewed for possible disciplinary action. The chrono serves as a warning to Norris, to stop these kinds of activities. Norris's outgoing mail (non-legal) will be sent to 'C. Bolles', for review, until further notice."

Needless to say, I was quite flabbergasted by his reaction! Especially — the information he "didn't" provide to "C. Bolles" on the telephone. Specifically that he contacted me and persuaded me to send him items to sell...and that he sells items of many other infamous criminals — alive and dead. Without the cooperation of such prisoners, he wouldn't have a business!

As a result of the phone calls, my mail is still being "reviewed." And I did receive a disciplinary write-up, but not for making derrogatory and/or slanderous remarks. Rather, for being involved in a "business arrangement" with him — in the first place. Though, I didn't know it was illegal (nor did all the countless 1st watch officers who inspected my outgoing mail to Mr. Sanders since 1994 <u>who looked at</u> and <u>knew the items were to be sold</u>!!); because this prison was still handing out 1994 rule books that didn't list the new rule. For <u>all of the hassle</u>, I only <u>temporarily lost</u> 30 days of "goodtime." (Goodtime is really <u>meaningless</u> to me. The loss of 30 days only means that instead of being "eligible" for parole "<u>consideration</u>" in April of 2010 a.d....I would have to wait until May of 2010 a.d. Getting a parole, is the <u>last thing</u> on my list of desires (though most people don't believe that).

The "<u>review</u>" doesn't inhibit me much — eventhough "C. Bolles" is female. Initially, in August of '96, she stopped three letters from going out — because I made references to money <u>for something</u>. A liberal judgement of a business-involvement...but again, that was before I'd received info about the new rules. Since, I've had no mail returned <u>for any reason</u>...though I've had a mailing stolen outright by an unknown staff member. Luckily, in this instance, "<u>Ms. C. Bolles</u>" <u>is a witness for me</u> — as she remembers the mailing and <u>sent it to be mailed</u>. I can prove it wasn't mailed out — easy enough! If confiscated by staff, I was supposed to receive written notification...and as I haven't, there's only one possible reason for its disappearance between Bolles and the mailroom; and only a State Employee had access to my mail after I submitted it for mailing. So...I think I'm now being ignored (a CDC method of avoiding responsibility), <u>for the moment</u>. (That will stop, soon)

April 21, 97

I'm back, finally. I've been swamped with letters from new people seeking correspondance. It's how I picked-up this routine of writing a bit every other day or so...on six or seven ongoing letters. Though I'm beginning to ease back on my prolific quantity of writing per letter.

I'm curious about how your husband reacts to your correspondence with criminals like Larry [Bittaker] and I? Is it a problem for him? Also...what do your parents say? I can imagine that it's rather frowned on?

Larry [Bittaker] has a tale. His parents were in their late forties (as I recall) when he was born. They'd never wanted kids and as one might apparently — the first time he got into trouble, serious enough to send him to Youth Authority...they packed up and moved away, being careful **NOT** to leave a trail to follow. When his "time" was up, no one came to get him. So he had to stay in YA until the court could arrange a foster home. From then on, it was one Foster home after another. (Foster homes — are well known to be little more than motels for troubled kids. The couple accepts a kid — only for the money the State gives.) Larry only spoke of this — once, but included that he seldom got any spending money...while the couples' kids got a weekly allowance. He spoke of being teased by such kids (usually in Spanish homes) and having to wear hand me downs, worn-out by the kids. Our last victim (his victim) [Shirley Lynette Ledford] had some spanish ancestry...and I discovered from investigators, that he'd asked her out a number of times. I suspect he'd been quite generous to her (I think she worked at a fast food place he frequented in Burbank or Glendale). This, is the same girl he claims to have been screaming "on-cue" for the tape. (I'd never seen her before that night, and wasn't expecting a victim.) It was already about 2:00 a.m. and my car was giving me electrical problems....and I lived in Redondo Beach and worked for LLOYD's Electronics in Compton, so I had a long drive ahead of me — after he gave me a battery boost, to get my car started.

There's much to be said about Larry's past — and the crimes. Imagine how you'd feel, being 'essentially' parented by the State of California's impersonal bureaucracy and greedy foster homes. Though not a justification, it does give pause — when considering whether or not he should be executed. And though you've not yet read all my major background segments, I'd feel better about my own involvement — if I had lived through such a nightmare past as Larry. Is it RIGHT(?).......that he be executed, and not me? Not LEGAL......but RIGHT? And though you say he is now — pure evil, he's still not the same person he was...nearly 20 years ago. I saw him give hundred dollar bill donations (3 different times) to the Salvation Army...and one evening in the downtown L.A. area — it was his idea to hand out sandwiches and pints of milk to the homeless and winos. He stopped at a closing "Jack in the Box" and bought every item they would normally have thrown away — and the same at a McDonald's near-by. We handed out food all night. Even some wine for the winos — after they'd eaten. Looking back, it's these events of humanity that may have also given me reason not to turn ourselves in.

I don't have "all" of the answers you want from me. But don't you even think for a moment that Larry thinks...'that the last girl (and probably all of them) enjoyed what happened to her.' That's Self-Serving Tripe!! For his ludicrous appeal contention that I'm the sole perpetrator of all the murders — while he only had minimal involvement with the victims and that all were alive when he loaned his van to take them somewhere. He wouldn't have loaned me his van — to go the corner liquor store!...without him! (He has an impressive I.Q. and intellect...when he wants to use it. I often felt like a candle flame in the beam of a headlight, around him.

April 25, 97

Would your freckle, under your chin...enrage me? Huh? Hmmmm? Maybe you're misunderstanding me about the moles that some men find erotic. I don't get angry. I simply (unconsciously) loose any interest I may have 'initially' felt. The person, becomes, just another face in the crowd and no longer gets my undivided attention. If...for some reason...I found myself in a situation where I had to speak to her (or even a "him"), I'd be friendly and affable. I just wouldn't...be interested. I could walk away without a glance back. Saying that I would be 'turned-off' is appropriate — but it's too strong for what feeling there is. Like redheads. I don't particularly like redheads (male or female). I'm not angry to be around them and I've even enjoyed their company on occasion...but I'd just never seek a differ-ent — more personal relationship. In the same vein...I find many black females to be exquisitely beautiful — but totally hand's off otherwise. I could be friendly neighbors, without so much as a twinge of desire. I think our (people in general) minds contain a key pattern of our ideal mate (genetically speaking) and that it is dependant upon the strongest ethnic dna code of our make-up. In my case, Scot-tish, Irish and German. The German being the strongest (with some Scandina-vian influences I suspect). I tend towards green-eyed (Scottish) blondes (German) with smallish (A-B cup — 34") breasts (Scandinavian influence) and narrow hips (34"). I especially like mouths like Heather Locklear's or Farrah Faucet's — in that the upper lip is an exaggerated "M" while the lower is thin and flat...giving a permanent "frown" (?) effect. Jennifer Runyan ("18 Again" with George Burns and "Up the Creek" — WOW! Great FACE & Lips!!) is the best example — and I expect her ethnic background is Germanic with a Scandinavian accent, geneti-cally. On the streets, I would go to extreme efforts to meet such a female — in hopes my make-up triggered her dna code. It's one of those instantaneous events that doesn't need to be acknowledged — as both would realize the kinzmanship. Obviously, the "pattern" can be over-ridden...and is, more often than not. Other-wise, Nicole Brown wouldn't have married O.J. Simpson! (Boy!, that was a case of an accident looking for victims! She, the bleach-blonde cheerleader — seeking any rich sports-star to 'praise' and 'cow-tow' to...and He, the black man seeking a white woman for status symbol envy. He, of course, retaining the right to screw anything he wants and she — just the reverse. She being, his posession. Her psychological make-up is as much to blame for her death as O.J.'s violence. She was a gold-digger — in the wrong mine...just like her sister and her coke-addict friend...Fay Resnick (?)!) I should point out — now, that I've never been inter-ested in kids...(teens). That was Larry's whole trip. At that time — my preferred age was 19 to about 23. (I was 32)...now, I tend towards 23 to 32 (?) — with exceptions (+10 or -3). While I might ogle a teen and secretly wish I was her age again...I'd never consider an actual relationship or assault (rape). My idiosyncracy isn't physical in nature (though, I have become physical when I lost control of events...due to a shift in power or control. [Drawing of a key] If she did something to grab the power away from me). And this just entered another realm...that I wish to save for a later letter...when you'll understand me better.

April 26, 97

I was incarcerated at Atascadero State Mental Hospital — for a time, as an M.D.S.D. (Mentally Disordered Sex Offender). Not RAPE or CHILD MOLEST. "Assault." Physical assault. Not until I left there, did I lose my virginity. A lengthy story for another time. I mention it now, because I think about the place a lot. It was a SAFE place to express myself to others. I miss it very much — (the place, that is) — and expressing myself. It's just not possible to do so in this environment. I often think about contacting old friends from there — to see how their lives have faired. Living vicariously through others is all I can do now.

Sincerely yours,
Roy L. Norris

✧   ✧   ✧   ✧

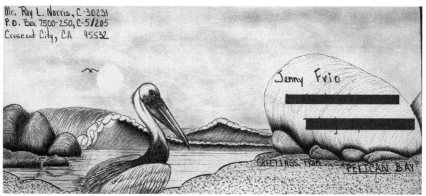

May 18, 1997

Dear Jenny,

Your letters to me aren't censored...and only mail that I try to send out...that seems to imply "business dealings".....have been refused for mailing (returned to me). You can say most anything, so long as it's not the directions for making bombs, explosives, poisons, etc.....or pornographic in nature. If you're interested, I'll be specific about what's considered pornographic.....but since I don't anticipate such a response, I'll leave it there.

I'm concerned about your husband. And does your husband ever get physical with you? I mean, violence? With the kids? And does your husband know you write to me? If so, does this displease him (I'm concerned not about myself, but for your...sanity).

Mood plays an important role in my addressing some of the topics you are interested in. In your very first letter, you suggested that you may have been a girl <u>we</u> would have wanted to have as a victim. I didn't address "that" at the time...because I've never had anyone suggest such an idea before. Do you......or......did you, think of yourself as a victim type of person? Such a remark would seem to me — to be an avenue to many possible meanings. Would you have ignored <u>unmistakable</u> leers from a guy offering you a ride in a van with another guy driving? And are you suggesting...when you were a teen.....or now? (This remark of yours troubles me...much!)

"Ellie Nesler"..........remember her? She shot a guy in a court room, because he was suspected of molesting her son. She's done three years of a ten year sentence, and has said that she'd do it again. I was enraged that she avoided a first and second degree murder conviction. Her story was just on "Hard Copy" again — because she's got breast cancer (she says....((?)) and wants out of prison. This is a person that "planned" an intentional murder of a man "in-custody" awaiting trial for a crime that he was surely going to be found guilty of. She shot him five times, after sneaking the gun into the courtroom. She refused to let "the law" mete-out its comparable justice for his crime (which wasn't murder) and with afore-thought and malice....she executed someone before he'd been proved to be guilty. Personally, I think she should be on California's Death Row.........with Bittaker and others...

I testified in court, that Cindy Schaeffer (our first victim) asked for time to pray.....if we were going to kill her. However, that's what Larry told me about that night, as I don't have a coherent — in sync memory of that night — — until about midnight. He also said I argued with him — about killing her (I'd like to think I did), but gave in for fear of a new — very long prison term, and its affect on my family. I see her face in my nightmares (her newspaper face) all the time. He said nothing about her begging for her life, but I can't imagine she didn't.

Again, in the case of the second victim [Andrea Hall], I don't have first hand knowledge...because I had driven [Bittaker's] van away from the scene of the crime (because there was no place to park it — safely). However, Larry took great pleasure in telling me "after the fact" how he'd given her the opportunity to beg for her life.....and showed me pictures he'd taken [of her begging for her life]. It's easy for me to imagine him doing just <u>that</u>, from the expressions on her face. And this <u>situation</u> is my current worst nightmare, as it's me...begging for my life. Great dispare, aching dispare, dread..........and hope, that something I might say would make a difference. I would say ANYTHING and, <u>do</u> (as I imagine Andrea did, as well).

The first time I had this nightmare, I woke up as Larry shoved the ice pick through my left eardrum and into my brain. For several long moments, my ear actually ached.......and since then, I have "tinititus" in both ears....but mostly in my left one. At times like this, I hear a constant 600 to 800 Hz sound in both ears — though mostly in my left one. I figure I've had tinititus for a while, but only became aware of it at Tehachapi's Ad. Seg. because the officers enjoyed kicking the tray slots [in our cell doors] closed (which is like a gun report in our cells). ((I can't say <u>for sure</u> that Larry didn't let her go, or that he killed her, for sure; but I believe what he said)).

I venture to say, that Jackie and Leah (victims 3 + 4) didn't know their actual lives were in peril.....and didn't suffer ® consciously. It seemed very quick, to me. From the time it took me to walk up to the van from where I'd heard a momentary....squeak like sound, Jackie was already dead and Leah was so "stoned" on Larry's Melaril, that she seemed to think she was home, finally. Larry hit her from behind, as she was struggling to step out of the van, with his sledge hammer. Not a great swing, but damn hard. I'd guess, she wouldn't have lived very long — even if taken to an emergency room. I recall (I think) hitting her in the head as Larry wrapped a coat hanger around her neck and tightened it with pliers (I didn't want her waking up!). ((A stress headache is beginning.))

The last girl, Shirley, I've touched on already (the [girl that we] taped). By the time Larry was finished with her, I was <u>just</u> <u>desperate</u> to get the living nightmare over, and <u>away</u> from him. When he said it was my turn.....I did only what I felt would be necessary to make him think I was also enjoying myself. I turned on the recorder and hit her right elbow only hard enough to make her continue screaming and the tape even picks up me saying...."please, scream." I did nothing more and didn't turn on the light, until I had produced a number of minutes of her screaming — for him. He'd been driving, like I had been earlier, and when I told him I was finished....he told me to kill her, since he'd killed all the others.

By this time, Larry had become rather paranoid (generally) and had begun to carry a 38 caliber police special, all of the time. I wasn't keen on an actual hands-on murder (I'll tell you!) but I saw no way to 'bumble' my way out of it (as I had other kidnap attempts & even letting Leah jump out of the moving van in Redondo Beach!). Plus, I'll admit, I didn't fancy Shirley [Ledford] on a witness stand — pointing at me and Larry — after what I'd heard for several hours before 'my turn' came. Mechanically, I did as Larry had done to Cindy and Leah...with a coat hanger wire and vise-grips...and turned away so I'd not see any reactions. She, too, had been "stoned" of her own choice before getting into the van. On what, I don't know, but she was really...."out of it"....from beginning to end. She didn't have any physical reactions that I'm aware of, though her eyes were open when Larry stopped on a quiet street and told me to drag her body out of the van.

As for how it feels to kill someone.........I can only say that it's a terrible feeling. For <u>me</u>, at least! <u>Hands-on-wise</u>, it was my second killing. The first was in Vietnam....a kid...a boy....about her age, also. Of course, it helps, that he was shooting at me and others.......but I watched him die. That memory, livid and vivid as technicolor....drove me to use heroin, cocaine and many other drugs while in Vietnam (opium and grass are my favorites, now). Vietnam is a whole different ball of wax — though.

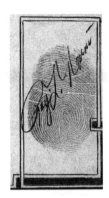

I told Larry, after <u>just</u> dumping her body, that I couldn't be involved in any more murders. It was a risk, considering how he'd enjoyed himself; but I knew immediately after ending [Shirley's] misery, that I couldn't see another girl die. A part of me....humanity-wise, also died with her. I think it was like — losing my soul, if you can imagine. But, I'd also experienced similar feelings after Cindy's murder. I found myself sitting in the parking lots of the Carson Sheriff's Station and the Torrance Police Department lot...thinking about turning myself in. It's a sickly feeling in my guts and glaring eyes, <u>when I close my eyes</u>, condemn me all the more. I seldom make eye-contact with anyone—fearing they'll see my great guilt. And, of course, I have no desire to receive visits...from anyone. I don't like leaving this cell, except to shower. If I had a shower in here, they could weld my door shut — for all I care.

Though I spend a great deal of time in the Bible...I don't seek personal salvation. I say prayers for others, mostly...and quarrel with "Him" over many things that occur. I will be happy — if I can be wholey and completely annihilated — soulwise. I'm definately not keen on bumping into any of my victims, on the other side! I shouldn't be here and didn't (as far as I know) wish to be born. Though everyone is in the same boat — so to speak, I <u>can</u> confidently state that life would be better off without me (my having been born that is).

It's easy to tell when I've been thinking about <u>all the life</u> we cheated our victims out of. I get morbid about God and my miserable life. Well...6½ pages are the limit!

Roy L. Norris

✧   ✧   ✧   ✧

August 13, 1997

Dear Jenny,

Your letter and photograph arrived this evening.

Suggestion......don't smile so broadly when being photographed. Whoever first said...."Smile for the camera"...should've been cold-cocked! Wide-grins, <u>especially</u>...ruin the real look of a person's face. They're also too pretentious...and hide the person's <u>self</u> — that's looking into the camera. A "pleased" expression...as if reacting to a somewhat funny or amuzing (amusing) irony..........is best. (As for your original statement — about your possible being someone we might want as a victim.......I can say that.........that wouldn't ever have crossed 'MY' mind. And, as Larry's preferred age is much younger.......I'd say you would be quite safe around us.* However, there are other S.K.'s out there.) So.....what color was your hair when you met your husband? (HINT: It's always best to go back to "that" color when trying to "come to terms" in a relationship.) There's nothing quite as disturbing to a true 'lover of blondes'...as seeing that a blonde was only a wanna-be/pretend blonde. To avoid that...most gals who decide to go back to the beginning — use a hair coloring that best matches her original color. It saves that embarrassment of dark roots appearing. [*I should probably note, that we didn't just offer rides to specific types of girls. Literally.... "ANYTHING" walking — gave Larry pause for consideration. I argued with him about this many times. Almost constantly, in fact. ((In my "then" fantasies...((NO KILLING))...it was the 'older' young women that had far more self-awareness, who literally chose to lead a guy on with no intentions of a real relationship (gold-digger mentally)................that I was interested in. I hated his 'anyone that'll get in the van' attitude. Such young "girls" (not "women") were/are too naïve and too inno-cent! My preferred age then, was 20-25. Larry and I shouldn't have been involved with one another in these crimes!! We have/had different interests and motiva-tions. I would've been keen on abducting a really hot sexy beauty for a month or so (taking great care that she not see me or others) and then releasing her. But only those young women that were hauty (haughty).....ah (?)...bitches! So-to-speak. And...I knew it was only a fantasy;..but enjoyable to debate the pro and cons of with other guys who'd had harem fantasies)) Yeah...neurotic chauvinism to the max! (But I went to prison for a rape I didn't commit! Yeah! I'm still angry about that — but I didn't go looking for her (a stunning blonde, by-the-way!) when I got out!!) OH!...for some wisdom of hindsight aforehand!!!

You contacted me as an individual seeking some insight into why the crimes occurred. I know of many prisoners that write to women (especially) with the disdain you mention (like a version of a porno magazine queen). But, they want something from the women. I only seek embossed envelopes for my return mail and occasionally — information, easy or cheap to obtain. I prefer remaining indigent...and I consider our correspondence to be temporary (30 days to three years — but still temporary). I do not seek an "emotional" involvement — since it leads nowhere fast (CALIF. LAW SAYS NO FAMILY or CONGUGAL VISITS FOR SEX OFFENDERS — EVEN WITH WIVES!). So...I don't run the "jive bitch" game on any women who only want a few answers. (I do appreciate, that you're not a memorabelia/criminal art collector, hounding me in every letter for more.....more!)

Well, I've gotten carried away and used up the space I intended to save...for your response to my last letter...so I'll mail this Sunday evening (the 17th). (Isn't there a prison in Bellingham?) It's 3:00 a.m. — the 16th and my religion TV programs are about to begin. So I'm closing.

Peace to you and your's!
Roy L. Norris

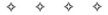

September 21, 1997

Dear Jenny,

Guilt isn't keeping me from making telephone calls. The rules of this facility and CDC.....stop me from making phone calls and getting photos taken. Reread "End of the World" photocopy I sent on February 23rd and understand that I'm in higher security housing than Larry [Bittaker] is — eventhough he is on Death Row. He has many priviledges that I haven't had in over fifteen years.

In your initial letter to me....you introduce yourself as....'likely a female that Larry and I would have liked to make a victim.' It has given me pause ....many times since then, as it's the first time any female correspondant stated anything like it. In my last letter, I wrote....that I didn't consider you as a victim type. I apparently should have added that you don't appear in the photo you sent, to meet the characteristics — to have been one of our victims. That's what I meant to express....rather than the general statement that I don't consider you could be a victim.

I never know for sure, why someone decides to write to me......and a big concern of mine is that I hope I never have a pen-friend that gets arrested for similar crimes. I go out of my way, especially with the guys, to make sure they understand I got no rewards from my involvement in our crimes. That the crimes have only caused me and everyone involved.....extreme misery!

Your 'victim' statement gave me much pause, because I don't understand your reasoning for having stated it. It set off an alarm, so to speak, that I still don't understand..........and it nags at me. Not yourself, personally, but the idea. But that's why I write to anyone that writes to me.....for the tough questions that make me delve into tough answers...and they usually come from women.

There's a new movie being advertised, entitled…"Kiss the Girls"...with Morgan Freeman and Ashley Judd. (BOY! Has she lost her looks!) Freeman has a line that haunts me...."he's not a killer, he's a collector".... When this film hits the VHS Tape Market, I'd like you to rent it and give me a synopsis of it. ((More later...when I know more about it.))

This mail delay thing and other concerns (mom's health, my health, disappearing mail, etc., etc. and even the deaths of Princess Diana and Mother Teresa) have cluttered my mind and I've forgotten what I've already told you in my letters.

Q — Why aren't AUTOSEXUALS given public-defenders in court?

A — Because they can get themselves off!

A joke, obviously. But with a ring of truth. I suspect that I've become an autosexual heterosexual. Without a partner...the idea is to stay aroused as long as possible (keep the adrenaline pumping!), because the climax or orgasm is the end experience, and for someone without a partner...it's really not so important. In hindsight, I've likely been an autosexual since high school (or even junior high school?), though orgasms were still important...as I remember. They say that sex...(the experience)...is 90% mental and 10% physical. I absolutely and emphatically agree. In all of my fantasies...the act of sex...is so rare, that it's almost non-existent.

In all of my life......I've had only one experience with a female partner.... that even remotely touched upon the IDEA of a higher-consciousness-mutually-shared climax.* And.....................she later <u>claimed</u> RAPE and sent me to prison to meet Bittaker. (She was/is (?) married and was caught in the act of douching by her mother-in-law/babysitter.) ((*After having been slapped in public — by her husband — and a long walk home.)) (((Our momentary fling was her revenge upon her husband — and claiming rape saved her marriage!))) And, yes, I am still angry at her!

The "non hands-on" idea is what I tried time and time again...to explain to Larry. But he's a hands-on immediate gratification person. I can sit on the sand at the beach, for hours, enjoying multiple fantasies with many young women.... remaining physically aroused most of that time, but with out the orgasms that end the adrenaline. Basically, I'm an adrenaline junkie....and if I could get aroused by terror.....then I'd love to jump out of airplanes, off buildings or bridges, etc..

The grist or fuel for the fantasies...comes from the past. And I recall my having written about that already (and your letter even responds to it). So I'll jump that and add........that, had I married someone..............I would likely have "Al Bundy's" attitude towards the physical act. That it was more work than it was worth.....considering that I could enjoy myself more.....viewing strange women. (While I may still LOVE "the ball and chain" person...the act of sex would have long since, lost its mystery and intrigue.)

The "game" then, remains the motivation in fantasies. Some men learned the art of charming women. And I've actually seen a number of men do this. The women get a glassy look in their eyes and it's...."wham-bam..thank you ma'am, time." It literally amazes me! I do not have the ability. Most of those fella's are one-timers, interested only in the total count. It's their 'game.' Other games are: baubbles (jewelry / $), sports, the smarts, cars, etc. In a sense.... forms of power. Force, also. "All's fair in love and war!" Who said that? And what does it say about women, to men? It sounds to me like...force is okay. In my head, however,

I am especially aroused by certain characteristics exhibited by some women....who are almost always, exceptional beauties. Not just attractive. Women who are so far beyond my normal reach....that all I can do (normally) is look and admire. (Not only don't I have what interests her, I wouldn't know how to act if she ever offered herself. And in reality, I'd never actually approach such a woman for a relationship.) She must exhibit... superficiality, greed/desire, and a hauty/pretentiousness. Other prerequisites exist also...but each can be compromised to varying degrees. (((My experiences in tapping into telephone lines, plays a big role here.)))

Roy L. Norris

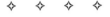

October 30, 1997

Dear Jenny,

Now, on to your letter..........................writing to someone female, who has read about our crimes is an unusual experience. I've written to quite a few women who have inquired about various aspects of our crimes. I imagine, that women are greatly affected by the recent Serial Killer phenomenon.* Not, like what I describe as regular crimes against women (assaults and rapes, etc.). As Robert Ressler says * 'personal crimes against women.' I imagine my correspondants....cringing with chills down their spines, when reading about Larry and I — and others. (I've met guys that I consider to be far worse psycho-pathic than myself...and they've made me feel very insecure and almost transparent as though looking right through me. Which is how I imagine you and other women, feeling about myself).

With that in mind, your very first letter seemed to imply (to me) that you considered yourself to be the kind (variety?) of female that Larry and I would have sought out.....and that you half expected to end up someone's victim, or felt......"hunted"......at one time.

I get strange and off-the-wall mail occasionally, as you might imagine. So I have to be very aware of what I'm writing to someone that may not be wholey sane. The very last thing I want is for my response to an inquirey to affect someone in a way that may cause them to react negatively. I see myself in a rather precarious position most of the time — with new correspondants... (women, especially).

I've been...tip-toe-ing...(or trying to) around that impression I got from your first letter. Initially, I thought you may have deliberately implied such — thinking it would excite me and open the flood-gates of my own psychotic mind. Further, the women who write to people like me...don't enjoy the best characterizations from society. I wish to avoid publicity — at all costs...and yet I know the day is coming when Larry's execution is at hand — which will attract media sensationalism like flies to a pile of shit! So, I've refuse all media requests for interviews — since coming to prison.

While you may not be a member of the media (per se), I question why a sane female would like to visit me. I have sent out two visiting questionaires to possible visitors. Both are men. One recently received his PhD in Criminology and is now working on a Master's Degree. I would prefer to answer all of his questions by mail and avoid the visiting room (telephone through bullet-proof glass). I participate with most college students because she or he may ask the crucial question that allows me to define myself — in such a way that others with my personality type might be discovered early on and be guided elsewhere ....plus what he writes will not become fodder for the media. His friend sought to visit as well, but he asked me about one of the women I wrote to for a few years — and admitted a desire to do a video on her, for cable. Needless to say, I've refused a visit with him as well. The other fellow I sent a questionaire to — most likely won't really make the effort. Especially as long as his excellent paying job holds out.

I refused your visit suggestion because I would feel overly uncomfortable.... and because you suggested it much too soon for my sensibilities....and aroused my <u>paranoia</u>. I don't make eye contact with the females that work here — unless forced to....why would I want to sit across from a female on a visit.

Don't misunderstand...that I don't like women. That's not true. I thoroughly enjoy talking to them. However, I have very little self-respect and I feel too humiliated and ashamed of myself — to put myself in a situation of feeling even more self-conscious than normal. (I shouldn't be here for these crimes! They're not what drives my urges!! I was too weak — as a personality — to refuse involvement. The crimes were too serious ® not to refuse, but I didn't. That alone, as far as I'm concerned, is unforgivable. I see enough....DAMNING EYES...in my nightmares and from staff, without risking more.

Sincerely,
Roy

P.S. — I think Louise Woodward (the British OPÉR-Nanny) was railroaded by an over enthusiastic District Attorney in Massachusetts! I wish I had some money to donate to her, but her community in England will meet her needs! Thankfully! I was stunned when the jury said GUILTY!

August 13, 1997

Dear Jenny,

Your letter and photograph arrived this evening. However, I just mailed you a letter -- last Sunday evening, the 10th. So, I'll begin this now and finish it later..... when you respond to my letter --- since you'll discover, I've addressed the very issues of this letter.

You'll note I've glued a section to a normal 8½"x11" page. This page now represents all the wasted space on your printer-paper. You should reset your margins and use as much space as possible --- and save as much paper as possible. Everyone should! I often use the back sides of old menus, used canteen order forms (twice a year, usually), and other incoming paper pages and salvaged envelopes. It adds a bit of additional interest to my letters. I abhore the waste that computer-printers generate. While you don't have to add additional postage until you exceed one ounce, I figure you could send seven or eight of your current pages in only four to five pages. Pennies add up when you write to a lot of people, as I do. For example ------ since 1992 (late April) when I arrived here — I've spent a total of $606.44, just on postage. Far- far more than I've spent at the canteen in the last 10 years!!! I don't waste anything. (I've still got coffee from my November annual package, deodorant, anti-bacterial Dial hand soap, and even jelly beans --- which I use for my colors.) Being so frugal — I'm astonished at the waste in the world! I'm extremely "PRO" recycled paper and other materials. ∟ Aug. 15 + 16, '97

Suggestion...... don't smile so broadly when being photographed. Whoever first said ..."Smile for the camera"... should've been cold-cocked! Wide-grins, _especially_... ruin the real look of a person's face. They're also too pretentious ... and hide the person's _self_ - that's looking into the camera. A "pleased" expression ..... as it reacting to a somewhat funny or amusing (amusing) irony --------- 's best. (As for your original statement - about your possibly being someone we might count as a victim .... I can say that ...... that wouldn't ever have crossed 'MY' mind. And, as Larry's preferred age is much younger..... I'd say you would be quite safe around us.* However, there are other S.K.'s out there.) So... what color was your hair when you met your husband? (HINT: It's always best to go back to that "color when trying to "come to terms" in a relationship.) There's nothing quite as disturbing to a true 'lover of blondes'..... as seeing that a blonde was only a wanna-be/pretend blonde. To avoid that... most gals who decide to go back to the beginning – use a hair coloring that best matches her original color. It saves that embarrassment of dark roots appearing. *I should probably note, that we didn't just offer rides to specific types of girls. Literally... "ANYTHING" walking - gave Larry pause for consideration. I argued with him about this many times. Almost constantly, in fact. ((In my "then" fantasies... [NO KILLING]... it was the 'older' young woman that had far more self-awareness, who literally _chose_ to lead a guy on with no intentions of a real relationship (gold-digger mentality)........ that _I_ was interested in. I hated his 'anyone that'll get in the van' attitude. Such young "girls" (not "women") were/are too naive and too innocent! My preferred age then, was 20 - 25. Larry and I shouldn't have been involved with one another in these crimes!! We have/had different interests and motivations. I would've been keen on abducting a really hot sexy beauty for a month or so (taking great care that she not see me or others) and releasing her. But only those young women that were haughty (haughty)... ah (?) _bitches!_ So-to-speak. And... I knew it was only a fantasy;.. but enjoyable to debate the pro and cons of with other guys who'd had harem fantasies)) Yeah... neurotic chauvinism to the max! (But I want to prison for a rape I didn't commit! Yeah!, I'm still angry about that — but I didn't go looking for her [a stunning blonde, by-the-way!] when I got out!!) OH!,.. for some wisdom of hindsight afterhand !!!

You contacted me as an individual seeking some insight into why the crimes occurred. I know of many prisoners that write to women (especially) with the disdain you mention (like a version of a porno magazine queen). But, they want something from the women. I only seek embossed envelopes for my return mail and occassionally – information, easy or cheap to obtain. I prefer remaining indigent --- and I consider our correspondance to be temporary (30 days to three years-but still temporary). I do not seek an "emotional" involvement – since it leads nowhere fast (CALIF. LAW SAYS NO FAMILY or CONJUGAL VISITS FOR SEX OFFENDERS - EVEN WITH WIVES!). So...I don't run that "jive bitch" game on any women who only want a few answers. (I do appreciate that you're not a memorabelia/criminal art collector, hounding me in every letter for more ... more!)

Well.... I've gotten carried away and used up the space I intended to save... for your response to my last letter --- so I'll mail this Sunday evening (the 17th). (Isn't there a prison in Bellingham?) It's 3:00 a.m. -the 16th and my religious TV programs are about to begin. So I'm closing.

Peace to you and yours!

May 10th, 1998

Dear Jennifer,

A number of things have forced me to put off a response to you, until now. Not the least of which, is your seeming insistence of finding excuses not to include 32¢ embossed (printed: Green Liberty Bell type — no paper-patch or hologram or stamps) envelopes for my return mail. After a year of being ignored — I shouldn't be surprized....but as our relationship has obviously taken a different track, I figured you'd adjust. Regardless, it rankles me to be ignored over any issue.

I have written my sister — about [getting] some photos from annual yearbooks and the family photo album. Only copies, of course, and you're not the only "interested party"....so she's said she'll get around to it. I've asked for photos of myself — roller skating (competing), playing the violin, in Cub/Boy Scouts' uniforms, old pets and me in my Navy uniform too! One of my pen-friends has my only picture of the house I grew-up in....and a negative of the only 'recent' photo I have of myself, taken here....and probably not as good a photo as my mug shots. (How did you obtain the ones you say you have? Are they dated?)

Another concern that has given me pause on all outgoing vital information is a rumor generated by a Mr. Sanders of "Crime and Criminals", a business concern that sells criminal memorabelia. For reasons too involved to get into here, I'll simply say that he and I are adversarial — now. In a remark to one of his clients and my pen-friend; Mr. Sanders let on, that he'd been in communications with a Mr. Stephen Kay (the prosecutor of Larry's case)... And that Kay had told him — I was in "hot water." Well.......as Mr. Sanders likes to grind axes, I first assumed Kay may have inferred some hostility towards me concerning remarks I'd made to Larry's Federal Attorneys; but on second thought — since Mr. Sanders did have his nose up someone's........well, just that if he was involved — it likely involved California's "son of sam" law.....rather than Mr. Kay attempting to void our mutual "AGREEMENT BETWEEN PARTIES" for my plea of guilty and cooperation in the case. However, I've not allowed any money to come to me — for any of the drawings I've generated since discovering that a Son of Sam law existed in California and that my previous involvement with Mr. Sanders — was a violation of the Prison's Rules and Regulations, for which I was........"dealt with"......so to speak.

Well, that...and my own continuing depression and the settling in of the full loss of my mom in my life.........and a myriad of smaller issues plaguing me, has put me off on more than a few correspondances. (My TV has stopped performing!)

I'm not a complete "babe" when it comes to book writers and TV interview-

Rape Crisis Centers, I was in mind of the usual arrangement whereby you, as the writer would be guaranteed a specific amount generated within the first six months to a year, usually, and profits thereafter — becoming subject to the percentage (usually only part of a percentage point → up to two or three percent). An amount that wouldn't stress you nor make the 'Centers' filthy rich — obviously. But, <u>something</u>, to ease the heavy load of karmic weight bearing down on me. I understand, of course, your book is about others you've written.....or tried to write......so my request may have been out of line — for what you've actually (as an author) asked for.

Hey! Men....and criminals....gossip just like wives and girlfriends. Criminals in every prison and jail — talk about how they got caught or errors they'd made in their lives. It's human nature....that we talk about 'that one other person we wish we had had a relationship with'....or....'the way foods seemed to taste when we were kids'...or....'what we'd do differently if we had a second chance — in time!' The subjects vary and one person may leave and another joins in. Is this "social dialogue" — the machinations of future goals? Well...according to Stephen Kay, it was equivelent to Larry and I scheming and planning "things!" Like politicians who will take <u>any</u> stand if there are enough votes, District Attorneys are putting on performances in front of an audience of jury members they hope to convince. They are <u>full</u> of dirty little "legal" <u>tricks</u> and will do most anything a Judge will ignore or overlook — to increase their 'conviction rate.' Stephen Kay is a Press Hound — cheated out of <u>the glory</u> in the Charlie Manson convictions by Bugliosi's now famous book "Helter Skelter." Kay was competing for MEDIA COVERAGE with the Hillside Strangler Case....and the Freeway Murders Case...not to mention Rodney Alcala's rape and murder case. Our <u>supposed</u> prison planning sessions...are a result of HIS fantasy, not our culpability. It makes "good copy." (And like diapers... Politicians and D.A.'s have to be changed now and then...and for the same reasons!)

Another error in [on your part]...is my charge and conviction in 1975. Kay, was also the prosecutor — by the way. I was charged with rape <u>by threat</u> and found guilty of the same. I was sent to prison at CMC-East in San Luis Obispo, California — where, after nearly 2 1/2 years...I met Bittaker a few months before our respective paroles. I had no idea upon my release, that we would eventually 'get together' again...and I didn't even have his address. He wasn't my first, second or even third choice in the kinds of people I would choose to befriend in <u>free</u> society.

A long yearned trip back home — ended my fantasy dreams of marrying one of the girls I'd grown up with...admiring...years on end. My 'hometown' didn't "FEEL" like the friendly small town that San Diego and Los Angeles made me want to return to. I sought out as many people as I'd thought <u>much</u> about in the want to return to. I sought out as many people as I'd thought <u>much</u> about in the past ten or so years...and to my utter amazement, some didn't even remember me. Now that, was a jolt of reality — I'll tell you!

Oh!, I forgot to mention above......in the previous paragraph; I DIDN'T RAPE MS. DIXON. WE TOOK "ADVANTAGE" OF ONE ANOTHER'S <u>MOMEN-TARY</u> SITUATIONS...IN A VERY MUTUAL EXPERIENCE! One, that I still cherish and appreciate — even though her circumstances forced her to lie about it. She had a husband of some worth and children to fend for, so I understood her priorities. While I've wondered how her life has turned out for her.... I've never sought to contact her again. I hope she's happy!

I once mentioned...whether or not...the social good of society should concern itself or even be aware of my feelings, unrelated to the crimes. I've cooperated with all law enforcement inquiries and many Psych studies of students across the nation.

If I could go back in time......with just an inkling of what's happened...to 1963 (after Kennedy's assassination), the world would never hear my name. At least — for crimes against humanity.

I've been asked for quotes — but never have I given one. This once....I offer this:

"In a few short months of utter insanity and indecision, I literally helped commit murder and figureatively committed my own suicide. I just haven't stopped breath-ing yet; as though in a nightmarish coma state. My mind is both.....sharper than its <u>EVER</u> been, but DULLER than <u>any</u> other with an ounce of common sense. What little wisdom I gain from growing older, is poor compensation for all the wonderful joys of life that I've overlooked or missed — in <u>my chaos of personality disfunctions</u>, <u>failed relationships</u>, and lack of <u>self-worth and self-determination</u>. The only reason I haven't already found the guts to end my miserable life — and give California tax-payers...and the collective psyche of the world...a sigh of relief, is simple......and it's the pattern of my whole life. And though I've tight-ened many a noose in the last nineteen years (nearly), I'm still the definative....coward. Sadly, <u>but poignantly</u>, my insight....is also my only good quality."

Sincerely yours,
Roy L. Norris

❖   ❖   ❖   ❖

-2-   3/14/97

I should add to the previous segment ... that my grandmother blamed me for many things I was led into - or talked into - by both of my older cousins. This occurred so often, that I got to the point of not even bothering to defend myself. I simply accepted the blame and punishment. (Note: 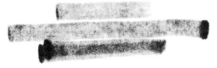 As you might guess, this was likely the beginning of many suppressed and angry feelings <u>in regards to</u> two female personality types.)

_____

3/15/97

Mood controls much of my life now. In the past, I avoided being a moody person -- by suppressing nearly all of my feelings.

Today is my sister's forty-sixth birthday. That sounds so strange to my ears! Because .... I never really expected to live beyond forty years of age.   To explain, I must go back to the summer of my sixteenth year....... While 'hanging out' with a friend who worked at a gas station down town (clean-up work mostly and pumping gas), I overheard some crude language about what a guy would do - if he ever got the chance with a certain woman <u>that walked past the station every evening</u> - in route to her parked car in the lot across the street. The fellow sounded quite serious to me and about an hour later, she walked past. This guy tapped on the window and when she turned - she saw me and waved. It was my Aunt Margie! The guy was surprised, as she'd never acknowledged him before.

Margie lived across the street from us for a while - then she and my Uncle - moved about a mile away (but still in town). Margie was a bit brazen. She was the first woman in our town to dare wear a bikini swim suit. Normally, she wore tight clothing ... mostly dresses, about an inch higher than the current trend and high-heeled shoes. Until I heard about Amelda Marcos's shoe collection, I thought Margie was eccentric with her collection. I liked her legs (great!) ... but I didn't care for the rest of her much. A bit too busty for my tastes and she had a mole just below the left corner of her mouth. (Why do women ... and some men ... like that? It's a nasty imperfection that makes me cringe. Many times, I've been in awe of a girl's face, until she turned fully towards me and I saw a mole. Instantly, she became invisible to me! I <u>adore</u> beautiful women!)

My Uncle Lee, was a semi-truck owner and driver; out of town a lot. He's the oldest of my father's brothers and he talked badly about Margie, in my early years. He felt she was running around on him - while he was on the road. I'm sure, his mom (grandma) was (again) responsible for his attitude. Because Margie and my mom often felt bruised by family gossip, they were friends.

Okay .... now back to events. I considered telling my Uncle about

A page from one of Roy Norris' letters.

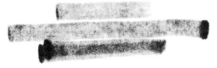

Harrison T. Graham

On a sweltering day in August 1987, Harrison "Marty" Graham nailed his bedroom door shut and left his North Philadelphia apartment behind. When police came to investigate neighbors' complaints of a putrid smell that was emanating from Graham's vacated apartment, they were sickened by what they found when they broke down his door — six bodies and the remains of another in such an advanced stage of decomposition that at first they couldn't even determine whether the victims were men or women. One week later, Graham turned himself in with the hope that police would believe him when he said the bodies had been there when he moved in. He eventually admitted that he had strangled all seven black women to death while he had sex with them — sex that had occurred both while the women were alive and after they were dead. Even though Graham pleaded insanity, the judge who was ruling (because Graham waived his right to a trial by jury), charged him with seven counts of murder and seven counts of abuse of a corpse. At the penalty hearing on April 27, 1988, the judge gave 30-year-old Graham 7 to 14 years for the abuse of the corpses, one life sentence for the death of one victim and six death sentences for the others, to be served in that order. In effect this means he has a life sentence. Today he is at Greene County Prison in Waynesburg, Pennsylvania.

No question, Harrison has had a sad and complicated life. He tells me: "I felt neglected unloved unwanted and no one really shown me true tender love and care! Even when (I) was more young, younger than my teen year's (I) still experience same mistreatment." As a child, he was sexually abused by a man. He was also emotionally abused. His mother drummed it into his head that he was retarded and he was teased and harassed by others: "Other's who knew of my mildly disorder meaning of retardation who only interest was taking advantage of me as a humanbeing and person who still hath human emotion and feelings."

Harrison is torn and confused about his sexual identity, and this may very well be at the root of his problems. Specifically he feels extremely uncomfortable about his bisexuality. He even made a promise to himself that by the age of 30, he would never have another relationship with a man: "Its not my cup of coffee...once any get involved with any Homosexual and life style its like a Drug. Once you get into it your hooked and its not easy to get off of it until you are strong enough to say NO. Even so (I) was tempted while incarcerated. (I) had to be strong for my own sake, salvation and Life. All (I) needed was a good woman."

Even though he confessed to his crimes, in his letters to me he seems to forget that: "So what if (I) may have lived inside One of the building's bodies of the dead was found...it don't mean (I) did anything. All it prove (I) failed to report what (I) discovered upon the day (I) was ask'd to move! Why do you keep Assuming (I) commited this Terrible 'crime' when (I) used to rent out the back bedroom unto others! A multitude are under the impression (I) sleep with the dead when it was only one person." Then again, in the very same letter he admits: "(I) made of Terrible mistake and if it come's down unto it (I'm) willing to pay with my own Life."

Today, at age 39, Harrison Graham has undergone a major religious conversion as a result of his crimes and/or his incarceration. And he is very serious about it. He even refers to himself as The Reverend Harrison T. Graham. God has become his way of dealing with his past. "(I) became a victim when (I) submitted myself unto the prince of Darkness 'Satan' which (I) became powerless even to resist the Temptation of Drugs Alcohol and everything which he has to offer unto the weak. But Now (I'm) strong Healthy and within my right state of mind. (I) was a slave to Satan But now (I) recognize (I'm) a child of GOD."

The Graham Letters

1-6-97

Extending only humble warmth of Greeting's and very best wishous throughout the remaining of your "Life" here upon this earth,

Received of your whole "Letter" And Trust this Letter may find you within the very best of spirit which its not uncommon for me to receive "Letter's" from a new individual or humanbeing! who hath of some common interest or concern about this whole humanbeing of man behind these lonely wall's, prison-life is very hard Likewise of it's Natural effect it has upon the human Heart 'mind 'body 'soul 'spirit: But am enable to handle this situation even with the support of concern 'caring "person's" along with faith and prayer! encouragement (I) receive Through the reciding of God's word "The Holy Bible" which give of comfort 'Hope within serving time behind These mighty wall's of prison! which am sure you have a Great multitude of Question's yet (I'll) try to answer unto the very best of my God given ability! which within reality amount many Prisoner's would question:

Behind the manner Thereof which you have interoduce of "self" Are you an investigator of Ann Rule when you first begin correspondance with Other's in prison

Because you did fail to give understanding based upon how you have come to abtain person's name' number' Address!

which (I) do understand your curiousity and willingness even to write of person's in prison in order to abtain information from person's unknown!

Am not frightened by your curiousity and desires to write or corresponde with me of whole. which (I) have know commit as it relate unto any crime: Because There is a great contribution of thing's which has happen'd in this case against me of whole, (I) don't worry about any man's Judgment about me as a person and humanbeing who has made mistake's within his whole Life!

which if any maybe without sin "Let him be first to cast forth the first stone."

"(I) have come under repentance" meaning, of whatsoever wrong's (I) have done in the sight of God, who see all Thing's and hear what we may say:

Actually (I) Think about every Thing as it relate unto my Life and Future:
Likewise of this situation (I'm) now going through as being here! Which (I) also
Think upon every Thing "That was wrongfully done" But also of the reality'
There is sinfulness Throughout this world and placed within the very "Heart" of
man, whoso refuse to go within the way of the Lord "Almighty" GOD' for God
is Love: Which There is of rebelliousness amount the nation's: whoso desiren't
to go within the way's and teaching's of the LORD of Lord's King of King's.
Who will alway's Look out and keep our best interest within his own "Heart"
which the way's of the "LORD" my GOD is best for me of whole, (I) refuse to
walk within the way's of this world: Additionally of those in this world'
meaning of man, "who aren't walking within the path of Teaching" example or
Love" who will apply God's Teaching's within there own "Life" which a
multitude don't know unto whom They "serve" God will not have any of his
walking in Darkness: But the enemy unto all men will try and keep us within
totally "Darkness" which you maybe in wonder why (I) have come out from the
Darkness into the Light by Grace Through Faith with courage and confidence'
"My Life is abit more better" Because am no longer involved with whatever
was in the past Am doing what (I) can in better of myself and this situation! By
Grace Through Faith prayer, (I) truly try to avoid "Trouble" 10 year's (I) have
been successful in staying out of Trouble: (I) listen unto the small still voice of
God who Lead me within the right way! Surely some correction has had to be
done first in me next within my Life! Which it couldn't be done while (I) was
out There within the free "world" Therefore (I) had to be taken off the street
and taught over again the right way's which (I'm) now living' according to
God's will' plan.
Please write back' from Harrison Graham

✧   ✧   ✧   ✧

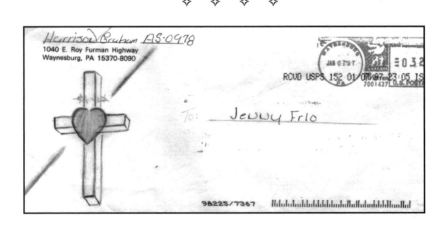

[Undated]

Am sorry but (I) want my day in court before (I) say anything to anybody. Other's may come unto there prison "cell" window and say what they want to do unto you "Behind what you have been Accused thereof "which (I) don't need be judged by any other person Especially a prisoner or inmate (I) don't have any friend's behind this situation

"Jenny has mentioned" (I) will not be Judgemental, which (I) can only take you at your word of promise, (I) had written "Because" this whole individual hasn't heard and was in wonder about my "friend" Jenny, which after knowing and receiving all this information about this individual, if your still interested within corresponding and writing please feel free Because (I) have been long longing to hear from Jenny which am still awaiting to receive of your "photo" "My reason for asking is (I) would not just have all your written letter's of comfort' support and encouragement But (I) would also have a face to go along with the Letter's "sent" (I) still try to picture within my mind the sound of your voice! (I) recognize this individual may ask not much: But if you feel personally (I'm) asking to much Just Tell Me
My love and prayers,
Bless be GOD' God bless Jenny

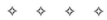

1-19-97

Jenny,

Within the beginning concerning my incarceration (I) was truly separated from the general "population" refering unto the other inmates while being in the "Detention" center personally (I) witness the very act of person's involved refered unto as homosexuality.

When (I) was transfer from the Detention Center unto Pittsburg "Penn" (I) was receiving a great multitude of mail from stranger's who later became of friend: Some where curious while other's ask "How do you feel being in prison and Death Row" which at the present (I'm) still on Death row but (I) didn't really recognize (I) wasn't serving my life "sentence" but my Death sentence handed down upon me by the Judge: who said (I) would have to serve the life "sentence" first and naturally (I) would mostly die incarcerated: (I) just thought in my mind (I) was only where (I) was for safe-keeping "separated" from the other inmates who would mostly cause me "Trouble" what is death "But to live again of new not to cause any confusment unto your whole heart or mind: But when (I) was brought and placed in prison (I) had to change the manner in which (I) use to think. Life in general is hard know matter if your out there or behind these lonely wall's of prison its hard and some time's very complex being here!

Once (I) even "Attempted" in taking my own life "But (I) heard the voice of an Angel" who spoke unto my Heart with words of comfort and Hope.

"Personally" (I) don't care if any may think (I) maybe "crazy" or out of touch with reality "But (I) heard the voice of my "beloved who caused me not to take of my life "which actually don't belong unto me even if any may think "my life is my own to take"

(I) know Jenny mayn't know me "But the door is open" which (I) welcome your friendship therefore we mayn't be stranger's unto each other but become "friend's"

Yes am very interested in getting to know "Jenny" Are you still interested in having correspondance communication with this man of whole: Am opening the door and welcoming of your friendship 'Love' letter, even of your prayers:

(I) hope and pray my first "Letter" didn't upset you or bring confusment personally (I) have had alot on mind.

Am sure you maybe "busy" with your correspondance! But please don't forget me who can use of your letter's of comfort and encouragment support and prayer's in our friendship of new:

(I) was in wonder how you come to obtain and receive my Name 'Number' Address!

Question do you visit any in prison beside through your letter. which (I) can only assume you may do herein "that" which is possible: Am going to bring this "letter" unto a close about here.

Harrison Graham

[Undated]

Trust this Letter may find you of precious "friend" in the very best of Spirit and Good Health, from reviewing of your recent letters sent (I) have take the opportunity to re-read them over and under line "Statement" Opinion and comment's made contain within your letter's. Which was interesting unto me of whole human being: actually "from reviewing all your letters sent and received" which you are very "curious" direct and determinable: meaning of Satisfaction in your curiousity about a person' place or Thing: Which within this case you are interested about the complete "person" who has become a victim, Even of Other individual's' Being objective unto there mistreatment and abuse' mental emotional and Physical "abuse"

"From The biblical perpective and point of view" "Sinfulness has alway's been within this world" Even before 'we hath so been born within this whole world" which at one point and time every last One of God's creation refering 'concerning of man" So hath had and some still have of very sinfulness' and

RebelliousNess in Nature!

Within general "past" Relationship has never really been considered as being Great or even nearly "perfect" Even if it may start out yet perfectly within the beginning But you know "yourself" if Drug's and Alcohol is a part or have any involvement thereof "which you have your Bible and what it say about the Outcome! There will be of confusement and mostly "separation" which (I) can remember living with this person' who had started in stop communication or even talking with me while living under the same roof we became very distance: which we had started in the beginning taking long walk's through the park's enjoying each Other's company and sharing of life: which Drug's and Alcoholism began to start taking over our life and emotion or feeling's which we once had yet within the beginning' which everything just went straight to Hell:

(I) don't have any good memories of my past: meaning of past "Relationship's" Am not realy concerned about what was "Because (I) have to focus upon with is now' There is nothing worthwhile behind me but pain! Actually the healing progress has finally taken "place" over the period of complete 10 year's. Which am now back within the unity and fellowship with God and Other's within the faith.

Next my lawyer has strongly advised me against speaking about anything "concerning" or refering about this case! (I) have to accept whatever my lawyer has said: But it will not stop me from being of friend or sharing a few thing or being myself, which if am to be judged of any thing's "Especially" of my performent's and you see its effecting of our friendship: "Judge of my wrongfulness pray and forgiveth"

"Personally" (I) do exceedingly Desire of your "friendship" Honest' Love' prayer's' Letter's support and encouragement

Based upon a personal and spiritaul level and Honesty through tove' care' tenderness sensitivity and patience 'with sound mind in understanding willingness of heart even to make of difference which (I) need of kind "caring" friend who would be concerned

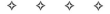

1-25-97

Hello precious new found "friend" Am very greatful you have been successful once more in getting another letter "written" and had time in sending it out unto me of whole "friend" Actually (I) hath been "praying" about abtaining "Another" letter from Sister Jenny of precious Thoughtful: individual of sweet! "Absolutely Sister you are correct" refering unto your "statment" it was quite necessary in reality in order of this whole "Child" to abtain and receive of my

salvation: which it was importance unto me personally in coming "clean"
Especially if (I) was to come unto the LORD Almighty GOD (I) refuse to lie
unto myself 'God likewise of friend Actually the Truth of any "person" will
alway's be brought out and revealed in the Light: The Choice is our's to make
'we can do it here and now upon this earth within our life or we can wait until
Judgment "Day" (I) perfer in being honest now Therefore (I) will not have to
worry about Thing's "That may come out of my mouth" which if any desire of
new person's must first "Change" from there old way's of Living' Thinking
Chance of Change will come when we hath of desire deep down within our soul
"Heart" Actually within my reality personally (I) couldn't keep living the
manner of Life (I) became accustom (I) was hurting myself and bringing
"Heartship" unto my mother who kept me within her "prayer's" along with the
rest of her "Children"
"But also try in understanding" God has called you to fufill his purpose and
plan within our Life! Which you shouldn't presonally feel whatsoever "That"
your using him in order of reaching me!
Am sure you know your "Bible" But its God and of the Holy Spirit that's
working his will through you of precious (I) never tought "Sunday School" But
(I) have been called from the very pit of Darkness and Hell to even share within
the Light and Truth of God's Love and rich blessing's with my Brother' Sister'
family and blessed of friend's, (I) speak the word of GOD: which (I) made of
"Terrible" mistake and if it come's down unto it (I'm) willing to pay' with my
own Life: which am not married nor any "Children" which the women (I) was
once involved with thereof had "died" while in her sleep (I) only discover of
this when (I) came in from working: we never had any children "together" but
she had a Daughter who (I) use to treat as my very own: which (I) really feel
bad about everything "that" took part within my past somethings (I) clearly
understand and other "thing's" (I) have been trying to make some kind of sense
thereof the situation even as a small "child" (I) was attack "sexually" abused no
(I) did not tell anybody for year's: But (I) have had very bad "dream's" about
the sexual abuse: which (I) never received any counseling until (I) was in prison
Next (I) began meeting other's who have gone through the same incounter of
experience sexual abuse' which someone male do hurt me and (I) was afraid to
open my mouth and share this with my mother only because my father was not
involved nor apart of my growing up in this life on earth (I) hate the wrong of
person but (I'll) alway's love people and care Greatly about them. Why because
the LORD "loved" me
as far as the sexual abuse you are the first female (I) have shared this with thereof

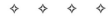

2-9-97

Extending only humble warmth within greetings unto you "Jenny" May God's peace be upon you of very precious "friend" of mine, who has made her way by Grace into this man's whole ♥. Please understand with our whole spiritual ♥ and mind personally (I) have taken into consideration "Acceptance" (I) base "friendship" completely upon Honesty and caringness additionally of willingness in taking a step of "faith" making a difference: Truth, love and understanding will bring of positive "Results" that we may share in the full blessing's of the LORD OUR GOD through our estabished relationship of friendship and correspondence: which you maybe under the impression this man has not open up unto you: but the "Truth" of the matter is (I'm) a bit slow especially when it comes down unto specific "Direct" question's (I) have to take my time in order of giving or providing the correct "response" But there is know right or wrong response! From re-reading your whole letter (I) see you teach Sunday School which the spirit of truth will not allow me to give bad information...that some day you may write an alternative "book" about why people become out of body or enraged: personally (I) know where mine came from: personally (I) have been alone which not many was willing to take the time nor had the patience to listen unto me.

Within my past (I) felt neglected unloved unwanted and no one really shown me true tender love and care! Even when (I) was more young, younger than my teen year's (I) still experience same mistreatment. Other's who knew of my mildly "disorder" meaning of retardation who only interest was taking advantage of me as a humanbeing and person who still hath human emotion and feeling's. Those around me didn't see retardation because of my progress and development in Christ Jesus! I don't hath a low (I.Q) anymore such as in the beginning because I'm teachable and hath of strong will in determination to learn, whatever is good acceptable "Holy" Right. But let us get back unto the other subject concerning enraged a multitude of person's mostly have or will experience some form of being "anger" which, in my past (I) never really knew how to handle being angery. The fact was (I) was "addicted" hooked upon what is called T's and Blues, cocaine and alcohol. (I) once lived within a "shooting gallery." Someone (I) was involved with there said "we need a place to live" and the rent was quite low!

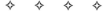

March 97

Dearest precious And Never begotten friend within Christ Jesus our LORD! Grace be unto you and of his peace remain Cherished deeply and pure As His Living word in your ♥ which most humbly (I) extend only warmth wishous of

God's very best be your's in abundance prosperously and Spiritaul:

There is know answer unto your "question" why death unto any person man'
women or child: which from my studies and yet understanding of God's word:
which a multitude of God's creation shall sin or rebel against Authority "which
its the opinion of this Disciple "That these Thing's was forth told" Actually
"these thing's would come to pass yet manifestation "that the word of God
might be fulfilled:
    "Which only now (I) have come to understand (I) was wrong in keeping
this unto myself" Because its been eating me up within the inside deep down!
How did (I) met my ex-lady friend well it was at the time when (I) was living
with one of my Homosexual "friends" which (I) had told him (I) had know
desire to live "Homosexual Life-Style anymore" Therefore neither party would
be alone it was suggested why not throw a party and from amount those, who
would come, we could mostly find someone special and thats when (I) ment her
The very first night we slept "Together" is when she had gotten knock up and
because (I) refused to sleep with the Homosexual we was ask' to move out of
his House! which we stayed "Together" with my once upon a time Homosexual
"Lover" while living with him under his roof: Is when she lost the child and my
mother didn't even know about the second child she lost behind "Drugs and our
Drinking heavy" which (I) have carried the burden and lost of my lady "friend"
But even so more of unborn child, (I) suffer deep down in my soul and Heart
behind the past yes (I) recognize God has forgiven me of all my wrong's, once
(I) have confess them unto him by faith "trust" belief and surely repentance! (I)
still dream of Death being upon the row: Jeffrey Dahmer was killed by other
inmates' Gary M. Heidnick had also received a death warrent But has received a
stay of execution "But now (I'm) awaiting Life or Death in result of what (I)
have been believing "GOD for within my life" by faith, yes (I) known Gary
while we was inside the institution at Pittsburgh because he was my next door
neighbor Even then he was talking that he wanted to die, (I) know if (I'm) put to
death (I) will be going unto a more better place "Than this earth" (I) wanted to
be with GOD in Heaven but also my Task is not accomplish nor finish here
upon this earth. Am totally attracted towards female's (I) made a promise when
(I) had finally hit my 30's (I) would never get nor allow myself, even to get
involved with any Homosexual's. Because its not my cup of coffee! Which once
any get involved with any Homosexual and life style its like a Drug once you
get into it your hook and its not easy to get off of it until you are strong enough
to say "NO" Even so (I) was tempted while incarcerated (I) had to be strong for
my own sake' salvation and Life: which all (I) needed was a good woman and
(I) was turn around and yet GOD who sew unto this man has gotten himself

straighten out and upon the right road of Happiness Love of God abide dwell within your very precious

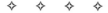

4-29-97

Dear Jenny most humble "joyously" (I) wish to extend warmth "Greetings" which quite abit of time has gone by before our corresponding or writting one Another!

Personally (I) have been experiencing of difficult time while serving my sentence Here within this ungodly place called prison or institution...it has its own effect upon the person's "heart" mind soul

(I) don't appreciate anybody pointing or passing any judgment upon me! Which was the same thing that happened "Before" (I) even went to trial and hearing (I) was found guilty before (I) even had a trial or went before a Judge in the county: "which within reality their is of Great contribution and reason's why individual's end up inside institution" surely (I) may have lived within a pit of Hell "filled" with Darkness which personally (I) had know Ghost of a real change to Truly experience and Live "Life" unto its fullness thereof, which again (I) was held back from being able to go forth! which (I) became a victim when (I) submitted myself unto the prince of Darkness "Satan" which (I) became powerless even to resist the Temptation of Drugs Alcohol and everything which he has to offer unto the weak "But Now (I'm) strong" Healthy and within my right state of mind

(I) was a slave to Satan But now (I) recognize (I'm) a child of GOD And what a friend we hath in Jesus Christ Our LORD "Amen"

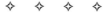

5, 23, 97

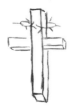

"Warmth wishous of my very best be with you indeed of whole friend" which (I) have almost given up all hope within hearing from a very precious special kind "loving of sweet" individual even after re-reading your letter's over and over again!

(I) was going through some old "letter's" of person's, when this whole individual has come across your's and began to read it over once more! Sorry it may take sometime with me of whole to truly unlock and express "feeling or deep emotion of pain"

(I) have never had anyone to share of my "painful" feeling's. "Detectives have suggested maybe it was Accident, while having sex you strangled individual's" which within the beginning (I) said No "Am not sure (I) don't think so (NO)"

That's when the Detectives and (I) over heard their converstance in the other room of the police station, yes (I) slept with a multitude of Different person's "female" and a few "Homosexual's" which (I'm) truly sorry and now ashame 'which at one point and time (I) slept with person's for different reason's money' sex and Drugs which is false

Yes (I) was employed But (I) had to do something to feed my Drug' Alcohol habit (I) felt within my past (I) could not make it through the day without my Drugs' Alcohol, Therefore (I) would get High before my ex-lady friend even awaken up and see me getting High "Before" giving her some food "first"

In Jesus' name, which am appreciative you have started "sharing" some Thing's about yourself a married woman and mother! Actually Am quite sure your

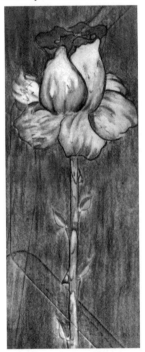

children and Husband truly appreciate all you are doing and hath so done!
Which my whole Life is complete within Christ Jesus my LORD and My GOD yes (I'm) married 10 year's now unto this ministry!
"We will become the very best of each Another's friend" which amn't ashamed of loving anybody "But even with my sure involvement with Homosexual's" personally (I) had to find out or try and discover who (I) was! Which (I) did discover (I) was attracted unto male' female, Even at a very young age! But amn't sure when this started being Attracted unto both: which while within my teen's (I) began to think "Is this kind of life-style will (I) still be involve with this form of life style' when (I) finally hit my 20's or 40's instead of using my body to get what (I) wanted (I) had to start using my mind that's when (I) stopped sleeping around: which Homosexuality has no place within the kingdom of Heaven! Which is non-acceptable of

The back of one of Harrison Graham's envelopes.

behavior even amount the people living within "Today" which even when (I) was inside this other institution my eye's was opened unto the reality how sick "sicking and unclean it was! which some other male was attracted unto me and (I) could only say "NO" Because (I) was not going down that road any more "GOD" didn't make me a gay man "But a straight man" "personally within reality and consideration (I) cann't really "Help" Herein, thereof what this man may feel deep down within his whole Heart' mind' soul' spirit"

Even as Tribulation' Temptation Test and Trial's "we will go through within this life here on earth, But may (I) put on the Lord Jesus Christ and make no provision for the flesh to fulfill its Lust, Experience incounter of my past Relationship's (I) left my mother "Mother's" home age 14 or 15 Only to move in with my "Lover" who treated me as a king and showered me with gift's or presence "car's" money' Drug's not knowing (I) could be brought" even unto slavery by these thing's of Satan who worked wickness Through That particular individual of Lover! Which unfortunatily (I) knew not what was forth of time nor future

(I) met this female indeed lovely and She was my escape "from a very bad Relationship" which (I) was within a very bad relationship often being past around from one person unto Another "Actually" (I) never thought much about it: being blinded by the gift's But when (I) met this women she took me away from that to experince of new "Life-Style" which (I) wasn't being past around anymore "Because" (I) made up my mind not to be past nor shared with any but one female

Over a period time, she was with child her's and mine! But one cold winter's night she came unto me with tear's in her eye's and softly said (I) just had a miscarriage and lost Our Child next (I) placed my Arm's around her to comfort her and said, we can try again

I often felt (I) couldn't make it through a day without taken a Drink or getting a hit "shooting up in my vein's" Actually (I) don't know what (I) had become within reality! Which it's not like any so hath come and pointed out "Hey you are an Alcoholic' Addict: which it's not uncommon within my old neighborhood for any to acknowledge the Truth: we often said "we are abuser's which we aren't "addict's" because Addict's will do any thing for a hit or cash. Which actually (I) did have of Limitation based upon what (I) would agree in doing

(I) did not have any "Desires" in watching individual's having sexual contact and intercourse which is not my cup of coffee! But not to say "someone" hasn't called and payed me to have intercourse with his wife while he watch us "which you can picture what he was doing" (I) didn't enjoy having someone set and watch me having "sex" or otherwise intercourse! Which (I) have be into this profession actually quite a long time within my life: This is not an easy subject even for me to speak about but it's a part of my past (I) have kept secret or hidden until now, when you came across my name and heard about this case. Sometimes (I) read your "letter" and you do sound like an investigator' more

than someone who has been called into a ministry! (I) know in reality we do
hath a multitude to learn thereof one another as time permit us to learn more of
each other by God's Grace and our willingness to share whatever of Truth:
Through friendship Love and concerness' care question will (I) be enable to
abtain and receive your picture yes (I'm) tall and thin short black hair "Brown
eye's! Well am going to close about here and (I'll) be looking forward of
hearing from Jenny God's grace and blessed peace with you!

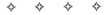

7, 13, 97
Grace be unto you And his peace remain upon your house: Greeting's be unto
you oh precious new found blessed "friend" Jenny which absolutely (I)
understand acourse you aren't able alway's to write right away "But" will when
you have the opportunity.
Am appreciative of "Honesty" in friendship and keep of opened mind about
thing's: which (I) learn abit from you! Actually within my reality GOD didn't
make man "for" man But woman for man and both for each other "even as its
written in Genesis "concerning" Adam and Eve which if God intented man to
lie down with man why would any need or hath strong desire of womans'
I was by-sexual not homosexual "Homosexual" males will only be or involved
with other homosexual's which within my past (I) was involved with both
Homosexual and by-sexual individual's "Because bothe had something to offer"
One of my main reason's of being involved with "Homosexual's" was to abtain
information based upon my question's "How you became this way and attracted
unto the same: which a great multitude who gave of response said 'Oh (I) was
very attracted unto so and so, while in the service while Another made
"mention" of being incarcerated and raped which (I) found this interesting of
those (I) ask'd "even" spoken unto thereof "There sexuality" The same can be
said about the opposite "sex" concerning of female's by-sexual 'Less-be-in'
Nevertheless unto me its "sicking" But must be recognized as a sickness and it
can be "corrected" Because its the state of person's mind in manner one maybe
Thinking" Of themselve's. God don't have in mind women to Lie down with
woman and have sexual intercourse, the matter concerning sexual 'intercourse
with the same God will alway's be against which my desire is woman "praise's
be unto GOD 'Bless his name" (I) may have been abit confused But praise's be
unto GOD am now "straight" by his Amazing Grace And of his Son "Jesus
Christ" Likewise of the power indeed both his word and Holy Spirit Thank God
for Jesus "Amen"
Correction "sex" can be beautiful and lovely "experience" when its with that
special someone of the opposite "Amen"

God loves me unconditionally yes he allow us to make mistake's "But"
Likewise he expect us to learn from them Actually everyone will suffer behind
the misdoing of wrong no matter if it may be of child molester or murder
"adulter" But it will not be to hard unto any who come unto repentance Blessed
is the man whom Thou chastenest Oh LORD. And teach him out of your "Law"
But Judgment shall return unto righteousness and all the upright within "Heart"
Shall follow it now may we move onward unto another subject:

The Bible may only be "confusing" unto those who will not seek' knock or ask
of his guidence and understand
(I) regret burning my first "Bible" simply because (I) couldn't read it
"Blessed be GOD "God bless you" indeed of precious, who will always have a
place of "Special" warm within my "Heart and prayer's"

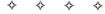

8-12-97

"God's Amazing Grace and blessed peace along with my prayer's remain
within in your whole   for am sure this Is not the response "Jenny" has
been awaiting upon But with heaviness of saddness deep down within my
own   This man's "Testimonial" cann't be permitted only for the simple
reason this man is awaiting to get back in court likewise to appeal the
complete case now against him.
Am privilege and greatful of your asking me within sharing my story with you
of precious friend and beloved "sister" within the faith and Heart of many"
Actually (I) have prayed very hard and listen quite closely unto the small still
voice of GOD:
Which its not unto me of whole to go against what he desire' meaning Christ
Jesus Our LORD. "He said let thine Heart retain my word and by faith keep my
commandment's and live"
"Especially when it comes down trusting of person's new"

My being imprisoned has its very own effect being surround by Other's, who
maybe my "enemies" (I) cann't "Help" what this Child maybe experience
within his life yet (I) would keep my Distance "Do (I) hath a real reason to be
fearful of person's while living within these time's behind these walls of prison"
which (I) have gone through enough' that will last even of Life time within this
man's whole new life!

Some other inmate's hath made "his desires or wish made known Based upon
what he want's to do unto me of whole! which my fear is what (I) would do

unto him: Out of defending of myself, which (I) have of "friends" while being
behind these walls, "person's want to end my life" But two wrong's don't make
anything better nor Right" "Murdur is not Justifiable" for a multitude within
position think "They are doing "God's service, when within reality they are
carring out the will of our life-long "enemy"
Amen.

1-98

Warmest wishous and Greeting's from Christ Liberty Gospel ministries
additional including upon behalf of this whole child and friend who hasn't
begotten of you nor family whom still remain within this child's "prayer of
faith" absolutely it has been quite some time since not hearing of "word" nor
having correspondence one with each other. But within the utmost excited name
Christ Jesus Our Lord this whole concerned friend can only pray this may reach
and find beloved friend including family within the very best of physical
mental' spiritaul. Blessed Good "Health" Trusting in the LORD with all your
giving unto God, Glory 'praise due unto his "name" for all thing's he hath done
within making of difference in each one of your lives by Grace through faith
'prayer blessed be GOD 'God bless you,

Dear friend "Hello" Jenny.
What have been going on with you personally? It was of blessing in receiving
your "letter" which (I) may be jumping unto conclusions, but (I) haven't heard
from Jenny in months, naturally whenever persons don't write, often (I) think
and feel maybe individual has lost interest within writing me! (I) maybe
assuming: There is more unto Jenny than what you have shared written and
spoken with me, which (I) may assume much within life concerning and
referring unto people! Who make me re-think and view things within a different
"light" manner!
Naturally, (I) shared "thing's" with you in confidence meaning whatever might
have been said or spoken ought to be kept between friend's for (I) cann't get
over the shame of what may have been the past: naturally we all have made
mistakes within life which (I) never claimed to be perfect: Amen, which (I)
cann't simply nor clearly understand why you need or have the desire to get in
touch with my "Lawyer" naturally am filled with questions and you are the only
one whom is enable to answer my burning "Questions," dwelling within this
child's ♥ this lawyer don't handle any of my importance "affairs" which (I) don't
allow when (I) truly don't know the person well enough naturally (I) don't have
"Trust" established between lawyer and person hasn't even tried nor shown care
or concern and interest within me: How am (I) physically or emotionally

'spiritually' doing which this hasn't been easy upon my nor my family: But also amn't unsensitive about these other "families" who has lost of loved one! Which once upon a time this whole child said he don't have desire to go through another trial now my attitude has changed "because the True of this case has to be brought out into the light" which am sure you have already formed your own "conclusion" of what might have been, personally (I) don't need any more of this upon me! Because (I) have suffered enough of this enough And (I) simply refuse to be subjective unto anybodies bull and mistreatment! Am getting to old for this

Slowly am dying behind these wall's of prison, (I) need a friend to care and be concern about me! Because am all alone: facing this situation alone with only GOD by my side. Honesty (I) began corresponde with Jenny simply because you are female and (I) though we could become "friends" and each other support strength through these hard times, But also be evable to ya! encourage one another within assistance one another building up each other within our most Holy Faith within GOD and fellowship! Well am going to bring this unto a close about here: please write if you are interested: GOD Bless.
Harrison Graham

✧   ✧   ✧   ✧

[Undated]

From viewing carefully the "notes" both comment's and statement's it was complex as Troublesome But sure enogh this whole really understand slowly the pain and very deep emotion running deep within your whole spiritual ♥ That which was expressed and shared through conversation you so hath had with inmates a Great multitude you have had correspondance "thereof" are considered by society and court additionally of "prosecutor"

"Serial Killer's"

Naturally you would be complex upset and out raged of person's comment and statement's through correspondence these individual's of prisoner's whom are Lost soul's filled with the devil and Darkness of Hell, which is spirit indeed "wickness" They haven't the Holy "Spirit" of God whom is Love!

Therefore you should understand they don't know what "They" Are actually doing: Because its not them even if they speak and believe in There own troubled "heart's" recognize its the spirit of Satan abide' dwelleth and rooted within there soul' Naturally the "principle" power indeed "Darkness' of Satan: who rule over the lost soul's! Which (I) hath hatred toward's Satan and very art of sin! Absolutely GOD "Almighty" Great he shall be justifiable, when He punish the evil doer: which none of us are "perfect" while we are still within the sinful "flesh" naturally after each and every one come up out of Darkness "flee"

from out of Satan's "power" influence' then the better off all individual's shall
be yet in this world: Absolutely we must hath Obedience unto the Lord "Jesus"
Christ and father of creation, which outwardly, we are made "perfectly" within
his image within appearance "sake" But nevertheless two wrong's shall never
solve anything Even as (I) reflect back unto the note's send and shared
comment statement's

The foundation and basis of your Book "fore public view" publication, Actually
(I) often "say" whatsoever we do: let us do it unto the Glory of GOD' That he
may abtain 'receive all Glory ' praises' love. Thanks!

When you started "corresponding" with the Rev. Harrison T. Graham what did
you espect to learn! Am sure behind your having of sure correspondence with a
great multitude of inmate's "imprison" Am sure its a change indeed: from
other's, who may hath ask or describe of breast or other part's "personal" unto
Jenny! Or person's who may have written what are considered sexual "letter's"
unto you! Which unto me its not right and its very disrepectful especially when
its not that kind of relationship: which if its your own husband asking these
kind's of personal "questions" (I) wouldn't abject but when its not your husband
or boyfriend (I) would have of problem with the person! Now (I'm) not going to
say here (I) have never ask'd of female but it was some one whom (I) was
involved and close unto within "life" But the spirit said what are you doing, and
(I) stop! Confessed and repentance which (I) have been imprison now 11 years
and (I) have not written those kind of letter

from Harrison T. Graham! Smile.

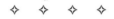

Dearest precious An beloved "Friend"
it was of privilege and blessing to hath received your whole "Letter" date 1-2-
98 which it has taken some time: Oh my beloved of precious "Friend" Greetings be unto you and peace be upon your "House" everlastingly with this child's
Their is no "question" what happen did "Happen within the past of this child's
life "Filled" Darkness around and about:
which abide deeply within my Heart' mind' body' soul' Spirit while within a
world (I) didn't understand Filled confusement! But far to many Jumped unto
their own conclusion yet Assuming what may have happened even you of
precious! So what if (I) may have lived inside One of the building's' bodies of
the dead was found naturally inside one of the Apartment's (I) lived within it

don't mean (I) did anything which all it prove (I) failed to report what (I) discovered upon the day (I) was ask'd to move! Why do you keep "Assuming" (I) commited this Terrible "crime" when (I) used to rent-out the back bed-room unto others! Now (I) started in remembering naturally unto whomsoever! which a multitude are under the impression (I) sleep with the dead' when it was only one "person" But (I) didn't have any knowledge this individual was dead until very late within the evening 6:00 p.m Naturally Literally (I) worked from 9 until 6 or 7 p.m

Even with this ministry (I) still work from sun up unto the going down of the same! which it was by "suggestion" of the police who said may be this or that "Happened" And (I) just went along. After over hearing their conversation in the other room of the police station which by following of their suggestion (I) also avoided geting beaten up by "police"

Naturally if you really want to hear and write my "story" let us work upon this "together"

Naturally it will also mean you will have to come visit because some words (I) cann't spell nor place within a letter! Absolutely if (I) cann't spell: which you may have already written the first part of your book "But (I) still hold the second part of the story to make it yet complete" understandable, which (I) understand your desire of my allowing Jenny to let others see me through your eye's: Next month we can set this up and put it into motion: which (I) like to see and read for myself, what the first part of this book sound's like you should have no problem in sending it here, which if (I) like it, we can go forth and work upon the second part of your "Book"

Please understand I have always had lack of trust within people "That" started back upon the day (this) case went to trial and other's lied, which is not uncommon' For any one who has gone throgt this "experience" within their own life!

Am prayerful you have had our blessed "Holiday" with your whole beloved "Family"
From your friend "Harrison T, Graham.

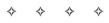

3-13-98

Extend heartfilled warmth wishous and Greeting's "God's Amazing Grace peace 'LOVE including abundance of joy's be with both family and friend whose Christian love + prayer's have been of blessing as the Joy which your being of concern "friend" has brought back into this Child's whole life and

Heart:

Additionally you should know me by now if any hurt my feeling's with "word" Amn's afraid to open my mouth and make mentioned of the wrong and how individual may have hurt my feeling's But that's not the case: Because we have gotten along quite excellently without any real major "problems" being the natural adult's which we have become in Christ naturally we have been able to discuss anything and resolve "situation" within adult manner reaching of positive "solution" we have of "communication" which within the past, we have had our "problem's" nothing quite major "but, Together we reached of positive "solution" Trusting GOD and each other "Amen"

By Grace Through faith "prayer"

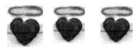

Which we are friend's forever in
    Christ Jesus Our Lord!

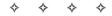

4-6-98

✞ Happy "Blesseth" Easter!

Greetings Jenny in the utmost exalted name "Christ Jesus Our Lord"
Appreciative of your kindness within concern and desire to make a difference in my whole, Grace and peace be with you along with his eternal blessing Am sure your kids shall hath of lovely time with the rest of your family "Easter"
(I) really appreciate thy prayers for me! Additionally of my whole "family" whom (I) don't get any visit's from which it's well with my soul: Because we can't force any one to care or be concern' they must hath within their own "Hearts" Personally amn't really close unto them only because am starting to get to know each one of them. Absolutely all over again!
Understand its not "Am (I) allowed to see them" They must have of desire to want to visit "me" my adopted mother was good to me But after my imprisonment everyone has changed: The truth of sure person's will alway's be brought out into the light: which its understandable.
God bless you indeed precious and beloved "friend"

from Harrison T. Graham.
"Shalom"

"Situation"
General "Rule" policies has Changed
Once again Upon Those upon the
Row : Naturally OF this Institution,
And a multitude OF thing's Once
within the beginning, we was
able to have in Our cell Or receive
has been Taken away !
Personally (I) don't Know, when
Any Upon the row will be enable
to have pictures Taken !
This institution has already ~~taken~~
Forced every Last One OF Us
without "Question" to send Our
Personal property 'Home'
inmates will be provide RHU
Jumpsuit and Footwear !
which we were given State brown
Clothing now we have these
RHU "Jumpsuits" personally within
reality its something you would
put On Over your Clothing
working under a car and believe
it's warm enough For this weather
my mistake its not warm
enough For this Kind OF weather
its Okay to wear while inside
the cell, But not Out door's !

"Situation"
Am prayerful Things will Turn
God go back to the way it was
naturally in the. beginning !

A page from one of Harrison Graham's letters.

Randall Woodfield

andall Brent Woodfield's childhood was not filled with horrifying abuse and neglect like so many of the men I corresponded with. In fact it was just the opposite. He was a cherished son in a close-knit and supportive family, a star athlete and an accomplished student who was admired and respected by most of those who knew him. Charming, handsome, brimming with possibility and promise, Randall Woodfield could have done great things with his life. Tragically, things didn't work out that way. He is now a convicted killer who will spend the rest of his life in prison.

The first sign that there was something wrong with Randall was when he was caught, at the age of 11, exposing himself to women. He also seemed to have a problem with anger. Even though his concerned parents sent him to see a therapist, no one seemed to pick up on the seriousness of his problems, or if they did, they certainly weren't able to help him. The "flashing" continued and before long, Woodfield started committing petty thefts and burglaries.

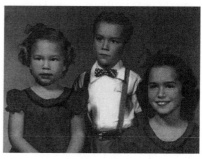

"My two wonderful sisters and yours truly, circa 1956."

At Treasure Valley Community College in Ontario, Oregon, Woodfield excelled in just about every sport, especially in football. But his problems had not gone away. He was arrested for breaking into a girlfriend's house and trashing her bedroom. (Due to a lack of evidence, a jury found him not guilty and all charges were dropped.) In 1971, Woodfield transferred to Portland State University where he became a born-again Christian. He took religion very seriously, but it didn't seem to interfere with his need to expose himself to women. He was arrested repeatedly during the next few years for indecent exposure.

Woodfield's dream finally came true in 1973 when he was drafted by the Green Bay Packers. However, once training started, he was cut from the team — a monumental disappointment that devastated him. Angry and depressed, Woodfield promptly dropped out of college — just three semesters away from graduation. At age 25, things didn't look too bright for Randall. He had no money, no job, no prospects.

In 1975, after being caught red-handed trying to rob a woman at knife point, Woodfield was sentenced to ten years in Oregon State Prison. Paroled after only four years, he was back on the streets. The crimes continued, but by now they had escalated far beyond flashing and petty theft.

In 1981, a spate of rapes and murders began to occur along the long stretch of Interstate 5 that runs

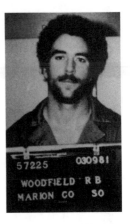

Randall Woodfield in 1981 as he was booked into the Marion County Jail.

through Oregon and Washington. The killer eluded frustrated police for a long time, especially because the attacks were occurring in so many different counties that it was hard for police to coordinate investigations. The first murders attributed to the "I-5 Killer" were in Keiser, Oregon, in 1981, when Shari Hull and Lisa Garcia were sexually molested and shot. Shari Hull died, but Lisa Garcia survived the attack, despite two extremely bloody gunshot wounds to the head. The next murder was in Redding, California, where 37-year-old Donna Eckard and her 14-year-old stepdaughter, Janell, were raped and murdered. Two weeks later in Beaverton, Oregon, Julie Reitz was found shot to death in her home. And there were many more victims that police suspected had died at the hands of the "I-5 Killer."

In addition to Lisa Garcia, there were other women who lived to give a description of the man who attacked them: white male, 25 to 30 years old, 6', 175 pounds, brown hair, short beard and mustache, Band-Aid across the nose, using a small nickel- or chrome-plated revolver, driving a gold VW. Finally, many victims later, the name Randall Woodfield popped up while police were investigating the murder of Julie Reitz. Not only did Woodfield match the description exactly, but subsequent investigations turned up enough evidence that police were sure they had finally caught the "I-5 Killer."

Randall Woodfield was 30 years old at the time of his arrest. All told, he was charged with sodomy, attempted kidnapping, robbery, attempted murder and murder. He pleaded innocent on all charges. In the end, although suspected in as many as 18 murders, Woodfield was charged and convicted of only two murders. He is now serving a life sentence plus 157 years, in Oregon State Prison.

Woodfield admits to a history of exhibitionism and robbery, but murder? "No way!...I'm really innocent of this terrible murder charge." Woodfield says that the "real" killer is a man named Larry Moore. Woodfield also believes that he is an innocent victim of a legal conspiracy. "Something [about my case] stinks of corruption by a resigned D.A., a demoted lead detective and a judge [who retired] soon after my case."

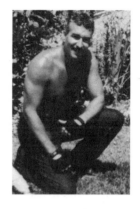

Woodfield didn't seem to hate women — that is, with the exception of true-crime author Ann Rule, who he unsuccessfully attempted to sue for libel for her book about him, *The I-5 Killer*. He wanted to make sure that I thought Ann Rule was all wrong in her estimation of him and it was clear he had read her book carefully. "You think Ann Rule lied about me having 'shark' eyes? Maybe I just looked a little scared or depressed in my bogus trial for murder? Ya think?" He also denies her accusation that he has small hands, herpes and a low I.Q.

Randy Woodfield in 1995 at Oregon State Prison.

Of all my correspondents, no one was more eager than Randall to get me to visit. When I finally did visit him, he was every bit as handsome as everyone says he is (he is gorgeous — and he knows it). He was also extremely convincing in his pleas of innocence. He even cried. I must confess that I had a hard time *not* believing him. He later wrote: "So you see Jenny, I may not be an angel, but I'm definitely not a killer, or rapist of women! I have confessed and repented my sins, crimes, etc. But I will fight 'til my dying day to show the conspiracy to convict me for murder, and that I was robbing people.... I never harmed people." If Randall Woodfield is telling the truth that he's innocent, then a terrible injustice has certainly occurred. If he's guilty, you just have to wonder how such a promising young man could have turned into a maniacal rapist and killer.

The Woodfield Letters

12/19/96

MERRY CHRISTMAS Jenny…

Thanks for reaching out to me. I am always grateful for anyone writing, or anything I have in life. Im not that dedicated Christian I once was in college, but Ive asked for forgiveness and want to be a better person now. I believe we all have "free will" to choose, and I choose to be helpful to others around me, and Juveniles in trouble who come in to our clubs here. And yes, I do have many different "pen-friends", but its hard to trust people, so I expect alot of communication and proof of who people are. So I work with people in selling my leathercrafts, and ignore the gamers. Who are you though? Will I ever really know? Peace to you & family….Randall

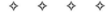

Dec. 20th, 1996, 10 p.m.

Hello Stranger,

Hope you receive my Christmas card and photo by 12/25. Sorry for re-creating my own card, but Id used the last cards in a box I'd purchased. Maybe you'll write long enough to see my talent in pressed, dried flowers I put together from our "Lifer Garden" here. And, maybe you'll be interested to see my leather crafts photos or Cichlid fish I breed in the Hobby Shop. (Smile) So you see Jenny — we really dont see or have much "barbarism" here, unless you call the practice of locking us in our rooms from (11:00 to 5:30 am), barbaric! Ha!

Nice to know you don't see me as the "monster" Ann Rule tried to show [in her book about me, *The I-5 Killer*], or just what a conviction may dictate, etc. Im really innocent of this terrible murder charge Jenny and the man [who is actually] responsible was arrested for mass-murder, here in Salem, just 5-6 weeks after my arrest as the "I-5 Bandit". <u>This man</u> (Larry Moore), is identical to police description and the police Hypnotic-Composite drawing, done by the victim-witness in the murder case against me! You wont believe it until you see the case files, which I could share with you, as Im still working on a new trial

126

appeal. And a "Break-In" at D.A. offices in 1986, prompted the Calif. Authorities to dismiss the murder charge against me. Go Figure!! ☹ something stinks of corruption by a resigned D.A., demoted lead detective, and retired Judge soon after my case. Comments, Jenny?

You're probably unaware that there is another "I-5 Bandit" suspect, who is pointing the finger at me, while he is facing a "Band-Aid" robbery in Longview, Washington, prior to my arrest. Officials in Salem & Beaverton and Clark Co. (Vancouver) dismissed charges against him for his testimony in court. But he lies, stating he made "No deals". I can now prove it.

So you see Jenny, I may not be an "angel", Im definitely not a killer, or rapist of women! You're probably disappointed, but Im not going down as some "scapegoat". I have confessed and repented my sins, crimes, etc. But I will fight 'til my dying day, to show the conspiracy to convict me for murder, and that I was robbing people in places in Oregon and Washington — maybe someone you know in Bellingham too, <u>but</u> I never harmed people, No Way!! Many victims told this to police, and many ex-girlfriends testified that I was <u>NOT</u> an angry, hurtful person.

In fact, some (ex) friends, girlfriends too, feel the need to stay close, and this is quite touching. It may surprise you, maybe not, but I do have a conscience and guilt over my crimes and hurting my family so much with my behavior. I am ashamed also and care to change for the better as well. And I cry in prayer times, and family visits, too, even loosing a girlfriend, lover or friend over time. So Im <u>not</u> the cold; unemotional person, people have been told that I am. Are you still interested in knowing me better? Im not shocked with strangers writing any more.

Actually Jenny, Im writing so quickly to you because Im not as busy like I used to be. Back in 1984 thru 1988, after I filed my federal lawsuit against [Ann] Rule and her Publisher in New Jersey [for writing a book containing false information about me], I was swamped in fan mail, or the well-wisher, and yes, even the hate-monger too. But thru it all, Ive found some life-long friends, and even been blessed with a child too. Sorry, I cant explain that to you. ☺

Guess we are both spiritual people Jenny, for I believed in marriage here with my (ex) wife, before we had our child. Now Im divorced, and beyond the pain, and as supportive to my child as I can be. Have you married or had children yet Jenny? And is Jenny Frio your real name? I wont be getting parole, so no need to worry about me stalking or finding you. Im not that kind of person...sorry.

You made a statement about "psychs" picking my brain? Well, I never spoke to doctors in trial, and haven't here for the past 15 plus years. I dont buy into their games and "psycho-babble", and only my "<u>convictions</u>" have been the basis for doctors to describe me. So you figure it out, Ive been painted and labeled and convicted of murder, based on a hypnotized (victim-witness) by detective (Kominek) in charge. The victim was told to look for her "attacker on a T.V. screen", (19-20 times) in a 45 min. hypnosis session. And never describing me or picking me out of photos, <u>PRIOR</u> to arrest and

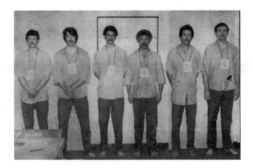

Lisa Garcia picked the fifth man from the left, Randall Woodfield, as the man who attacked her and killed her friend, Shari Hull.

publicity on T.V.! ☹ So why change their case to fit me — now picked out of a "line-up" by hypnotized witness? Blood types are wrong and thrown out of the trial. Evidence in semen & hair shows (A/B) blood-type! I am a rare (B Neg.) Jenny. Does anyone care to investigate the scandal? I guess my case is too old or too messy for people to bother with. Hell…I was even "shackled" in front of my jury for 5 weeks and made to walk in leg-shackles to testify, without official records (transcripts) showing it. A mistake, or planned corruption on my appeal? Most defendants are <u>NEVER</u> handcuffed in sight of any jurors, due to prejudice and impartial jury! So why me? Why the cover-up?

Okay, enough about all that. Maybe you are sincerely interested in me as a person. Maybe you're collecting information for (Rule), or another person. Time and our meeting will tell. And we do have special, private booths (security-glass) to keep us apart. Or we could be in a crowded room for coffee and snacks, or even picnic outdoors in warmer months by the "Wall" ☺ See how confidant I am? Ha! Actually, I just like to explain how I can show you legal files, even in a private, attorney room for "lawyers" only. (wink) This room has its advantages of course. Ha!

Have you ever written or visited anyone in jail or prison? And do you believe the "BS" written by fiction writer Ann Rule? I spent $2000 over 2 yrs. in suing her for libel. Would you care to read over the lawsuit and news of it? Or the burglary on my file only in D.A. offices? Let me know —— K? You made me smile reading you make a companion of "lyrical sorts", and fun to "play ball" in pen and paper, and you can match wits with anyone. Are you sure? Will you prove your identity and be open to share photos with me? "Hmmmm" ☺ I have to doubt all who write…sorry. But I feel you <u>may be</u> who you say, and genuinely interested. Would you be open to talk by phone sometime? We can call "collect" any time until (11 pm) and direct thru clubs, for business only. Such as in our Athletic, Lifer or Chess clubs. I could call for information to be put on visitors form, for records check. (police) Any record and we would only receive a window-booth visit. Clubs would not allow you in to speak or watch at night visits. And clubs allow one annual (party), with a guest on a visitors list! This special time is given to inmates on best conduct over 2-yr. period, and are given dinners and dancing. (Smile) I will enclose a visiting photo or club party photo to show you the setting. Please return any pics. marked for "return" — Thanks Jenny. I will return your pics requested also. So, may I see who this attractive, 29 yr. old? Come on…you did speak of the challenge and no fear too. I promise not to bite, after I grow wings and fly to your bedroom in my black cape! (Ha-Ha)

Your offer of sharing your view is nice. I have a view thru bars, but open window into my room here, of a courtyard and peacocks, pheasants and pigeons soaring and roaming about. I even see over the 28' wall to the eastern "Cascades" & our last (Moon Eclipse) frontview! Unreal, too…Did you see it too Jenny?

Oh yeah, is that your handwriting at the end of your letter? You said…"Sorry for the typo's" & you used a smiley face too. Coincidence, or something you read that I use? "Hmmmmm" Come on —— 'Fess up now. ☺ What did you mean by saying you are "hopeless without the help that you can provide to me." (unquote)? Care to explain please. Are you writing a masters thesis or doctoral paper? I could help, but only if honest and willing to meet me halfway. Only fair Jenny. (Smile)

One more personal fact for you Jenny. I have no such disease as (Rule) mentioned, and my girlfriend and prior dates testified to knowing my body, primarily the LOINS & manhood area, never showed signs of sores. This was evidence for my defense, since the victim-witness developed this disease (Herpes) and said her assailant gave it to her. This should have exonerated me, but the jury believed her identification of me in court. She was very confused and hypnotized lady. You have to see her hypnotic drawing of suspect, she agreed police should put in newspapers, prior to my arrest! And since my trial, I have had documented, regular check-ups of my privates and this will be evidence for my new trial. For I am not a carrier or have any lesions on my body. I have been a body-builder and exhibitionist and very proud of my physique and manhood prowess. So Im very open about showering and sharing myself with those I feel close to. Hopefully, you wont be shy about questions, because Ann Rule has been a viscious liar and fiction-writer for years now.

I find it amusing that female guards are so nosey and dont mind watching men in their naked, aroused states, or urinating too. I cant believe they allow women to work such areas in all male institutions. Male officers are not allowed to "frisk" or watch women bathe or use toilets! What a double standard — Huh?

Oh well, such is life in prison, and there are many romances and affairs not talked about in the press. Care to know more Jenny? Are you going to share equally? "Hmmmmm"? ☺ Dont be afraid with a "pen-pal"! Ha!

Now —— is Jenny your <u>REAL</u> name? And may I see who you are? May I know you better too? Hopefully, we can help one another. Im just as curious about "women who write men in prison."

So tell me your thots on my reply here. Are you surprised? Put off or intrigued more, or disappointed? My ego can handle rejection and your honesty. Im not the maniac (Rule) tries to depict. And I write to people to get this message out and to make friendships and to even sell my crafts. I make a pretty good "KEIKO" (Free Willy) whale on leather, and have sold many to coastal stores thru my family. Want a (key ring) for a sample by chance? Would you use it? Ask and I'll show you more Jenny.

You write a well, thot out letter. I tend to ramble here. Maybe I wont be that challenge to you, what do ya think? At least give me your honest thots on my poem. Return only the two photos here please. You may have the yard "Chess Set" pose with friends. Now its your turn to show off Jenny. (Smile)

Thanks for writing and reaching out to me. Im grateful for the time we can have here. Hopefully we can grow closer and know one another better.

God bless you and your family this special holiday season. Hope to hear from you in the New year.

> Sincerely,
> Randall W.

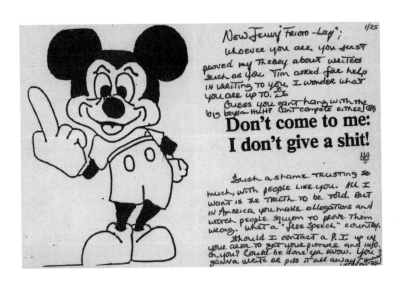

Feb. 5th [1997]

Hello Again;

Okay, truce it is. I really wasn't upset or angry, it just came across as such. Im always very defensive, and it is natural in this "Walled City". So chill & accept my apologee. I was just preturbed about going behind my back to Timothy [Aikens, a fellow inmate], and you never answered <u>my</u> questions or cared to share any pics. too. Can we even talk?

Give me a some credit please. I did share a lot with you. But are you <u>really</u> interested in the corrupt, frame-up case for murder? You became upset with my first reply, you didn't even ask about it? So what's up with that?

Tim showed me your letter, and it sounds like you've written to me earlier? No letters reached me. So I just "ASSUME".

At least you acknowledge Im not a "weak" person —— thank you. But will I ever <u>really</u> know who you are?

Im sorry you expected <u>more</u> in my response. You have no idea how much abuse and ridicule I get from fiction-writers. And the sad part is my Civil Lawsuit was not accepted after 2 yrs. What discrimination we have in our so-called "Justice" (Just-Us) system!

Now, to relieve your fears Ms. Frio, Im not having any investigator follow you. But will that be the <u>ONLY</u> way I will get to see who you are? Just curious is all.

And no comments about the pics. I sent you? No questions about anything? Just an angry response Jen?

I apologize for the wise-cracks. I was just wondering why you wrote Tim & didn't say why or even answer me. Care to explain?

Cute phrase you used…"Mickey flipping me off". What does it mean exactly? See, Im not that smart after all. (Smile)

Can we now communicate both ways now? You answering my questions too? You know about "Quid Pro Quo" right? I did help Tim with that one. So are we on now or what?

I'd just like to feel more at ease with you —— a total stranger picking my brains here. Ha! I see ya smiling…

Lets start over here and dont be so reactionary and I wont either. And how about pen & paper letters now and then just to be more personal. May I have a photo of you please? No stalking, following you ever!

My word is my bond too —

"Ciao"
Randall

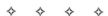

Feb. 20th 1997

Dear Ms Frio;

Okay — Truce. We are both right, and we need to find a middle ground. Im not angry with you, just disappointed in your style, or possibly "hidden agenda". Whatever. I will never really know. And you will just use me for your own purposes.

Ive shared a lot with you, now its up to you to "ASK" the right questions. And to be open-minded as well. You make statements like…"All the inspectors and courts disagree", etc. Not so Jenny. Read the police report first filed by Det. Kominek, lead "Dick" who hypnotized the victim-witness, who helped police draw the composite drawing of "I-5 Killer" suspect!! Go figure….

Now ask yourself why they would fight my defense counsel, to keep (Larry Moore) out of my trial for murder. Because they __KNOW__ they messed up, and arrest this mass-murderer 4-5 weeks after my arrest in the "I-5 Bandit" crime spree. Even the blood-type evidence doesnt match my type (B Neg.), so Judge throws state's blood evidence out of court! But my jury had a right to hear how the first blood test revealed (A/B) typing, and after my arrest, it changes to a plain (B) type. No "negative" enzyme can be detected. Maybe (Larry Moore's) blood type is (A/B)?

The 1986 "Break-In" at D.A. offices, stinks of an "Inside" corruption case! Only my file is ransacked —— so go figure Jenny. They only charged me because of a "Line-Up" identification by (Lisa Garcia). But she never __ONCE__ picked me out of color, close-up photos! Or did she describe me in any police report! Even the ambulance attendants testified for me, they state Ms. Garcia was slightly wounded, with scalp wound, but clear thinking to describe a shorter, sandy-haired fella matching the mass-murderer (Larry Moore).

Justice prevails on appeal as my trial judge's ruling to bar defense from seeing (Larry Moore) in court, under cross-examination, etc. He said it was…"Irrelevent and immaterial" (unquote). Appeals court also agreed! Ha! Where is my right to call defense __WITNESS__ & get a __FAIR TRIAL__?? I believe this is info. that (Walter Todd) knows, as he was Deputy D.A. and law clerk under my prosecutor (1981). Today he is covering up what he meant in his (1993) letter to me. (see both letters enclosed).

Now, Im trying to show or prove a frame-up in my only murder trial. God knows they (state) wanted me bad enough to violate my rights to fair trial. Now the __TRANSCRIPTS__ dont reflect the truth of [what actually happened during my trial] — "leg-shackling" & blood type errors in State Testimony!! Even the other "I-5 Bandit" (state snitch-witness), testified that he made "No Deals" with prosecutors. Today we prove otherwise. But the transcripts omit his statement!!! Corruption to the core, Ms. Frio!

Okay, enough crying on your shoulder. You only care to know "why murderers strike out in anger or rage"? How should I know? ⊗ What a question Jenny. Care to write more personally? Share a photo? Talk once by phone? Your choice.

"Ciao"

Randall Woodfield

✧   ✧   ✧   ✧

April 23rd 1997

Hello Again;

Yes, it was a surprise to hear from you. Although you do feel somewhat intimadated, and a possible "victim" too, I cant help but wonder if you really are this pretty, young and vulnerable woman. Now dont get hostile please, Im being honest with you.

And as you can see Jenny, I have enclosed a visiting form for you to fill out. Now is the time to volunteer your info., because Im offering you your choice of ways to visit. Check the (Basic) visit preference, and you will be given a security (window booth) to visit. We will have more privacy to talk, and maybe just relax and be ourselves. You will be able to walk back over to "Contact" side for drinks or bathroom, but Im stuck on the other side. Your choice Jen.

But I take it you are planning on seeing someone else, and you cant visit but one inmate. Should you decide me, Tim [Aikens] told me to tell you he takes photos in the visiting room, so he could be out there to socialize with us.

And Tim also wanted me to tell you he's not into writing, but he would like to get paid some to afford the envelopes, etc. Now, of course we talk and you know he told me he would tell you certain things, but he was hoping you would help him more. I can't speak for him, but Ive told him to not go this route with you. Regardless, I spoke with him and we each shared our letters from you. So naturally you are playing both of us for your own reasons. Im not angry with you —— nor will I be should you quit writing. I just think you have your own opinion about me, your own judgments, and your own boundaries within this game you have set up. Correct?

Anyway, we both can psychoanalyse people, and I guess we are both curious people by nature. So will you allow me to <u>see who</u> I will be meeting here? Why keep yourself secret? Havent I been forthcoming with pics. & info.? Havent I given you my word I wont use your photo for any wrong motives?

No matter, you have guessed wrong about my anger, my writing you, and my working with any and all to get released. Im <u>NOT</u>! I just hate the unfair so-called "JUSTICE" system our forefathers fought and died for to preserve. I only

wanted a fair trial Jenny. Because…from that wrongful murder charge I have
been framed and trashed by writers. Do you see my point? Can you even
understand?

We may never meet or see eye to eye on issues, but at least I tried to show
you the scandal in my prosecution for murder. And the suspect is LARRY
MOORE!! Not me, or someone running loose. Although several more .32 cal.
killings on women, here in Salem – 1981 & '82. You can learn about that from
records too.

But you dont care to read the record, just fiction books? How come Jen?
Do you justify your rationale or opinion with knowledge from an ex-cop,
turned fiction-writer? "Hmmmm"?

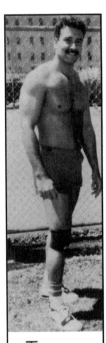

Why did you say — "You will never write to me"?
Cant you accept that I dont care if you believe me or not,
its what I know, and can prove that counts for anything.
Well, Ive written back to you, and appreciate your reading
of part of my case file. Trust me on this one fact Jen. If
officials are willing to alter transcripts, they are capable of
doing ANYTHING!!

So to me Oregon doesnt care about a defendants
constitutional rights. So we are ALL in trouble, Jenny.
When our government starts to tear down the protections
our Const. guarantees us, then Democracy itself is in bad
trouble. Do you not agree?

Enough about all that. I appreciate your honesty even
your flattering remarks too. But will I be able to know
(see) a photo? You say you are willing to visit, but not
share a photo-copy pic? Go ahead — humor me. Just be
more real and open to share. Can you?

Hopefully you will understand about visiting rules.
So if you are planning on visiting, who will you visit?
What is important to you? Would you prefer an "open-
contact" visit, which is (priviledged) or more private visit
with me? You will be safe and more likely to have me
share more with you in our own private booth. I promise
to not bore you or be disappointing! Ha. And you will feel
the powerful one, with me on the other side of the glass.
(Smile)

Do you really think I enjoy overpowering women?
Why? You don't even know me! I find you quite an
amazing, judgmental type of person. Unbelievable!

Jenny

Your Caged
"Dream- Lover"
Want A Hug!
Not Afraid
Are You? HA

I'm Not Angry….
Peace To Ya, Randy

So tell me who you're writing, or visiting here besides me and Tim. I'll know sooner or later anyway. Are you truly interested in knowing me better, or is this just your game? "Hmmmmmm"? I suggest you call (OSP) Visit-Supv. about rule of visiting only one inmate. And you could speak with Tim and I, should you decide on returning the form for me to submit for a police (record) check. Will you please reply sooner this time? Id like to know your answer.

Are you glad that Ive written back? You mentioned being sincere in your hoping to hear from me. To be honest Jenny, I normally dont trust this much with a writer and one who is not very open to share about herself. So you can be lucky or feel special. Something tells me that we will meet here one day. 'Cuz the only way you can truly know someone, is meeting and being truly interested in the person. Now, do you wish a private booth visit? For private talks and personal sharing? Or picnic type, with a chance to have photo-sessions, etc. Tim will be making us laugh with his Elvis impersonations. Ha! Well Jen?

Are you afraid or sincerely interested? I will enclose one more photo for your collection. Do I get one of you? Please? Ive tried to be trusting and open with you. I promise to share much more should we visit Jen. And you do not anger me with your "guilty" opinion either. Sleep easy…

Take care, Randall

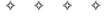

July 14th 1997

"Jenny";

Received your two short notes in one letter. Now why do you ask me what is going on with no letters? It is YOU who has not responded to my last letter, and not-so-impressive-photo. So ask yourself, why — not me.

I have no intention of writing or publishing your letters, and I cant stop you from publishing mine. I knew all along you could write whatever you chose to write…I saw Ann Rule get away with libel [in her book about me, *The I-5 Killer*] and the trash (1st person) style, etc. So you are on your own, I have no animosity or anger in me. Im disallusioned with the word of "JUSTICE" — I prefer it as "Just-Us" ! K?

So please don't be afraid of me. I have no intention of suing or seeking any revenge. I will just continue to pray for peace in my life & in others Ive touched too. I believe people can change and work at being better human beings. So do what you wish. I can only share from what I know to be true.

And yes, I would enjoy seeing (who) you are, just to be on a more personal level. And you may sign your letters too. I wont do anything with your visiting info. But you will need to submit your name for visit-approval. Unless you are with police or D.A. too, then you can arrange for visits without my assistance. Up to you "Jenny". (Smile)

So, if you ever plan on visiting, contact me or Visit-Supervisor with info & your wishes to not share your personal I.D. with me. Tim [Aikens] won't write [back to you], dont ask me why, he just isnt a writing person ——— K? But he will be in the visit-room to take our photo together. Would you be too scared? I have never given any visitor, or lady friend, reason to fear me. Only Ann Rule and the media/police have scared you. FACT!

I understand your own theory and feelings. But you only know what police & D.A. wanted you to know. How can you trust a government that break-ins and ransacks the D.A. files, and who alters the court transcript?! How can you?

Now explain how you will be seeing me? Tour or visit thru Psych. Dept., or whatever? "Hmmmm"? Care to share please?

Ive shared openly and as honestly as I dared to with a total stranger. Maybe the dangerous ones are with long legs & hazel eyes? ☺ Well? Should I fear you stranger?

And you are <u>NOT</u> setting yourself up for a "mousetrap" — okay? Maybe Im being set up too? I just tried to explain who I am, and how unfair "justice" can be. Im lonely with feelings and regrets, heartache & sorrows. But life goes on here, and I do my best ——— K?

Yours truly, Randall

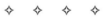

July 24th 1997

Hello "Miss Blonde-Human";

Guess you really are for real, huh? Nice to know Im more human to you now too. We both had our own reasons for doubting, so maybe the ice has been broken and we can converse more openly in a visit. Thanks for the photo Jenny. I appreciate your trust and openness to meet. You wont be disappointed, I promise.

Okay, here is another visit form. For peace of mind, you may mail this directly to my counselor: C. Abrams, and request a "Basic" visit, which will give you more security and privacy to ask personal questions too. Is that satisfactory to you? Later on you could request the open-contact visits, and even picnic with me outside (but inside the WALL! Ha!) Should you stay over night in Salem, you could even be a club guest for dinner (6 pm – 9 pm). But only yearly events for each club.

For now I will agree with you to have the Basic, non-contact visiting. You would still be free to use snack & coffee vendors, and see the adjoining open-contact room. Tim works there as cameraman, so he could say "Hello" etc. I will be stuck on the other side behind thick glass. You will be more at ease this way I'm sure, yes?

Anyway — it will be best to plan our meeting to not interfere with work or attorney, or family visits. Comments?

And you are very pretty. Guess Im somewhat relieved too, because you're not some ugly, fat person, who is playing a game. See...we both have had doubts about reaching out to strangers. You may be new at it, but Ive been trying to reach out and trust people for over 16+ years here. And there's always a risk Jenny. I know (Rule) didnt write about the weirdos and sickos taking advantage of a hostage behind bars (walls). But there are a multitude of lying, con-artists and hypocrites wanting to take advantage of a "con" locked-up.

So your trust with a photo and desire to visit is appreciated. Sure, Im just a "Guinea Pig" for your study or writings. But being human, means to desire human love & understanding. The world may not understand someone like me, but to read a "slash 'n trash" fiction, paperback sure isnt the proper way to know **ANYONE**!! Writers can be responsible for destroying someone or painting them into an "image". You agree?

So thanks for taking the step toward meeting or knowing me better. I wouldnt abuse the priviledge of your friendship Jenny. I live to make new acquaintances, and hopefully friendships too. Life is as full or boring, exciting as we make it. So I never stop trying to reach out to the community or vast world around my "little-walled-world" here. I have made fascinating contacts in my quest, and I now have someone new to share with in you. Hope your expectations of me arent too wrong! Ha! Just kidding....

Now, you do have a sense of humor, yes? Sometimes you read into my thots wrongfully and I have to re-state myself. Ive learned it is easy to misinterpret someone in a letter. You agree?

I showed Tim your photo, so he is surprised at my persistance and trust with you. He doesn't have writing skills, or the patience I have too. Maybe thats why I can play chess so well. You need alot of that "patience"!

Ive enclosed the visit form. By mailing directly to my counselor, same address, you can feel better about not giving me your (SSN#) & (DOB) too. Just my way of helping you feel at ease. Just as with the Basic non-contact meeting too. You can just <u>LOOK</u> me over, you cant <u>TOUCH</u>! Ha! (Smile)

See? I have a sense of humor too. But can you appreciate it? "Hmmmmm" ☺ Im smiling with ya. How am I doing so far? More interesting to you? Feeling safe to visit? You can write me a longer letter detailing your feelings, if you want. I wont reject you because of those feelings. You do have a right to feel awkward or scared too.

Care to explain where you plan to print or publish my letters? Will you be

advertising my name and SID #? Address too? You might bring in a few
interested writers — ya think? Comments?

I keep looking at your photo here. You look like someone with patience and
poise too. Must be difficult working with kids. I always wanted to be a teacher/
coach to H.S. students. I did some work for my (PSU) professor at a middle
school. Was for extra credit my senior year. I hope you dont believe any "BS"
that (Rule) wrote about sex with any girls! How low can a writer go to attack
one's character. I did try to sue her in Fed. court for $12 million. Time
restrictions against "Lifers" only, prevented me. I think I told you that already,
huh? Okay, must be the 1st stage of Alzheimers disease…"Sometimers"! Ha!
You do like jokes don't you?

Hope Im not boring you here. Do you think we could talk by phone
sometime? Prior to meeting? I can go "Dutch" with the bill. Dont laugh
now…I'm just trying to help is all. Will you
send me your waist size for a belt? Id like to
gift you with some art work— may I?

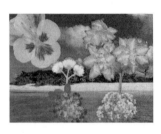

I can look out my window here over my
desk and see the moon rising and planes flying
about. The Salem airport is a couple miles south
of us here. Down below in our courtyard, we
have colorful Pea Fowl and Pheasants. So I can
A card of pressed flowers   find solace when writing, and seeing some of
made by Randall Woodfield.   Gods creation around me. Im not one to stay in
my room alot, except for privacy in my writing
and movies too. I like to make tapes too, so maybe you'd like to hear my voice
before meeting? I just cant mail it out until our "shop" is open for work again.
Repairs and remodeling is going on for 2-4 more weeks. Write again soon now.
Dont be afraid to sign your letters. ☺

Sincerely, Randall

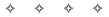

Mon. Eve

Hi Jenny.

Received your more personal letter today, explaining your call to Abrams
and your application for visiting. Thanks for opening up more Jen, it means alot
to know you better. I hope you can understand me better in visiting, since one
can easily misconstrue the meanings behind the jokes, or feelings expressed in
writing. Seeing one's eyes and facial expressions makes it much easier to read
someone. You agree?

So we will have only 1-2 hours to talk in the (Basic) non-contact visits.

But, you will have the privacy to be at ease, and for you to request favors too. But "Open" contact is across from a small coffee table and we can share in conversation and coffee, etc. Even take a picture together too. (Hug is optional Jen!) Ha.

But no need to share your photo & info. with others here, you cant visit but one inmate, so Tim will be at work to talk with me. [Dayton] Rogers is on "Death Row" and [Jerome] Brudos doesn't visit anyone anyway. So good luck with getting their approval to publish. But Ill let you in on a secret too Jen, since you asked me to not talk about your name, etc.

So ask me when we meet, about the secret info. Ive gathered for you ——— K? Im sure you will appreciate the info.

May I ask what your intentions were in writing, if it <u>WASNT</u> a book? And why did you just write to only a few [inmates] here? I hate to be in the same category [as "serial killers"] Jen, because I had only one trial for murder, and I proved the victim-witness was so confused and described [the attacker as] (Moore), also here in the area. And blood tests didnt match me to crime-scene evidence, thus Judge threw it out of court! So why include me Jen? Because (Rule) says I killed people? Im confused...help? ☹

Anyway ——— do let me talk with ya prior to our visit, may I call? Can I pay you in leather crafts? You may want some gifts, yes? No? Or would you prefer a visit first? You can purchase "tokens" for vending machines at front desk. And you can only bring in a small coin purse & tokens. (No money or pen & pad!) Paper & pencils in our visit-area. Comments?

Later friend... (Smile)

Randy

✦   ✦   ✦   ✦

Friday pm

Dear Jenny;

Thanks for talking with me. I was hoping we'd be able to iron out all the details about meeting the first time. You mentioned your comfort zone, so just request the no-contact (Basic) visit in the (AM) and speak with visit-desk staff after we visit about your comfort in a contact visit for coffee & snacks, etc. Dont mention Tim, he will just arrange to be there while you are. Rules sorta prohibit visiting two inmates, etc. You can converse with him in our afternoon visit. We can sit right by the Sgt. Desk and Tim's photo station too.

I'll call Wed. night to confirm everything. And I hope you will feel alright about our private visit, since you can imagine how I might be a show off or tease you some. Ha! I dont mean to scare you away at all. Im just trying to come across as easy to know and not to be offensive in any way. Think you can handle my easy-going manner? "Hmmmmm"?

Let me know when we talk next — K? Im not asking for monetary value for anything I can help you with in your writings. But will you be understanding of this prison setting, and how lonely a place it can be! Hope so Jenny.

Had the family mail you some "KEIKO" key fobs and a checkbook cover [that I made] for you to have. I enjoy creating art on leather and look for business contracts in stores around the U.S. & the world. Maybe we could do some business together too? We can talk about it in visiting.

Sounds like your husband is very understanding of you, your project, etc. Hope you wont share everything I share with you. It will be awkward to think about it. Do you really know "why" you started this writing project? And how did it evolve into a book?

Anyway, drive careful and dont be too nervous Jen. I'm not the person portrayed by an ex-cop turned fiction-writer (Rule). It's sad to think how people can trash people and print lies, all behind the "Freedom of Speech" in our <u>Bill of Rights</u>.

See you soon Jen. Hope you enjoy your time here, and will feel comfortable one day to take a photo together and be my dinner guest at an annual club dinner party. Comments?

Later On....Randy

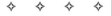

Sat. Eve

Hi Jen;

Really enjoyed our time together. Hope you werent too disappointed in our conversation. I was impressed with you and found you sincere, as well as attractive too. So let me know if you felt comfortable with the private visiting, and with me too. I wanted to share more with you, being so lonely and finding you so attractive. But I wanted you to know I didn't want to ruin the chance of our future project with a book. So let me know if you can handle everything I want to share, even being the show-off you undoubtedly know that I am. (Smile) I still have polygraph to show — yes? And more materials. Hope this helps you more in showing what a frame-up for murder they did on me. Any questions Jen?

Tim was disappointed that he couldn't be out there too. He said he would write and send transcripts, but he wanted you to help him find his father. Maybe you can talk to him about it next time you can visit. Next time lets have you request a morning, private (Basic) visit and then change in the (pm) for picnic & a photo? If you would feel alright with another Basic visit, Im sure I'll be more relaxed and myself to show off more. Ha. In fact, I never mentioned the tower shooting did I? I should show you the bullet hole in my thigh, can you handle that too Jen? I bet you can — huh? And more, yes? You appear to be strong-minded and capable too. Like I said Jen, I was definitely impressed with ya.

Hope your trip home was safe and peaceful. Glad you enjoyed the crafts too. Do let me know if you need something, maybe you could show off my (key fobs) to local shops? I sell those at $1.50 ea. and have a larger (fob) with key ring $2.00. Would you care to look around for me?

Were you questioned a lot by the "Hubby" or your kids? And did they worry about you? Will you keep our visit somewhat confidential between us too? I understand your project now with "letters" but will you not write about our private conversation or sharing? "Hmmm"?

I noticed your eyes on me and especially when I was stretching to relieve my knees. (wink) May I share more with you and will you understand my situation and loneliness? Please be honest about your feelings and thots on this — K? Thanks Jen.

Best close now. Any questions about all the paperwork? Charles Burt passed away in 1996, and maintained his support in my innocence for the murder case he defended me on. Check out the '93 letter from fired law clerk (Walter Todd). He knew something about my case, but lied and clammed up on my Appeal Hearing for new trial. Go figure…

Take care, Randall

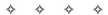

Thur. AM

Hi Jen;

Good to talk with you again. Hope you like the flowers. Just my way of saying "Thanks". Spending the time with you in visiting meant alot Jen, and I hope we will again. I think you have quite a good husband. Reminds me of the married women here (guards), who work in an all-male institute and watch men bathe, shower, and do personal bed or bathroom relieving, etc. I wouldnt have my wife working here with such degrading daily situations. Just like I wouldn't have or approve of my wife stripping for men, etc. So your husband must be a strong, understanding man — huh?

Anyway, nice to know we both enjoyed each other's compliments on our looks. You are attractive and I think I became too interested in looking you over as you modeled your dress. So please dont think of desiring thots as "disrespectful" — okay? It's only natural in this prison situation. So can you accept my lonely desires, as natural & understand my needs? I would not want to create any problems with us working together, but will you accept me as I am? "Hmmmm"? I think you know my meaning, huh?

Please dont think of me with any thots of rape or assault. Im not like that Jen and have looked for and found several relationships with women here, over the past 16+ years. One such romance ended in marriage and a precious daughter too. Maybe if we do our own book together, you will want to know of her & my wonderful parents too.

I'd like to see pics. of your family and hubby too — may I? Your parents too? "Thanks" And should you make it out to Philly, would you care to talk to my ex-fiancee from there? She is married to construction/contractor, name of Sands! She was quite a woman to walk into my life. Ill show you our visiting pics. later ——— K? She reminds me of you alot. (Smile) She is a singer/song-writer.

The reasons we do things wrong, probably can never be explained. But in my life, I will be forever living with remorse, heartache and regret. Plus, many, many wonderful memories and accomplishments. Im even glad I stuck it out thru all your verbal attacks! Ha! Not every day I meet someone like you Jen. J Have a safe and peaceful day. Talk to you soon then.

Randy

✧   ✧   ✧   ✧

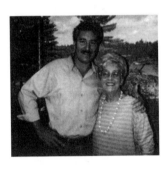

1997. "Visiting with my Mom! This isn't intimidating, is it Jenny? Hmmmmm?"

Feb. 3rd [1998]

Hi Jen; ☺

Thanks for the letter and answer to my visit-question. I really wanted to hear from ya, since your last letter was a photo-copied (note). Sorry Jen, I just felt it was an attempt to get me to respond in an "emotional" way. And we <u>both</u> know how you can push buttons to illecit a response — huh? <u>**Yes We DO**</u> .... Ha! ☺

So, all is forgiven and hopefully come spring you will have a book and time to share in a second meeting. And you can request your (non-contact) visit too. And we both will be more at ease to share in private. I promise to not be so shy with you. I guess your beauty and my respect for you moved me to be a bit shy. (Smile) Do I get a family photo of you all? Hmmmm? Hopefully you'll feel more comfortable after we meet a second time here. No doubt you were nervous the first meeting, yes? Will you be nervous or upset with me if I feel attracted to you and want to share more openly with you? I will respect your position of "writer" and married person too. Will you respect me in the morning (after)?! I see ya grinning. Just my way of being my own person, and trying to feel closer to ya.

What do ya think about our President? Think he is "Slick Willy" or an innocent victim of a false accusation? I believe his past history is finally catching up to him. Your thots on it?

Tim [Aikens] read your "Hello to the non-writer dude" ☺ He laughed and says he'd like to meet cha next time (Monday is best!) Okay with you Jen?

Check this out. I made a couple sales to (2) guards here before X-mas. One was a 3-ring binder photo-album cover. I made $100.00 on it, nice, huh? So things have been looking up for me. My latest project was some biker side-bags. I have done Harley biker wallets & purses too, and am selling them in L.A. area. Maybe you know someone with a bike? (wink)

Well, blondie-friend, I will close and get this off to you. Be well and safe always. Take care,

Randy W.

April 13 [1998]

Jenny;

Guess our meeting wasnt that important afterall. For all you had to do was call the visiting desk to confirm your approval. You have been on my list since last visit! You could have taken the time to stop by — even if you werent on that approved visitors list. Ya know?

Nice of ya to compliment my mom on her love for her kids. We always had a lot of love in our family. And it breaks me up, if I dwell on how I broke my parents hearts. I sometimes have a hard time living with the painful memories. See — convicts do have a conscience and souls, too. Every human does, and will answer to God one day.

Oh yeah, you think Ann Rule lied about me having "Shark" eyes? Ive had the same kind of eyes all my life. Maybe I just looked a little scared or depressed in my bogus trial for murder? Ya think? Probably a little sad too?

Peace, Randall

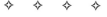

5/8/98

Hey "Bat Woman";

Good to hear from ya. Glad you accept my apologee. I believe ya when ya say ya just didnt know [about calling my counselor], etc. You tried, and that is deserving of credit.

And what's this about going "Ala Natural" on the hair? It is natural, yés? I will be curious to give my opinion, but if you look better then you did as a blonde in blue dress, will you forgive me for acting out, etc. I do express myself, in not so "normal" ways, as I know you have figured that out by now. But who says what is normal in the world, anyway Im just me... Will you object to my sharing such things as my <u>new</u> scar & 1984 gun shot (leg wound)? The shoulder scar looks better since the re-cut! So will <u>YOU</u> be prepared too? Hmmm? Give me your open thots now.

And no, Im not working out on the body, yet. I can hardly use it let alone, take the "manhood" out with "Ma Thumb & Four Sisters"! Ha! You know how us men are, yes? No?

Have you read —— "Men Are From Mars, Women Are From Venus"? It's on the Best Seller list. Good insight into relationships & opposite sex. Comments?

I just hope we can visit on a Tuesday, so Tim will be able to take a photo of ya (private side), and we can still share privately. Just be prepared for my sharing <u>more</u> with ya in private. And your opinion is important about all I share too. I think you're with me on this angle...No? Yes? Smile then!

Gotta go.

"Ciao"
RW

✧　　✧　　✧　　✧

"LOOKING OUT AT THE RAIN"

by

Randall B. Woodfield

He's spent too many years in prison,
As his brown eyes look out at the rain.
He is all alone in his cell,
But never revealing his pain.

So he writes to all who will listen,
And hopes someone will hear him someday.
About crimes he knows he didn't commit
And how they're making him pay.

Still, he is not a bitter man,
Accepting all the time he had spent.
In a cell with so many pictures,
The cell where he must repent.

And he knows he is no Angel,
Maybe jail is where he should be.
But to pin on him crimes he didn't commit!
Oh, why couldn't society see?

And why doesn't someone believe him.
The truth that he wants to be known.
He pieces together what's left of his life,
And accepts the old prison as home.

Each day seems like a repetition,
Many changes he does not see.
As he works for his dollar-a-day job,
And wonders how this could be?

But the walls are now so familiar,
He knows each crevice by heart.
He stares through bars that are locking him in,
And keeping the "free" world apart.

Now he lays on his bed on cold, lonely nights,
And wonders why he took all the blame.
A tear leaves his eye when he remembers,
His Trial! The Corruption! The Frame!

And each new day comes early,
As he moves towards a future with strain.
His memories linger on of a past, hard life,
As his brown eyes look out at the rain.

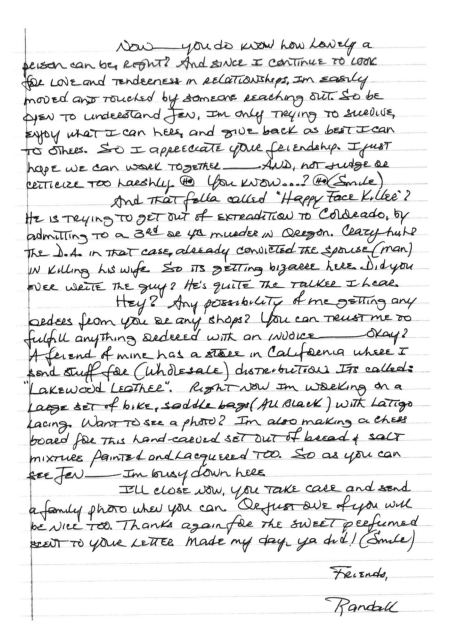

Now — you do know how lovely a person can be, right? And since I continue to look for love and tenderness in relationships, I'm easily moved and touched by someone reaching out. So be open to understand Jen, I'm only trying to survive, enjoy what I can here, and give back as best I can to others. So I appreciate your friendship. I just hope we can work together — And, not judge or criticize too harshly. #@ You know...? #@ (Smile)

And that fella called "Happy Face Killer"? He is trying to get out of extradition to Colorado, by admitting to a 3rd or 4th murder in Oregon. Crazy huh? The D.A. in that case, already convicted the spouse (man) in killing his wife. So it's getting bizarre here. Did you ever write the guy? He's quite the talker I hear.

Hey? Any possibility of me getting any orders from you or any shops? You can trust me to fulfill anything ordered with an invoice — Okay? A friend of mine has a store in California where I send stuff for (wholesale) distribution. Its called: "Lakewood Leather". Right now I'm working on a large set of bike, saddle bags (all black) with latigo lacing. Want to see a photo? I'm also making a chess board for this hand-carved set out of bread & salt mixture painted and lacquered too. So as you can see Jen — I'm busy down here.

I'll close now, you take care and send a family photo when you can. Or just one of you will be nice too. Thanks again for the sweet perfumed scent to your letter. Made my day, ya did! (Smile)

Friends,

Randall

A page from one of Woodfield's letters.

Robin Gecht

After reading about the savage crimes of the "Chicago Rippers," there was something I just had to ask Robin Gecht, the gang's alleged leader. *Why was he so obsessed with women's breasts?* In almost every murder his gang is suspected of committing, there was grotesque mutilation of their victims' breasts. "Well, in answer to your question on obsession with breast," Gecht replied, "It is a thing with my entire family going back as I'm told to great grandfather." Gecht explains, "Each of us men have married large breast women. My ex-wife is a 39D and yes she was very satisfying to me." Then again, Robin later told me: "As to your question about having sex with breast...I have no real obsession with breast in that form. Only a very sick person would even think that." Edward Spreitzer, Gecht's alleged partner, claims that Robin once became so furious with his wife that he cut off her nipples.

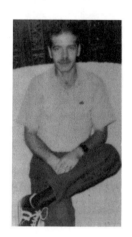

The Chicago Rippers had four members. At age 30, Gecht was the only adult and assumed the role of mentor and leader. Spreitzer was 21 and the Kokoraleis brothers, Tommy and Andrew, were only teenagers. In 1981 and 1982, the group reportedly committed dozens of murders involving rape, torture and mutilation.

Even though Robin Gecht denies slicing off women's breasts, he does admit he has a thing for large-breasted women.

Gecht claims that he is innocent of the murders, innocent of any murder for that matter, and that he didn't even know the other members when most of the victims were killed. "First mistake...is considering me a serial killer...am not considered one...I have never killed or took part in any such acts nor ever charged in any murders of anyone." And this is true. Of the four men supposedly responsible for these killings, Gecht is the only one who was *not* charged with murder. The other three not only confessed to their involvement, but claimed that Gecht was in charge and they were only following his lead. Edward Spreitzer is adamant about Gecht's guilt and offers detailed descriptions of his sick escapades: "A black female was picked up, blindfolded and gagged. Robin shoot her point blank in the head. Put chains around her neck and legs, attached two bowling balls and threw her in the water. I understand her body was not found."

In the spring of 1981, the "Rippers" found their first known victim, Linda Sutton, behind the Brer Rabbit Hotel in Chicago, a well-known hang-out for prostitutes. According to Spreitzer, Sutton was gang-raped, sodomized and her left breast was cut off while she was still alive. About a year later, a red van pulled up alongside Lorry Borowski as she was

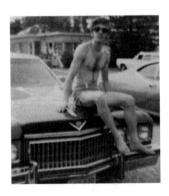

Gecht as a teenager.

walking to work. When she declined the driver's offer of a ride, two men jumped out of the van and grabbed her. They took her to a hotel room where they gang-raped and beat her. A wire was wound around one of her breasts and tightened until it was severed from her body and fell to the floor. According to Spreitzer's sworn testimony, Gecht "had sex" with Borowski's breast and then finished her off with an ax. Only days later, the "Rippers" abducted a young Chinese woman named Shui Mak, drove her to an isolated wooded area where they raped her, cut off her breasts, sliced her body to ribbons and buried her in a hole. Apparently, Rose Beck, a businesswoman known for her independent mind and outspokenness, was a victim who was not willing to go without a fight. When her body was found, a pool of dried blood lay beneath her anal cavity and her face was crushed beyond recognition.

The "Ripper's" last known victim, a teenage prostitute, lived to tell her tale and was able to identify Gecht's van. After Edward Spreitzer went to the police and gave them a full confession, police closed in on the group and arrested them. By that point, many, many women had come forward with chilling tales of the tortures they said Robin Gecht had inflicted on them. Most of these tortures included some form of breast mutilation with needles and knives. Several women said Gecht had asked them to cut off their own nipples because Robin wanted to see "how they worked." Not surprisingly, Robin denies this.

Gecht was charged with kidnapping, rape and attempted manslaughter of this last victim and incarcerated in Menard Correctional Facility in Illinois. The kidnapping and rape charges have since been dropped. Gecht is still desperately trying to obtain the DNA testing that he is certain will clear him of all charges. So far, he has been unsuccessful; no one will budge on the issue of DNA testing.

"I don't only face the injustices, but the nightmares that follows. You have no idea the pain and hurt I face and feel every single day I sit here and loose hope. I'm not an angel... but I never intentionally hurt anyone unless it was to protect myself or my family. I could never live with killing or knowing I was responsible for

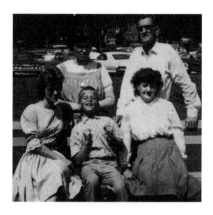

1963. Robin, age 10, with his mother, aunt and grandparents.

taking ones life." Despite powerful eyewitness testimony, there is simply no hard evidence to prove that Robin Gecht is guilty of anything but attempted murder of the last victim. Gecht's family, especially his wife, are 100 percent behind him, believe in his innocence, and look forward to the day when he will be eligible for parole in 2022.

The Gecht Letters

June 7, 1997

Dear Jenny,

Hope my letter finds you & your family well.

Receved your letter. When firist receving it, I thought to myself, how nice for someone to take the time to be concerned. Until I read it & realized it not to be the case here.

I sat here thinking to myself. Where would she get so badly misinformed to write with judgement? After a few minutes it dawned on me. Your reading the book DEADLY THRILLS [by Jaye Slade Fletcher]. THAT woman should write for Steven King. I'm so sorry you've wasted your money. But if you enjoy fantsy. You got it!!! "News flash"! The book was wrote to sell!

However you don't know me only what you have read. So please don't judge before you have facts, not fiction as you've gotton!

I have enclosed a legal Court Petition. It is a request by me 4 years ago requesting D.N.A. testing. Please note what I was charged with. Only!!

Not going to tell you I'm an angel. But I can tell you if I was guilty of murder or of what [Fletcher says in *Deadly Thrills*]. Question? Would I request for D.N.A. testing? Would be pretty stupid on my part if so. Read up on D.N.A. then think on my question.

I can't tell you why some choose to kill woman. I love & have alot of respect for them & life itself. Your right to believe as you wish. As I said, know me before judgement.
My conviction is based on one persons word. Nothing more.

I'm sorry if I disappoint you here but I'm not going to write you just to defend myself. If you've made up your mind I'm guilty as charged or more so, as your

150

reading, then I'd rather not get into being friends or penpals. I'm not going to add to fansity of others.

I do hold a lot of remorse for all that suffer needless & for my children & what this system put us all through the past 15 years. But faith in God above keeps me fighting. I'll have the last say. Anger? DAMN Right. There wrong. Would you be mad??

As for woman. I love woman & I hold a lot of respect for them. However you wouldn't know that would you? You read otherwise. Take it as truth. I do respect them. I too one day would like to know why, most are threated as they are. But not by me.

I don't enjoy letters or phone calls filed with judgements that says "What a Monster"! I'm long from the fanisty that woman cop [Fletcher] choose to write about. Nothing she wrote is based on Court records or family. Thank you for your letter however. I would of typed this but, recovering from a mild heart attack on 5-15 & was to tired to dig the typewriter out.

If you choose to write back, I'd enjoy it. But no judgement. Unless your 100% possitive I'm guilty of all stated. You might be shocked to see your wrong here.

I've never been charged with murder nor ever asked about it. & my out date now is at 2002. In 96 2 charges were dropped. DEVIATE SEXUAL ASSAULT & KIDNIPPING. Shock YA?

Sincerely your's

Robin.

P.S. Sorry so messy. Was really rushing to get this out to you. Was a little upset. I'll get over it. I'm sure you ment well. I wasn't going to answer but felt you needed truth. Enough misjudgements & hate in the world without addin to it.

June 23rd, 1997

Jenny;

Hi! Received you're letter & was nice hearing from you again, however still being somewhat obtuse, aren't we?

When I read your letter, it sure seems I've been down this path before! Only to soon find out she also was a writer. I don't mind, but if you want to really know ME & not what's in a book of fairy-tales [*Deadly Thrills*], I strongly suggest you visit & then I'll be thrilled to answer these ill questions, if I can or as truthful as possible & not as your reading as too someone's fantasy.

I will answer what your asking here however! My heart-attack on April 14th had nothing to do with HATE or Prison. Smoking, lack of exercize & stress caused it. At 43, I expected worse behind these walls. It was a warning from above saying, take better care of myself or DEAD DUCK CITY I go!!! I am today!!
I dis-like some people due to STUPIDITY, but never HATE.
There is much too much hate & judgment in our world today without myself adding to it.
I have in 14 years learned to FORGIVE, but not forget! What's happened to me today & these past years will not go un-answered! Everyone will have their day in Court. I'm not bitter, but YES very much without understanding to why our justice system is only for the rich not middle class people cuz if it was, then fairness would apply here. I do blame YOU the VOTERS. Not for the crime, but for those you vote into office as to Government elects.

As for [your question about my fascination with] breast ect. I had to laugh here!!! HOW can you draw opinions from a book [*Deadly Thrills*]? Isn't that a one sided opinion? More so for profit & gain other than facts? Know me first then form an opinion if it's that important to you & for you to understand whatever it is your seeking. Are you afraid that you might be wrong in thought here. What have you got to loose by seeking truth before judgments? You are doing that, regardless what you tell me. Sense it well just in your letters. I take it as meaning to be direct & cold. Please forgive my saying, but I can do without it. I have that here in this zoo.

Well in answer to your question on obsession with breast! It is a thing with my entire family going back as I'm told to GREAT GRANDFATHER & his. Each of us men have married large breast women. I as well! My Ex-wife is a 39D & YES she was very satisfing to me. As to shit your reading about breast being removed or having sex with breast BULLSHIT!!!! That came ONLY from the very ill child Andrew [Kokoraleis] during police questioning in 82. He felt it was a joke & was saying all kinds of shit & laughing afterwards. However our NEWSPAPER REPORTERS had nothing better to do so they printed it. As time passes, It's been added to & sold over & over again... WE live in a very sick world & shit as your reading all the way back to lies at Raswell or the 1800 Jack the Ripper murder in London. Amazes me how people get hard-ons reading fantasy.
Better & more ill things said about Mr. Gecht, the better is sells. Did the same for John W. Gacy & made him a model to most. NOT to me of course. He was a very sick person.

However NO ONES DEAD here & yet I'm this awful monster. Why is that? I can't answer or take credit for what these other guys say they did. Believe it or not, with the exception of one murder where they killed a guy at a phone booth, I didn't know them when these others they say were commited. Truth to why I was never charged.

Of course [Fletcher] hasn't told you that.. Has she? Opinion huh?

I'll leave you again with my question I asked before! IF I'm responsible as charged... Why won't they run the D.N.A. on me? Would prove I was or wasn't! TRUE??? I offered to pay even the cost.. Thats 24 hrs... so far it's taken the STATE 4 yrs & still won't comply.. SOMETHINGS WRONG!!! You consider that FACTS OR FICTION!

As to police framing me. Or why me? I can fully answer that question, anymore then the 17 men here in Illinois ALONE that's been freed in the last four years through D.N.A. cuz police made a HONEST MISTAKE as well as STATE'S ATTORNEYS ECT. Took only from 10 to 15 yrs to find out. Or ask these 7 men accross the states that were put to death for a crime they later are to be found not guilty of, only cuz police & State made a mistake & covered it up. I can't answer to, why me? Can you? I can answer why they have refused to act on giving me some fair justice here!!! To much B.S. has been added in this case, Media can't let go! Police are scared what will happen when they must answer to why I've been convicted yet they knew otherwise... Look into the CRUZ case now going on in DU-PAGE COUNTY ILLINOIS. 4 States Attorneys. 5 DET. & INVESTAGATORS are all being indicted for the CRUZ MURDER CASE. ASK HIM WHY POLICE FRAMED HIM & THEY KNEW THAT THEY HAD THE REAL KILLER ALREADY IN JAIL MONTHS LATER. CRUZ Spend 15 yrs here at Menard on Death row to be PUT TO DEATH late this year. Today he is FREE & CLEAR, Why cuz a lawyer didn't get scared of our State & dug in & through D.N.A. found he & his partner was not guilty. A little more digging, they found the REAL police reports. ONE BIG COVER-UP, cuz the Media & the public had been made FULLY awear CRUZ was their KILLER of a 10 yr old girl. NO ONE MAKES MISTAKES HERE, WE'RE ALL GUILTY! Know why, Judgamental assholes that know shit about laws, & feel if <u>YOUR CONVICTED & THEY WRITE A BOOK OR YOU COME TO PRISON.. YOU MUST BE 100% GUILTY OF THAT CRIME... TELL that to those that were put to death for NOTHING or us that still pray for fair justice.</u>

UNTIL THEN, easy up on the judgment & opinions. Your welcome to them, their yours, just keep them to yourself. They hurt when you don't know me to those being facts. Do I sound like a man of guilt? Guilty people don't get angry! I'm not angry at you. Your not the first or the last, I'm sure.

AS to your question to having sex with breast. What your reading is a fantasy of [Fletcher's] I guess. I have no real obsession with breast in that form. Only a very sick person would even think that. I have rubbed Jr between my wife's large breast & had orgasm. Hasn't your husband ever did that to yours when making love? My wife enjoyed it, but NEVER EVER EVEN considered hurting her or anyone as you are referring too!

As I stated in my first letter. THAT BITCH IS ill that wrote that book. However again I say, <u>SHE SHOULD WRITE FOR STEVEN KING</u>. Sure would be a movie seller, huh? Books like that cuz others to comit crime much worse. Trust me here! I have a guy here that watch PHYCO at the show & got turned on by the shower stabbing scene & stabbed his girlfriend 25 times in the shower while making love to her. When I asked why. I'm told the Movie didn't do it right & I wanted to see what it was like doing it right?
She's dead & he got life. Over a movie.
I have even got a letter asking how he could OFF his wife. Wanted it to look like a sex attack. Of course I NEVER replied.
Other than that, I get wonderful letters of Love & support from all over the world. And a lot of visits.. FRIENDS.
Bet you'll today, not find one of them that will agree with your opinion why cuz they know me for myself, not whats written. Most have to read the book.

I can help add to your fantasy if you'd like me too. I can think sick too. I watch enough horror movies & have a range of fantasy too! But honestly between us here. What do you get out of this. Spice up your sex life or what...?
As you say, we all have our calling…. Still waiting on finding mine. No I haven't found mine yet. Never thought on it!

Now a few questions for you… Who are you really? Husband, kids ect. What do you do & look like? And what is your real reason for these questions. YOU SAID HONESTLY... A GOOD START HERE. AGREE? I could check but I'd rather ask you instead. If your not writing a book, you should!
But if so, you'd be like others, & never print truth & facts. Might not sell! Their books sell cuz they care less who they hurt in the process. What makes them better then those they write about then?

As for normal obsession with Womens breast. WHAT NORMAL MAN OUT

THERE HASN'T? Not sure if your large on top or what. But if so, am sure you've walked down any street & some guy notices you & your tits. Why? WE'RE MEN, but that doesn't mean we cut them & have sex with them, cuz we have a obsession with large breasted women. 65% of men are obsessed with big tits. I'm sure you already know that. I'm not obsessed otherwise or for any other reason then a normal joe. MEDIA FOR YOU, IT SELLS!!!

For a home bond mom of 2, you sure write well & into deep questions. What did you or your husband do at one time or now, Work for the C. I. A.? (JOKE) (Grin here)

NO, NOT AN OPINION, A FACT!! Never killed any one nor ever considered it. Have you?

Over the weekend my kids were here to visit. Had a great time. Played with my grandson. That child wore holes in my neck for going on 3. Adorable but spoiled. Of course I have added to that. Kids were fine & we had a nice two day visit.
Hot there? Hope your dealing with the heat. Was 89 here today. Makes it 105 inside these walls. WE NEED A.C. here, but ZOO'S don't have A.C.

Well before I answer anymore of your question if I can, I want to know about you.. NOT I'm JENNY & 20 something... You can do better then that can't we??? Maybe a picture. Will send you one if you do! DEAL? Hey you can at least throw darts at me then!!!
Well I gotta go. YARD time & DR. Said I need exercize. Not getting sex so I must walk. Ha Ha!

Take care of yourself & stay well. WRITE IF YOU CHOOSE. JUST LIGHTEN UP SOME HUH? You want to understand things [about serial killers]. fine, not on paper. I'd love to understand a lot too. Care to learn togather. MIND WISE OF COURSE. I've sat & asked the same question over & over again. WHY did they kill or hurt others. I never got to ask these guys. I to have studied those as you do. But I can devide facts from fiction.. CAN YOU?
Later,
Robin

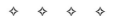

July 12, 1997

Hi Jenny;

In answer to your question on this book you've considered writing, I just can't
give you an answer [about whether I will allow you to print my letters], just like
that! This is again my life your choosing to write about. Could you if I wanted
to write about you & not know anything about you? I do remember just a few
weeks ago, your opinion of me was pretty awful & you had already made your
final judgement. "QUOTE".. "Guilty as written about"!
Why the now change of heart? Whats your motive for wanting to help me
today? Can you be honest with me, after-all your asking I be with you & I have.
Yes I agree it would be nice to allow the public to hear facts not fiction but
what GUARANTEE do I have from you that you WILL print what's given
as truth? Please forgive me for not having faith or trust in most these days, for
you've seen what happened to my life already by having faith & trust, even in
our justice system more so people. Would you, for I am trying!
Again what you write could as well hurt me more. Why would you care what
happens too me one way or another? Your writing this book based on money
not cuz you care about justice or my welfare, cuz if so, your the first in many
moons.

Okay, maybe I'm being a little obtuse here as well. Not my intentions!!! Before
I can give you my answer, your asking, <u>however you really don't need my
permission here</u>, you could be like others & write bullshit & it will sell, but
then that make you no better than the trash that's written what they have already
& yet know nothing about truth or facts. So I suggest that if your going to be
straight with me, before you can write about any subject, you first must know
it. TRUE?
First off, first mistake you'll make is considering me a SERIAL KILER.. I am
not considered one, & wherever it comes from is very well misinformed here. I
have never killed or took part in any such acts nor ever charged in any murders
of anyone. A sick rumor that's needed to be corrected. It would be a great
injustice if you wrote & considered me as such. So bottom line here is, <u>if your
writing souly based on serial killers in general, I don't belong in your book if
your going to be fair & honest with your readers</u>.
If your book is based on serial killers as I think your suggesting it will be, I
rather not be part of that project. Enough lies has been said if I'm listed as a
serial killer & I'm not.

Now if you are considering write about my life ect. I'm willing to listen & we can talk about it. If you decide on that idea, I do have an offer for you depending on your answer. No question the book will sale & money & justice can be made. Again can you write with all fairiness if you don't believe in what or whom your writing about, cuz if you do & don't believe in the subject, you than will write as this other bitch had already & not even know shit about me other then in the media & her cop friends. Follow me?

Bottom line is.. <u>KNOW YOUR SUBJECT YOUR WRITING ABOUT FIRST IF YOUR TOO BE FAIR & JUST</u>.

OKAY, MY QUESTIONS. If your honest with me, I'll know, for I have a reason why I ask these questions. If you lie to me, promise, I'll stop writing. Remember, NO LIES OR JUDGMENTS BETWEEN US.

I do think it will help my case very well & make a fool out of a lot of assholes that choose to write non-sense as well as the STATES case, but only if TRUTH is printed. Why would you be willing to do that for me?

If you think what I sent you in COURT DOCUMENTS is all there is, guess again!! I have appeals, petitions that were filed & they'll shock you into knowing that some that were filed still to date, (YEARS LATER) have yet to be answered or replied too. Talk about cover-up.... People only refuse to answer questions when their hiding something or it's very privite, but in this case, they made this conviction public knowledge, therefore no reason to hide a thing or reply if all is within facts & truth. However their hiding.. They've gone as far as too scare Lawyers away from this case but only when it pertains to me needing legal advise or help. Kinda makes one think!

There's so much bullshit the STATE & lawyers pulled as well as CITY POLICE that once you heard about it, would scare you enough never to come to Chicago more less Illinois. But this doesn't stop here we have it in every state in our Union. In all case's money is the key word here. ASK O.J. Simpson. With it you get fair justice.

I needed you to know what was facts & what was bullshit, cuz for some strange reason it mattered to me that you had the truth. Most I'm sure would of cared less what you felt or thought, I did & still do, but I'll not stop with the truth, for lies will get us nowhere & I have nothin to gain by it.

QUESTION: In your opinion why is it that US HUMANS find it easier to believe the awful things about people, yet find it very hard to believe in any good about another? Also why is it easier to most to believe a LIE then the simple TRUTH. Is this what we've become or as God intented for us? Is this human nature or what?

Am glad I learned to look at both sides of any coin. Everything & everyone has two sides, yet we often find only one sided opinions. STRANGE, we are.

By the way... where is my picture of you? I have one for you. Hey, just think, YOU CAN THROW DARTS AT MINE!.
Suggestion here! Before you start your book. Look for a book called <u>TRIAL BY MEDIA</u>. It will help you in writing & understanding how some high profile cases that are unfair & injust still get convictions. I say that cuz the MEDIA plays a big part in all high profile cases as this was. What you've read was based on that MEDIA coverage. I know, due to I have all the COURT TRANSCRIPTS & RECORDS & SEEN MANY NEWS ARTICLES. Book takes those word for word in many area's through out her book. Try finding the book, you will find it interresting reading & helpful knowledge.
I'm sure there's a few others alike out there, I haven't read or advised too.

Changing the subject on hand here a moment, if I may... Just been advised that a long time close friend of my family & I has passed away. She was 59. You might know of her in [*Deadly Thrills*] as JERRI. She lived on LINDER AVE IN CHICAGO at the time of my arrest. That was the house I was working on the night in question. She passed away of Natural causes in her sleep in Greenbay WI. In talking to my kids today over the news, their taking it as us, pretty hard. They knew her as AUNT JERRI.
She will be missed. We loved her dearly.

I was also just informed by mail from BERRY SCHECK (D.N.A EXPERT — SIMPSON TRIAL) out of New York, that there was no evidence to support RAPE in the Washington [not her real name] case. During the testing of her alone in 82, nothing was found that said... ROBIN GECHT WAS HERE! Rape conviction is now based on her [victim Washington's] word alone as the Attempted murder was. How does a conviction stand as this yet be called justice?
This happens only 3 ways in any State.. THINK ON THIS...!

If your ever called upon to be a jurier your asked if you ever worked for any justice departments, have you ever been in law enforcment or any members of your family, also any lawyers in your family or friends that are? Last ever been in jail or prison? Bottom line, your life history here! If it contains anything to due with law... YOUR ASS IS OUT OF THERE! WHY?
Simple.. You know to much!
THE STATE WANTS DUMMERS ON ANY JURY. Then the jury doesn't know law & except the STATE as GOD. When in fact the Judge in any Court room is

GOD if you think on it.

So if the STATE can talk good bullshit as a salesman selling cars can, you got a conviction, GUILTY OR NOT. What does a jury that knows nothing about the laws of evidence do or how do they determen evidence from bullshit? They don't only go by what their told by (GOD) the State's Attorneys who tell them about this crime as if they were RIGHT THERE as it was commited.

And we all very well know YOUR GUILTY TILL PROVEN NOT, cuz you'd not been arrested otherwise to be in that COURTROOM. What bull!

Lawyers (most) if not all, only care about two things. Money & their future. So if you got money, you go free like O.J. guilty or not. Even if NOT guilty, your going to prison. Money talks in politics. Next if the State can offer him a better deal to sell you out to them, & it helps his future. YOUR ASS IS THEIRS. Oh it's done legally but only on paper until a smart Attorney, that 1 out of 500, decides something wrong & starts digging for truth. Then we that don't deserve this, go free.

Last of all most judges in most court room is behind the STATE'S ATTORNEY'S 95% of the time. Like PUBLIC DEFENDERS, they ALL work & get paid by their State. Where does that leave us that doesn't & can't afford fair justice? PRISON & YOUR LIFE TRASHED. Says a lot huh for our justice system. WELCOME TO **POLITICS AT THEIR BEST.**

Oh I did forget to tell you that while this Salesman is talking shit, we have a jury that's in a hurry to get the fuck home. NO JUSTICE, why should they care? Their forced on you to serve as a jurier to start with, taken from their family jobs & loved ones for days sometimes even weeks. Would say, I'd be pissed! (Follow)?

Very few exscape our jury more so when they can read newspapers. TRAIL BY MEDIA. WORKS EVERY TIME. WELCOME TO THE 1st AMANDMENT.

Know what really pisses me off? I'm in this alone! After 18 million dollars to defend John Gacy for 14 yrs till his death & some of the best lawyers out to save his life as guilty as he was, I can't have that & haven't killed anyone!!! JUSTICE. Shouldn't I be angry?

With that note, I'll say goodnight. By the way, I'm doing fine since heart surgery in April. Thanks for asking!

Take care of yourself & maybe you'll answer my questions. I won't again, till you do! Meet me half way if at all. AGREE? My best to your family.

Later:
Robin.

July 26, 1997

Hi Jenny;

GREETINGS AGAIN FROM MENARD ZOO.

THANK YOU for the photo of the children & yourself. Your very pretty & the children are adorable. how old are they, for nothing on the backside of the photo saying their names or ages. I too have enclosed one for you. Again.. THANK YOU.

I guess I could understand as a woman how you could of hated me after reading that headline, how-ever again it came from the News media. I had noticed the hate in your first two letters, more-so your first. I almost didn't reply, but felt the need too, for I'm not even sure why for I normally don't respond to ignorance. I guess I needed to get my point out to you that all things WRITTEN in BLACK & WHITE aren't always within truth or fact, but sometimes nothing more then this is, <u>SENSATIONALISTIC BULLSHIT</u>. "It sells books." I'm glad that maybe your willing to look closer & realize I too believe as you feel. I too love life & family, I can hurt, feel remorse, & I cry as you do. Most of all & may not agree on many things I see, but I never learned to hate, to want to take another human life without cause.

I will trust you here & give you what your hopeing for! Maybe you can reach the public more possitively. Hopefully your willing to do this, is important here as to truth, if not then this project becomes nothing more then what others have done in the past only in a different form & your only adding to the already sensationalism & not in truth or fact. What you need to ask yourself is... What if, all Robin is telling me is <u>indeed fact</u>, & one day set free!? If so Jen, then your book becomes a lie. Now lets look at the credibilty you would gain if you trust me enough to give you truth & it's printed to the world to read & later you become responsible for my release saying <u>GECHT WAS NOT GUILTY AS CHARGED & RELEASED!!!</u> I am willing too trust you & give you that. I only in return ask that you trust me & not judge. As I stated, you can't write in fairness about something you don't believe in. Not & be objective. If your willing to write this book, do it with an open mind & self pride & within fairness. After-all what have you got too loose? There is another well known case, Cruz, that after 14 yrs on death row here he too was released. He was well judged & hated over the Rape & murder of a 10 yr old girl. He never committed the crime. Police & Attorneys knew the real killer & covered it up. Someone like you took time to write about what was fact & people too interrest. A 3rd trial freed him with help of D.N.A testing. Those responsible have since been indicted in Du-page Co. IL. Indeed law enforcment as well. Maybe reading that case will help open your thoughts to possibilties here to what I'm telling you. I'm asking for nothing but you too write with fairness that it may help.

Will you consider my point?
I do have a major concern here as before stated... SERIAL KILLERS... I'm NOT! I'm again asking I not be place or noted as one in your book. Can you do that? That is truth & fact.

Well, one thing I'm not, is STUPID, please don't treat me as such. There is money to be made here, or you'd not be doing it. I'm good at Money values & making it. Trust what I'm telling you. People will buy what I have to say if about souly me, or as your planning. You will make your investment back here to whats put in it. If you think Negitive, you get Negitive. FAITH MY DEAR & THINK POSSITIVE & possitive things happen...

I follow well on what your telling me as to <u>People are very rarely born to kill.</u> I too have study them, up until I started getting a lot of judgements here at the prison to why I wanted to learn about as they call them ANIMALS so I had to stop because it was being taken out of context as always to my motives in wanting to learn human nature & it's misdeeds. I'm sure you've ran into this or will. As you say & I agree. <u>NARROW-MINDS</u>, or as I call some..<u>JUDGE A MENTAL ASSHOLES</u>.

I have a print out from the computer my friend has that list SERAL KILLERS & THEIR CRIMES. Ever see or read it?
I am again not listed. THANK GOD.
NO I can't see you doing anything that might put your family on the line here. A REAL HUGE SACRIFICE, I'd say!!! No I can't imagaine! PLEASE BE CAREFUL. You & I do know as facts to what we read & see, THERE ARE SOME REAL SICK NUT CASES OUT THERE. I do know meaning of sacrifice well. I did my life for my families safety in 1982.
I know people will read this book in academic circles to study. Yes I'm sure like anything that is never looked at in a different respective, you will face the conservatives & narrow-minded of this world.
Definately an alarm system for your house is suggested.
Not sure you face hate, not from me at least.

I'll be willing to trust you, PLEASE don't give me a reason to regret it.

Who else have you written about in your book since you state this isn't all about me. Been in touch with Andy [Kokoraleis] & Edward [Spreitzer]? That should of been interresting, if so, or should I say "Scary" that's if either learned to read & write in years past.

Please forgive my lack of compassion here towards them. Would you have much if they put you here & took your life & family away from you without cause? I'm sure not. I'd just love to know why!

I'm sure if not telling me, they'll soon advise God to their reason. Maybe GOD will forgive them, I won't.

Well gotta run. just got my oldest daughter College scores, & need to read them. It cost me a lot to send her to college, SO I must be up on how she's progressing.

My best to your family.
Regards:
Robin

August 18, 1997

Dear Jenny;

Hope all I sent you was of interest. Now you have my side [of my case], the STATE'S side as it is.. & the appeals to date. Understand... we are only allowed to appeal whats part of Court record. A LOT the jury was NEVER made aware of. Feel if so, I would of never got a conviction. Am 100% possitive on that. However in any case as these, you first MUST have a good Attorney or you 99.9% of the time lose. I was free game to the State.. So far... I still am. As long as People look at me with Guilt, no one will defend me with honestly.

Well the good news is.. There is this Law student that just finished & received her bar, that may be interested in taking on this case. States to much not said that points to my not being guilty, but she is willing to handle this case as my attorney FULLTIME, at the cost of $100.000.00 & a final payment of $20,000.00 upon my release if cleared of these charges.

A lot of money huh? Again it isn't when we're talking one's life! Haven't met with her or given her any answers just yet. If I decide, it will take a lot of checking before I give her a final answer. Will take every penny I have & leave nothing for my kids future. That's most important to me today. My children always comes first. What do you think? Remember she finished 2nd in her class, I'm told but just out of school. That is a concern here.

State refusing to test me, cuz they have nothing that say's, "Robin Gecht" other then MS. WASHINGTON [the woman who identified me as her attacker]. They can run D.N.A on materials they claim to have in impound, but refuse too. Cuz their hiding the truth here. THEY MADE A MISTAKE & D.N.A would put their butts in HOT WATER. What other reason could there be?

D.N.A. is being done on 100 yr old subjects today.

Like the CRUZ rape case I told you about. That case was 14 yrs old & D.N.A was used to free him. Same I'm asking for & can't get help in my quest that the State doesn't seem to get too & scare off. Last attorney gave the State 4 yrs since filing for D.N.A. to wait on a law that they could get the Judge to dismiss & denied request using that law against me. Had it been stood on 4 yrs ago as it was intended.. I'd be free or had a new trial. Now have to be hopeful that Appeals Court look at it. So far.. no attorney has been appointed only Notice to Appeal has... Am working on a lawyer but my letters don't seem to get much notice, I guess. Guess I would have to be O.J to get anywhere in this system. However.. was justice served in that case?

Should of watched THE MAURY POVICH SHOW today 8/18/97. Titled A MOTHER SENTENCE TO DEATH. About mother sentence 2 die for killing her own children. REAL SAD, but my reason for saying you should take interest in this program was their was two juriers that were on this show that found two people GUILTY & sentence them to die, only later to be set free for they were later proven NOT GUILTY. The jurier's state they were never given the full story in each case. ONLY THE STATES SIDE. A lot is always held from jury's.

Maybe you can write for a TRANSCRIPT OF HIS SHOW OR A TAPE. Would be an intrest to your work.

Also fits as to what I've pointed out as to this case I'm fighting. I'm sure there are others. I'm not alone!

So your going to visit O.S.P. [Oregon State Prison] next week. Who's held there? Please let me know how it goes & why. Be careful!!!

Just heard a Comic book was printed on [the Chicago Rippers]. What's next? what people will do to make money.. A comic book. Don't see the humor here. Do you? Requested a copy. If I got it, will advise.

SMILE. . .YOUR THOUGHT OF... Sweet dreams, FRIEND.

Robin

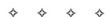

August 25, 1997

Hello Jennifer;

Well the courts are doing their best to screw me AGAIN... They once again appointed a STATE APPELLATE DEFENDER too defend me on appeal regarding my POST-CONVICTION & D.N.A that was denied in May. Once again there is a huge conflict of interrest here & their aware of it. They did this to me in the early years & I filed to dismiss & was granted. Then in 94 when I filed my P.C. ect. The same Judge again assigned the PUBLIC DEFENDER & STATE to defend me knowing the conflict... Guess what? This Judge just did it again. I'm on it. Will file to dismiss them A.S.A.P. Will soon send you my Motions for your records along with a few other interresting items.

In case your asking what the conflict here is... It is as followed. Both offices defended Andrew K. & Edward S. in their murder convictions & appeals. GUESS WHO they place ALL the blame on for these guys actions????? ME. So how could either office of the State defend me with any fairiness? Can't be done!!! This Attorney I just had was forced to have sold me out on my D.N.A. Gave the State 4 yrs. to find away to dismiss.. This was never done before till I. They know I don't have the $70 or 80,000.00 to defend myself with a REAL ATTORNEY if I could even find one. I do have a few thousand aside but no matter how many lawyers in chicago I wrote, NO ONE will take this appeal. Never going to get a fair shake, as I see it. The State has been allowed to hide to much & to many assholes would have to answer as in the CRUZ case.
I am thrilled you see there's something not right in this conviction. Sure wish I could make others see what you see.
I can't behind bars.
Want you to know from the bottom of my heart. I'm glad I have you listening with an open mind.

My news is the letter I received from New York stating the State had nothing on me for the Rape they charged me with. Nothing was found by hospital Rape kit that SAID Robin Gecht. That's why I was never tested... Yet they got a conviction of 60 yrs based on her [i.e., Beverly Washingon] word. How can that be?
It was cuz no one raised it on appeal until my request for D.N.A. These people knew on appeal it would get reversed. That's why the 4 yr delay here in not wanting to test me. They needed a way out of doing so!
However, Jennifer... No one here's listening.
I don't only face the injustices, but the nightmares that follows. You have no

idea the pain & hurt I face & feel every single day I sit here & loose hope. Like I once told you, I'm not an angel, I had a few afares ect. but I never intentionally hurt anyone unless it was to protect myself or my family. I could NEVER live with killing or knowing I was responsible for taking ones life. I don't even believe in the DEATH PENALTY. Should say something.

I had this strange idea on doing a tape of songs for you, that might give you an idea of whats in my heart as to feelings, but I held off in fear that you'd recent it or your husband would take the songs wrong & I'd cause problems for you. I never want that to happen. Hopefully we're friends.
I guess the tape would give you an insight of the love, NOT HATE that's within by these songs. Up to you. I don't mind, if you don't! The tape also saying, if I feel the way the songs are done, I couldn't hate or as evil as I'm being pretrayed to be. Your Choice, I'll await your answer if one.

SWEET DREAMS FRIENDS
Robin

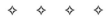

August 27,1997
Wednesday

HELLO AGAIN DEAREST JENNIFER;

YOUR PAIN IN THE BUTT'S HERE AGAIN! Miss me!!! <u>NOT</u>...

As promised here are two Motions I just filed with the Courts. This is in regards to this Judge appointing the State to defend me, & AGAIN the 4th motion to obtain my COMMON LAW RECORDS. This records are if all the Police & hospital notes before & during trial. BY law I am intitled too them, yet for 14 yrs this court has refused to give them to me. One would think there are things in this record they hope I not see.
If no reply or denied, I'll file again with Federal Court.
These records can show us just how much investagation there was in this case if at all.

Also enclosed is the booklet I got from the Net on Serial killers. Felt you might be interrested in reading it. There are some REAL ill people in this book. Funny if you look at their crimes yet people trip on me? Figure that!

Not sure you can get a copy of Edwards or Andrews murder convictions but there's two you should look close at.

There is so much false information in this book by this woman [i.e., *Deadly Thrills* by Jaye Slade Fletcher]. Du-page Co. finds a body at a motel in mid summer of 1980 or 81, I forgot. First off for the record, I didn't know [Spreitzer and the two Kokoraleis brothers] at that time. I believe she stated I had. Not true.

Body is of a female. Noted in her book that Du-page Dr's. state females breast was missing when found.

I can't say this is fact, but [Fletcher] wrote as such... One or both of these men were convicted or plead guilty to the females murder in Du-page as they did in the Washington case.

Okay.. now lets looked at the night in question October 5th 1982. Midnight to 1:a.m time Washington states she was picked up in a red van. However a time lapse Video tapes said otherwise, jury wasn't allowed to view it. Another subject.

Back to Washington... Edward [Spreitzer] & Andy [Kokoraleis] were convicted of Murder & Attempt murder of 2 men that were standing at a phone booth about midnight — 12:30 a.m on Oct 5th when they were shot by a passing Red Van. Within 20 min's of that shotting B.Washington is picked up within 5 blocks of where this shotting took place. Both the same night. Both vic's state a red van.

Now I lived 45 min's from where all this took place. You read my statement I gave lawyers & State's Attorneys, I tell where & what I saw & where these two men tell me what happened. Now mind you. Both cases a red van... Andrew fits [victim Washington's] discription well before she is allowed to change it once seeing me in person. How is it, I too had this red van at the same time they had it to shot these men & not charged with them in this shoting? The state does state I WAS NOT THERE!

The jury was never told of this shotting.

I'm not pointing fingers at anyone here. Just 2 more things the jury wasn't told to look at. I could give you a whole list.

One last good one. Washington states she was forced to have oral sex with me. State states the light in the van was bright so she knew what I looked like. First off not true. NO BRIGHT LIGHTS. Back light never worked.

Anyways... She states she did oral sex & saw me well. Yet, stated she never saw any scars down below..!!

On my right side at the hair-line I have a 7 inch scar from a HERNIA surgery done in 1979, & it is clear as day & would be seen if she had her head

anywhere near that area. NO question whats so ever. She never saw one.....
I showed the STATES ATTORTNEY'S & Lawyers, yet the Jury wasn't allowed
to know shit.

Next time I'll tell you about this so-called i.d at this hospital. It was bullshit the
way it was set up. Lawyers do raise the issue, but not as needed.
It was suggestive, big time.. This is all based on the fact the State & police felt I
knew about the killings these guys claimed to of done. I still don't fully believe
Edward killed anyone, but might of helped the other two. Just wish he'd tell the
truth as to myself. I never did a thing to him to deserve this..
Whats going on here is Police felt after being pissed off by Andy K. I knew
something & refused to talk.. **I KNEW NOTHING**. So they couldn't
hold me on murder so they got Washington to say it was me or made her
believe it was me. Wonder what kind of deal they cut with her back then. She
was wanted by police on warrants, I was advised at that time. Wouldn't surprise
me, but again she was the Angel on the stand. Don't get me WRONG HERE. I
feel very sorry for her & what she lost & went through. A living nightmare I'm
sure. I just can't help feeling angry as well. I too became a victim. Again her
being Black sure didn't help matters here.
Just something more to share with you. Confussed yet? I have been for going
on 15 yrs. Don't feel alone if so. There is an answer here. Trust me!

Sweet dreams:
Friends, Robin

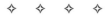

Oct. 7, 1997
Jenny:
Just a short note to advise I just received the Court records on the D.N.A &
Post Conviction Proceedings throughout the filing till it was denied in May
1997.
In this record, my Lawyer tells the Judge that I was cleared of any involvement
with other men in the Du-Page county [murder] through the D.N.A. that was
taken from me in 95 or so! I was not aware I was under any investagation, till
that phone call. (All on record.)

As stated, I was never involved with [Spreitzer or the Kokoraleis brothers].
Now we have it in Court Print..
Public Defenders office state they now lost Original POST-CONVICTION
PETITION... How can they appeal if they have NO copy of what they filed or

was denied???? Playing games with me again. WHO'S GUILTY HERE?

PLEASE BE CAREFUL WHO YOU TALK TOO. NEED YOU ALIVE &
WELL. OKAY? I FOLLOW WELL IN FUCKING THE SYSTEM..
Question... How can this Rape charge [for which I got] 60 yrs stand without
supporting evidence if Berry Scheck is correct?
Chances are that's why the State is fighting NOT TO ALLOW TESTING! It's to
be appeals. Will keep you up to date as I know more.
Keep in touch. I WILL!

Robin

December 5, 1997

Hi Jenny:

Hope you & your loved ones are well. I just now received your letters & was
thrilled to see your writing & still my friend. I have been real concerned.

You are most welcome for the ELVIS tape. Know that feeling WELL! No one
remembered my birthday either last week except Rosie & the kids. It was awful
regardless for I spent it in Chester hospital. I was once again admitted for chest
pains. It seems I was suffering from what is called ANGINA another form of
heart disease. It comes following a heart attack as in April.
I spent 3 days in I.C.U. & no one cared nor was I allowed to even advise family
of my whereabouts. So I spent my B-day there. Guess that too comes with
prison life. Anyways... A lot of tests, change of medication & God sends me
back to HELL.
JUSTICE FOR YOU AT IT'S BEST.

Jenny, if your my friend, Stop using the term SERIAL KILLER, towards me. I
hope you feel otherwise in thought & not as these stereo types here & out there
do. Far from facts or any truth. I love people & couldn't kill anyone without just
cause.
I hurt so much just hearing that word & all the lies I hear & read yet no one has
taken time to know me, but 1st to judge me. I'm ill of the concept.

I hope too I agree with your writing. I have trust & faith in you & it's hard not
knowing you as much needed to feel safe with as a writer when so much
bullshit has already been written just to sell. Does anyone care about Robin

Gecht, should they be wrong? NO!
I feel your different & you will write what facts not bullshit. Know this... You gain the chance to do good & become a name as a writer if truth is used not fiction. Up to you. You owe me nothing, but have a chance to either help me with the truth that will one day free me or help all these other assholes continue to barry me as they have for 15 yrs. Still no-one has the guts to talk to me face to face. Why is that? Ask your readers, whom judge & our legal system, why

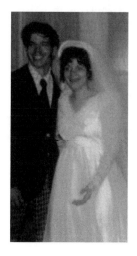

they refuse to test me if I'm as guilty & the Monster they pretray I am, or the Chicago police why they had to try beating a confession out of me if they knew 100% I was guilty! Amazed how they cover-up & people feed on it.

Regarding what I would want to say to people. Nothing really... would it change anything? NO! Those who wish to believe whats said & not know me, will feel as they will or do, regardless of what I say. To them truth by me would only be looked at as a lie. I face that here with Staff each day but only again only from stereo types.

Robin and his wife Rose at their wedding in 1975 in Bellwood, Illinois.

I never killed anyone & I love woman. Ask anyone who knows me as me! Was married to Rosie for 22 yrs, sound like I hate women? Jen. Maybe if you want to really write truth it might be better coming from someone who knows me WELL. Call & talk to Rose. Even though I haven't talked to her in months, she will give you your answer to write about, then the readers can't say I'm lying.
I love woman & Never ever gave any thought to men type relationships. I become ill just with that thought of gay life. Not judging them, but not for me.

They got shit but this B/W [i.e., black woman, victim Beverly Washington] saying I did it to her. Murder was never brought into this case. Media had. From my hearing in DU-PAGE Co. it tells you I've been truthful. I was never involved there nor in Chicago. If I was, count on it, they ran my D.N.A for that reason just as Du-page had. Be stupid not too, don't you think. They just don't want the Courts to know they tested me also to B/W or they'd have to clear me here too. If I'm wrong, why would they test me for the record or the public. Same reason till I showed you the public is unawear I was cleared in Du-page in any murder cases. Amazed they didn't give those findings to the Media...

WONDER WHY?

Jen... Most important, I was tested & cleared in Du-page Co. as starters. It does back up some of what I've said to what being said. Also ask the question, what is Cook County afraid of in not wanting to test me as Du-page has??? Need to stress Guilt or not here?

Jen... Must ask something... WE need to talk face to face. Can we do that soon? I don't understand how you can write about me or for me if not knowing me as a person not just in letters.
I'm me... in letters or in person & you need to see that.
Not a game or any bullshit here. I just need for us to talk, due to I have to watch what I write here & can't say as needed in letters. At times our mail is read... more so going out. Follow?
Nothing to hide, but rather this stay on a personal level till print.
I am willing to pay your air cost & time here if necessary, just say so. I feel you'll come away with less bias & a better understanding to who I am... not what others choose to lead you to believe. I know your not affraid. Nothing to be of. Please think on it but soon.
I realize you often see anger here in my letters. Not aimed at you. NEVER. But do you blame me for feeling so betrayed or filled with hurt. I feel I'm a victim here too.

PLEASE have a wonderful X-mas & a GREAT NEW years. Hope 98 brings us both some joy & hopefully for me freedom one way or another. Meaning this world or the next.

Take care & SWEET DREAMS,

Robin

March 17, 1998

Hello Jennifer,

ENCLOSED are the latest briefs etc. Their now in the hands of the Court & the State's Attorney's Office & we are awaiting the State's reply before oral argument & the Courts decision. The law regarding D.N.A testing is pretty cut & dry in my favor, however as you've read in the past the State is well known to re-write laws in their favor if it will fit regardless if it's just or not. We can only hope for the best out-come. As always, I will keep you advised to it's outcome.

I had tears in my eyes as I read your letter as to wanting to place me aside as a human-being other then the crimes itself. Heart warming I must say! My question often to GOD is what did I ever do too deserve someone as you as my friend after all that's been said. Most if not all would hate me as you once started out doing. I am happy the results today are different between us.

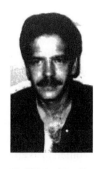

Gecht today. He claims he's innocent and wants DNA testing to prove it.

I'm sure you've again taken on another task parting me from the lies. Showing me as a caring human being, isn't hard if you know me as myself. I am in person as I often are on paper. Maybe just much more in showing love & concern for others.

I treat those as I'd want others to treat me, nothing more. I haven't changed much in my person, except being more less trusting to most or the valuable lessons I've learned during my stay at Menard. Not only as to prison life, but personal. I have learned to value many things since taken away, & had years of thinking to all in those years as to relationships, marriage, business etc. I could of changed or done better as to being a better person.

I also look closely at the victims families & what they must face or have, even though I'm not totally responsible for their loss or in Beverly's case. I feel the guilt for I ask myself often, why was I blinded to not knowing what was going on with the other two guys. There had to be signs that I didn't or maybe refused to see in order to stop their horror. After-all Rose sensed it, & I not, or maybe as I look back not willing to except it was possible.

But to involve me in their horror was way beyond any belief till it happened. Even a week after knowing what they did too Beverly, I still kept quiet in fear of my family being killed or hurt. I ask myself over & over again... "WHAT WAS I THINKING?" & guilt sets in. I hurt knowing I may of been able to change things, & didn't. You have no idea how much I wish I could just say I'm sorry to their families even if not involved, but saying sorry doesn't bring back their loss or what was done to Beverly Washington. I must live with that thought the rest of my life even if freed.

Does that make me a monster?

Now you know something others don't. Another true & honest feeling I hide from most here. They in prison call it weakness. You don't live long with other inmates knowing that.

I'd like that as to being friends for many years to follow. I hope one day you might be as proud of me as I you, for all your doin today & giving me the chance to prove whats said is not I. As often stressed, you'll never regret all your doing to see justice is done here & showing the awful nightmares of injustice that I've faced. I can only pray your book will share light on it & hopefully I'll then get fair justice as deserved.

I hope you've stress my meaning to BREAST. As stated in my letters their are millions of males out there whom love woman with simi or large breast. Women also are aware or most implants wouldn't be. I to am human, & attracted to such women, but if I loved someone, it would not matter if they had them or not. What is inside makes the person she is not whats out. It doesn't mean women should be subjects of harm for any reason as I stressed, nor did I ever think or feel otherwise to do such harm to anyone.
If you look into my years as a teen & school years & during my young & stupid years I have always loved women, large or small breasted, never treating them any less. I have a lot of respect for women, for all they do as to child birth, care & mates, even though I have once stayed away from what relationships as in marrige is truely meant to be, & I hold LOTS of regrets for all I put Rose through with another woman, but as said a lesoned learned well from those days as today. Still doesn't mean I did whats said based on this conviction or I hate women. NOT TRUE & I have never ever had a relationship with any man other then women sexually as I read. No idea where that again even came from. Any that knows me as myself would tell you that. I hope you will stress this issue well as to my meanings & thoughts as to all woman.

Note: I am reffering to relationship as to Tina. One has to think why would this woman spent two long years with me & my family if I was abusing her as stated, if at all true? She had two years to part, not continue to beg me to stay & have a child. Her reason for such Bull was the states idea. She told them that Rose & I were looking into taking my child from her at that time due to drug use & her giving her first child up to her parents due to her lack of concern in being a parent. Drugs & her whoring around as that was more important. With me in prison, there would be no chance of gaining this child. However no one was given the truth behind her reasons to all said in court or otherwise. They only seen her as a Victim, not the reasons for her lies.
Again, I'm making no excuses for this affair, I was plain & simply stupid not to realize what I had at home & where the love was. However Jennifer I never lost touch with my responsibilies as a parent to my children. Rose & I in most couples had our problems, & I guess I felt the grass was greener on the otherside. How wrong & stupid I was. In all Jennifer I must of done something

right all these years of 23. She has still refused to let go of the monster many choose to read about. I'm sure you might ask why. Only she knows & knows Robin Gecht as I one day hope you will.

Anyone can write, true or false & even though it hurts, I'm a good person at heart, even with my many past mistakes. Life is much like a chest game, you play, make mistake & learn from them. Not to repete is only when you've learn something with hopes for better by learning from them. I have that many times over.

I can with honesty say I would never dream of hurting another human-being unless it was to save my life or protect my loved ones. God teaches us to love & be kind, not kill one another without cause as in war etc. but never in cases as this without cause. How incruel that is. My belief in life was always if you vaule life or your own, what gives you the right to take another? It's only when 1 doesn't vaule his own life or it's meaning, they don't vaule other human life. I see that to often here, & I'm without understanding & become ill just to the thought. Senseless acts. These people that take life or cause harm without cause aren't human. I can't stress it any other way, but as I see it.

Well I'll stop here on those notes, I think I've taken up enough of your time today. Just another insite to Robin Gecht.
Keep in touch, I'll do the same.
Kids sent their best as I.

Friends, Robin.

P.S. My sister in the enclosed photo is the sister talked about. Makes one think why would she visit if I was to ever abuse her? Hmm. Would you? She, Mom & Nick in this photo were killed leaving here that same day [they came to visit me]. 11-16-88. This is the last photo of my sister, Nick & I that final day. I miss them.

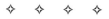

4/20/98

Hi Jennifer,
I must say I am somewhat scared to how the public will take my words to the truth. Will it open up a window to attorney's that are willing to find justice or will it simple go in deef ears as just a story the writter or I wish to tell?

I also saw the T.V profile on Cruz in Illinois. Sad, but fact. I knew the little girls parents that Cruz was to of murdered. As I studied & followed his case, I never once doubted he was being framed. My thoughts paid off as D.N.A & another inmates confession played into place. He was within a year of execution here at Stateville Corr. Center. Like I, 15 yrs on death row for something he didn't do. We simply must find better ways in our justice systems before others are executed as in the Limburg case years back & later proven innocent of the crime in which he was convicted to die for & did. There have been others who sit in these rat holes & our lives taken from us as to being human because we inpower those who simple care about getting to be a judge one day & have a number of convictions he or she must have to be noticed for such jobs. It's simple politics with other peoples lives. It works the same with Police officers etc. More arrest or traffic tickets given out, the better they look as to job promotions. Strangely enough our judges are WELL WELL aware of it. How would they get elected otherwise or promoted? I fight every single day of my life here just to stay alive & more so now once that [Jaye Slade Fletcher] WANT TO BE WRITTER wrote her book [*Deadly Thrills*] yet never knowing me, but written by the words of her friends on the force. These people read that book & took it as the gospel written by God himself. I also felt for Cruz, for he too received that same treatment over the death of a innocent child. The Police, the State & other attorneys knew without question he as I was not guilty from the start but it maked job promotions & it sold newspapers. I pray now those whom as in my case will one day know what it's like being on the low end of life through lies & the simple lack of concern in the lives they help to destroy by their deeds in convicting the innocent.

One day Jen, you really need to sit in on a murder case etc. You will see first hand the STATES ATTORNEY'S run our court rooms, not the judges. And of course you might hear on how our fine POLICE DEPARTMENTS & OUR STATES ATTORNEYS NEVER EVER LIE. BULL!
MANY OF THEM BELONG HERE IN MY PLACE.

Once again I stress, thank you for all your doing but mostly for being my friend. I hope for many years to follow. Keep in touch, will do the same. Stay well.

Robin

Henry Lee Lucas

Born in Blacksburg, Virginia in 1936, Henry Lee Lucas' childhood was about as grim as it gets. His mother, Viola, was not only an alcoholic and a prostitute but she was cruel and viciously abusive to Henry — sometimes forcing him to put on a dress and watch as she serviced her customers — and curling his hair and making him wear a dress to school. She also beat him regularly, once so savagely with a two-by-four that she knocked him unconscious for three days, leaving him with permanent head injuries. Lucas' father, a double amputee, only added to the family's dysfunction. Legless, he spent his life in a wheelchair, sometimes selling pencils on the corner, but mostly saturating himself with alcohol to dull the misery of his pitiful life. To make matters worse, Lucas and his brother fought constantly, sometimes seriously — like the time Henry's brother stabbed

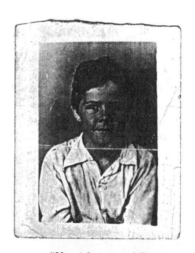

"Me at 8 years old"

him in the eye with a knife. In keeping with her total lack of responsibility as a mother, she couldn't be bothered to take him to the hospital, so by the time her boyfriend finally brought Henry to a doctor, his eye had withered away and had to be removed.

Henry was not what you would call a typical teenager. By the time he was 13, if he wasn't having sex with his half-brother, Harry, he was busy killing animals and sexually gratifying himself with their dead bodies. Bestiality became a favorite way for the brothers to pass the time, as was igniting and torturing animals.

By the time he reached his twenties, Henry was out of control. After an

175

argument with his 74-year-old mother, he stabbed and killed her (although he now tells me that he has no memory of the murder and is not even sure if he is the one who killed her. However, because he has been told that he did it, he accepts responsibility). He was found guilty of second degree murder and even though he was sentenced to 40 years at Ionia State Psychiatric Hospital, he ended up only serving 16 years before being released on parole in 1970. Lucas has said that he protested his early release, warning doctors that if he was let out he would surely kill again — but unfortunately for all of the many people who would eventually die at Lucas' hand, no one listened to him.

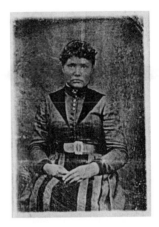

Viola Waugh, Henry Lee Lucas' mother, was a prostitute and an alcoholic. He ended up killing her when she was 74 years old — though he now says he's not really sure if he did it.

Shortly after his release, Lucas struck up a friendship with Ottis Toole, a psychopathic lowlife who liked to sexually assault children. Soon they became lovers and together they drove across the country, going from town to town abducting, raping and killing randomly chosen men and women. Toole eventually took off, leaving in his place his 12-year-old cousin, Becky Powell, who soon became Lucas' new lover and later his common-law wife.

Soon after the two lovers took jobs as live-in caretakers for an 80-year-old woman named Kate Rich, she disappeared. Within a short time, Becky Powell also disappeared. When police searched Lucas' cabin they found the charred remains of Kate Rich's body in the stove. As for Becky

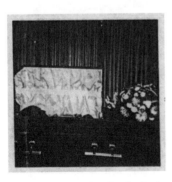

Inscription on back of photo reads: "Moms and her kaskit in Michigan."

Powell, investigators found pieces of her body scattered across various counties surrounding Stoneburg.

After Lucas' 1983 arrest, he admitted to police that he had killed Powell, Rich and a female hitchhiker who, because her identity has never been determined, is referred to as "Orange Socks" for the only article of clothing found on her otherwise naked body. Inspired by an unusual stroke of bad conscience, Lucas told the prison guards "I done 300 bad things," leading investigators to consider the alarming possibility that he might have killed 300 women.

In a two-day taped interview, Lucas confessed to hundreds of murders, but after a year-long investigation in 1986 by the Texas attorney general's office, it was determined that there was not enough evidence to support most of his confessions. In fact, once considered the most prolific serial killer in history, in the end, Lucas' confessions led authorities to only ten bodies. Lucas has since changed his story several dozen times, sometimes saying he killed 600 people (although in his letters to me he says it was over 3000) in as many as 26 states and sometimes admitting only to the murder of his mother.

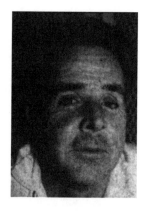

Once considered the most prolific serial killer in American history, Henry Lee Lucas ended up recanting most of his 600 confessions of murder.

Lucas now openly admits that he lied about all of the confessions with the intention of confusing authorities. "I set out to break and corrupt any law enforcement officer I could get," Lucas told a Fort Worth newspaper. "I think I did a pretty good job. I feel I've accomplished what I set out to accomplish. I'm not proud of it. There are 600 killers walking around out there. That's how many cases they took off the books. It's not a good thing. And that I'm sorry for." His confessions precipitated a massive wild goose chase that left surviving families bereaved once again and investigators stymied.

Lucas has ten murder convictions, nine of them in Texas. He has pleaded guilty to eight murders and he has one death penalty (for the murder of "Orange Socks" — ironically, the one murder he may *not* have committed), five life sentences, one sentence of life without parole and 210 years in prison. Lucas has had two stays of execution, one in 1985 and the other on June 26, 1998. Four days before his scheduled execution by lethal injection for the slaying of "Orange Socks," Governor Bush of Texas issued a reprieve for Lucas because there not was enough evidence to tie him to the murder.

Although no one except Lucas knows the exact number of people he killed, the murders he did admit and those he falsely confessed to caused an enormous amount of societal alarm about serial killers. His lethal attacks on one innocent victim after another instilled a chilling fear in the public, underlining the urgent need to understand serial killers.

The Lucas Letters

Feb 18, 1997

Dear Jenny,

    I recevied your letters and wanted to write but it's hard to get letters sent out from here with out a person's full name. You didn't shair with me that so I'm sorry you didn't recevie an answer on your Birthday but know I wish you the best ever.

    You don't realy understand what I have said all these years about not being guilty of what I confessed too.

    it took me two 1/2 years to make enough friends to findly get them to look at the truth about my case.

    I didn't have any attorneys who wanted to do their jobs of being my attorney instiad of wanting book rites so I could never trust them.

    as for Being a Killer I might have taken my own Mother's life I'm not sure of that. I have been told by my Family members that I did not kill her. But instiad was framed by my 1/2 brother in law and Half sister who Confessed on their dieing bed they killed her and why. I wasn't their so I haft to take their word for that. I only know I did 15 1/2 years for that. so I dont know. You ask how a long time in prison feels like. Well their is no words that can tell that because unless one goes through it I dont see where they could go through the Hell one suffers in a prison.

    I confessed to the cases I did because of drugs and Being charged with things I did not do but could not prove at the time I didn't. it takes money to prove a person didn't commit the crime he's being charged with.

    I relise ever body beleves that if a person is not guilty that a Court of law will free him that's Bull S. the court is no longer intrested if one is not guilty but only how to punish him or her. The legal system has fallen apart because of crooked police and DA's and Judges. and the people are not intrested in justice any more because of the crime that has hit this country Hard. because the Goverment keeps comming up with ways to distroy the work place in america.

    Jenny I dont care if you are a book writer or not it doesn't matter to me. I have nothing to hide from any one if you have questions you are always welcome to ask me any thing.

I use to have a friend I could depend on but any more she doesn't seem to want to corspond with me all she's been doing is useing me and I let her do it I know she isn't intrested in a good relationship.

so whats new. I got locked up Thursday by the Big shots here at the prison unit.

They clame I stuck my middle finger up at Jerry springer of the TV show who come here to Interview me Wensday. Well that a lie! I didn't. and even the officer who was right behind me listening at what was going on by Jerry Springer has stated I did not do what I was accused of and he was a wittness to that. He did say I got loud with him but that was Springer fault. and not mine. because he was provoking me into it.

I dont like the way I have been treated by this. I want to contact my attorney about this and see if Civil Rights Charges cant be filed in Court. since I did nothing to be done this way. they denie my visits and are doing me like I commited a crime.

it hurts when a person doesn't do anything wrong and is treated like this. I'm in a 3 x 9 Cell counting the open area in the Cell. the bed takes over half of the cell up so that only leaves 3 feet wide section to walk. I have got no yard since Thursday. and only one shower. today is Tuesday.

anyway Jenny I wish I could get an attorney to do my legal fighten for me. I don' know any Civil Rights attorneys here in Texas. Mr. Eddie Mays is the officer who knows I did nothing wrong.

Well I better let you go now. do me a favor write and let me know your full name and that way I can write more often.

> A Friend in the Lord Jesus
> and your Friend in Life
> Henry Lee Lucas

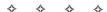

Dear Jenny,

I recevied your letters am sorry its not that I dont want to write but when I'm limited on my cash flow it makes it hard to write as I want to. Yes if you want to let others read my letters I have written thats fine. I have nothing to hide in them. The reason I never responded to one of your letters you wrote I should on up to what I did instead of covering it up. first Jenny I have told you the truth in my letters. I explained to you ever thing. And NO I'm not a Killer of Women as ever person says I am.

True I told lies in over 3000 confissions I gave and cold and lies was the reason I did start those confissings. But just because I confessed doesn't make me a killer or a searl killer as I have been labeled by so meany.

Even Jerry Springer come here with his lies and pissed me off. I told him what I thought of him. and will do that again if people keep trying to force crimes on me I never did.

Yes, I'm your friend as I said and would like to visit with you. If you want to come. You need to send me the following Information. How old you are your married name and maden name, your present address and your current job. so I can have you placed on my visiting list if your children are small and not over 12 years old they can come with you. I would love to meet them. if they are over 12 I will need to get age and names so they can come in with you. Well I don't have much time now because of working hours. So please dont give up. I will get back with you.

Your Friend, Henry Lee Lucas
in Christ Love.

✧   ✧   ✧   ✧

March 29, 1998

Dear Jenny

You ask me if you could be a pen pal or friend the answer is yes if you want. I have been realy busy trying to get a new tryal and am asking you to be paitent with me at this time. I don't know if I will live past June 30 of this year or not since I have this date to be murdered so hope and prayer will help at this time. I'll keep you posted.

Well I must go now take care till we meet again

best Regard.
Henry Lee Lucas

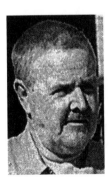

In June 1998, Lucas escaped execution when Governor Bush granted him a reprieve from lethal injection for the killing of the woman known as "Orange Socks."

Feb 18, 1997

Dear Jenny,

I received your letters and wanted to write but it's hard to get letters sent out from here with out a person's full name, you didn't shair with me that so I'm sorry you didn't receive an anwser on your Birthday but know I wish you the best ever.

You don't realy understand what I have said all these years about not being guilty of what I confessed too. it took me two years to make enough friends to findly get them to look at the truth about my case. I didn't have any attorneys who wanted to do their Jobs of being my attorney instead of wanting book rites so I could never trust them.

as for being a killer I might have taken my own mother's life I'm not sure of that. I have been told by my Family members that I did not kill her, But instead was framed by my ½ brother in law and Half sister who confessed on their dieing bed they killed her and why. I wasn't their so I haft to take their word for that, I only know I did 15½ years for that. so I don't know. you ask how a long time in prison feels like. Well their is no words that can tell that because unless one goes through it I dont see where they could go through the Hell one suffers in a prison.

I confessed to the cases I did because of drugs and being charged with things I did not do but could not prove at the time I didn't. it takes money to prove a person didn't commit the crime he's being charged with. I relise ever body beleves that if a person is not guilty that a court of law will free him that's Bull S. the court is no longer intrusted if one is not guilty but only how to punish him or her, The legal system has fallen apart because of crooked police and DA's and Judges. and the people are not interisted in justice any more because of the crime that has hit this country Hard. because the Goverment keeps comming up with ways to distroy the Work place in America.

Jenny I dont care if you are a book writer or not it doesn't matter to me, I have nothing to hide.

from any one if you have questions you are always welcome to ask me any thing.

I use to have a friend I could depend on but any more she doesn't seem to want to correspond with me, all she's been doing is useing me and I let her do it I know she isn't intrusted in a good relationship.

so what's new. I got locked up Thursday by the Big shots here at the prison unit,

They claime I stuck my middle finger up at Jerry springer of the TV show who came here to interview me Monday. Well that a lie I didn't and even the officer who was right behind me listening at what was going on by Jerry Springer has stated I did not do what I was accused of and he was a wittness to that. He did say I got loud with him but that was springer fault and not mine. because he was cross being me into it

I dont like the way I have been treated by this I want to contact my attorney about this and see if Civil Rights Charges cant be filed in court. since I did nothing to be done this way. they denie my visits and are doing me like I committed a crime.

It hurts when a person doesn't do any thing wrong and is treated like this. I'm in a 3 X 9 cell counting the open area in the cell. the bed takes over half of the cell up so that only leaves 3 feet wide section to walk, I have got no yard since Thursday. and only one shower. today is Tuesday

any way Jenny I wish I could get an attorney to do my legal fighten for me. I dont know any Civil Rights attorney's here in Texas, Mr. Ellie mays is the officer who know's I did nothing wrong.

Well I better let you go now. do me a favor write and let me know your full name and that way I can write more often.

a Friend in the Lord Jesus

& your Friend in Life

Henry Lee Lucas

David Gore

W hen David Gore was a young boy, he liked to fantasize. But unlike other kids, he didn't dream about becoming a basketball star or dating the prettiest girl in school. David Gore fantasized about violence, terrible acts of violence — with himself as the star inflictor. When he was only 13, David and his cousin, Fred Waterfield, whiled away their days fantasizing about "how we should just take women and do things to them." These sadistic thoughts of sexual violence — "bad seeds," as David calls them — just "needed to be watered" before they would become the real thing.

Apparently, that didn't happen for some time. Gore eventually got married, had two sons and became a relatively respected member of his community — that is, until he separated from his wife and she told him he could never see his beloved children anymore. Fueled by the boiling rage he felt toward his wife, David's "bad seeds," now a fully infected jungle of fury, were turned loose — not on his wife, who he grew to despise with a vengeance that had no boundaries — but on other women. Raping, torturing, mutilating and murdering women became David Gore's deranged way of venting his pain and anger.

For years, no one had a clue that it was Gore (sometimes with the help of his cousin Fred Waterfield) who was responsible for the disappearance of so many women in his home town. In his letters, Gore explains in grisly detail how he abducted, tortured and killed women — sometimes raping with a stick or a shovel, decapitating, scalping, skinning and even feeding body parts to alligators. David explains that even though killing relieved the suffocating pressure of his hate, eventually the pain and fury inside him would swell, forcing him to kill again.

Finally, a few of Gore's and Waterfield's victims managed to escape. In June 1976, after spotting a young woman, Diane Smalley, at a gas station, the two cousins followed her onto Highway 60, shot out her tires and forced her to get into their car. Terrified by what she could only imagine these men had in store for her, Diane decided that she would rather die trying to escape than allow these maniacs to hurt her. She jumped out of their moving car, miraculously avoiding severe injury and the rape and death her abductors had planned for her. On another occasion, Gore, posing as a detective with the sheriff's department, stopped Diane Sturgis for speeding. Gore explained that in order to file the necessary report, he had to take her back to the police station in his car. (Gore actually was a Reserve Deputy with the sheriff's department at one time, and he still had his ID and a badge.) Sturgis had the presence of mind to refuse and suggested that she would drive to the station in her own car and Gore could follow. Realizing his plan was foiled, Gore quickly backed down and suggested they just forget the whole thing. Relieved, Sturgis agreed to drop the matter, but she went straight to the sheriff anyway and reported the incident. When the sheriff tracked Gore down, he chose — of all things — just to take away Gore's badge.

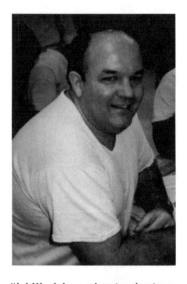

"I killed in order to destroy women. I mutilated their bodies...I **HUNTED** Women. I hunted opportunities. I rode the highways looking for hitchhikers, and I picked them up and abduct them, take them to one of my groves, rape them, sometimes torture them, then kill them...and it was all driven by pure RAGE and REVENGE."

Sturgis managed to save her own life, but others weren't so lucky. Another intended victim who lived to tell her tale was Marilyn Owens, who called the police after she spotted Gore hiding in her car. Gore was arrested and sent to Belle Glade Correctional Facility in August 1982. Clearly, no one bothered to conduct a thorough investigation into the daily activities of this deranged killer or else there wasn't enough evidence to hold him; he was released only three months later.

In 1983, after years of raping and killing, David Gore decided to call it quits. He had had enough. On the day he gave himself up, Gore and Waterfield had picked up two teenage girls, Lynne Elliott and Regan Martin, and had taken them to Gore's house. After the two men raped both women, Gore chased Elliot, who was naked, out into the street and shot her to death. She was the last woman to bear the brunt of David Gore's fury. He turned around, walked into his house and called the police. He received the death penalty on March 10, 1984 and was sent to the Union Correctional Institution in Raiford, Florida. (Waterfield was sentenced to life in prison.)

David Gore feels intense remorse for what he did. He has turned his life over to God — the only way he has been able to find relief from the nightmare of his past. He has also made a concerted effort to work with law enforcement officers to help them understand how a serial killer thinks and to show them how he was able to get away with so many murders right under their noses without ever getting caught. He is very concerned about women being such easy prey to people like him. "When I was out and I was abducting women, I pretty much could get who ever I wanted.... If I saw a Woman I wanted, I just waited for the perfect opportunity.... This is why I am so adament now to <u>WARN</u> people to not trust even someone they think is a cop.... Then there are [men who] disguise [themselves as] repairmen and such. You see these are disguises of <u>NORMAL</u> people. The main goal of a serial killer is to <u>NOT</u> bring attention to himself, but to FIT IN. You should feel frightened, but not so much from the men in prison, but just of everyday people around you, still walking our streets."

I appreciate and respect David Gore for his honesty and willingness to discuss these very personal, shameful and ugly subjects. I'm sure that most readers will find his letters *extremely* disturbing, as I did, but the information — even the revolting descriptions of raping and mutilating women — sheds much light on the workings of a mind twisted with anger and hate. And even though Gore says his reason for giving the graphic descriptions is to warn people about men like him, you just have to question his way of doing it.

The Gore Letters

Dear Jenny

Greetings. I do hope this letter finds you well & doing OK. As for myself, I am fine. I am glad you took the time to write. How did you get my name & address?? I'm assuming you got it from some book or tabloid, as I have been aware that I've been in them.

I do very much appreciate you writing & wanting to hear <u>my</u> story & get to know <u>me</u> as a person. Most of the articles & all I've read concerning me, really are distorted. It use to really bother me, but not any more. I know who I am, & that is what matters. When people do write, I try to be as honest & up front with them as I can be.

I'm not really sure what you want to know, so if you'll point me in the direction you want to go, I'll be more than happy to answer ANY & all questions you have, & I promise to be as honest as I can.

First let me share a little about me.

I was born & raised in a small town called, Vero Beach, in South Florida. I was married for 10 years, & have two Sons, who I love very much. The oldest is Michael, & the youngest is Jonathan. When my Ex

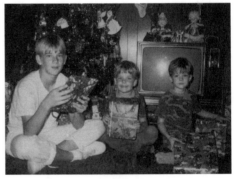

David Gore was thrown into a murderous rage when his estranged wife threatened to prevent him from seeing his beloved sons ever again.

Wife divorced me, it was a <u>very</u> traumatic time for me. She took my Sons & vowed never to let me see them. Well thru many Court battles I did gain visitation rights, & was able to establish some sort of Father & Son relationship. But it took an enormous emotional toll on me.

I have one sister who is married, & my Parents live in South Carolina. They have stood by me through it all.

Just before I was arrested I was in the process of starting my own citrus management business.

So what led me to where I am now? Gosh, I've asked that question a thousand times. I've had lawyers & judges tell me, my case makes <u>NO</u> sense, simply because of my background & the person I was.

I have witnessed the most horrible aspects of life, & I have witnessed the most beautiful aspects.

Do I think of my crimes at night? Yes, all the time. I've seen death as close as a person could ever see it.

You mentioned that you are FULL of questions. Jenn, <u>please</u> feel free to ask <u>ANY</u> & I do mean <u>ANY</u> question you want, & I promise I'll answer it. Just give me some direction you want to go in. Most people don't want to <u>know</u> the details & all of my crimes, so unless a person asks me specifically about something I usually wont volunteer the answer, because as I've mentioned it's ugly. I really don't have a problem discussing details no matter how graphic they may seem. I have nothing to hide, & if I can answer questions that people generally have, I will. So please do ask as many questions as you want.

How many Inmates do you write?? You said you <u>WONDER</u> about death. What is it that you WONDER about?? You asked how it feels. Are you referring to death or causing death??

You are so right, most psychologists DON'T have the answers. They have <u>their</u> theories as to why. But they dont have the truth. And this is one reason I <u>DO</u> talk about these things, because there has been so much <u>MISCONCEPTION</u> on these issues.

I really do look forward to hearing from you again, & like I said ask any questions. Please share a little about yourself if you want to. Anyway, please take care, & I hope to hear from you <u>SOON</u>.

Sincerely,
David Gore

<u>PS</u> If you would like a photo of myself I'll Be happy to send you one.

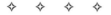

2-19-97.

Dear Jenny

Hi. I hope this will find you well & in the very best of spirits. As for myself, I am doing fine. I received your very nice letter this evening, & I'm really glad you wrote.

Please let me begin by sharing a little about myself with you. Also I will enclose a photo of myself in with this letter so you can put a face with the letter.

You mentioned that there is SO much I could help you with in your quest for knowledge. Could I ask, what is it exactly you would like to know? Jenny, I have absolutely no qualms in answering any questions you may have. If I can in any way help someone to understand what causes people to act irrationally, I will.

As far as MY case goes, Ive never hid from my responsibility. I know a LOT of people will cry & scream how they didnt do anything wrong, but Ive never done that. Ive had to face my own demons, & my actions, & I am certainly not proud of anything. But maybe something CAN be learned from my mistakes.

All I ask is for you to point me in the direction you want to go. It might help if you can just write out a LIST of questions & I can answer them. And please dont worry about how graphic or hard the questions are.

I can certainly understand you wanting to know & understand WHY people kill each other. Gosh, there is probably 1,000 of answers to this question. And I suppose it all depends on what type of crime you are dealing with.

When another person <u>kills</u> another there can be many reasons. You dont have to HATE the person even. That person may just have something you want, or you may be mad at them.

Rage is a pretty destructive force, & it <u>will</u> carry anybody, given the right circumstances, to murder.

Hatred will truly destroy a person. And if there is one lesson Ive learned thru all this, it is that.

Jenny, I normally dont go into a lot of details on my crimes, not because I just dont want to, but because I dont know what the other persons reaction will be. After all it isnt pleasant, & so this is why I asked the person to write down some questions as to what they want to hear. I can probably give you as much knowledge as you want. My crimes were pretty brutal & there were a lot of reasons behind them, mostly <u>ANGER</u>.

How much have you read about me or my case??? I can send you articles about me, my case if you'd like. I really appreciate the fact that you do want to learn. Most people could care less. By the way, how old are you?? What sort of job do you have?? If you dont want to answer any of the questions I truly will understand. I just ask so I can know the person better.

Please write back <u>SOON</u>, as Ill be anxiously awaiting your letter.

Sincerely
David Gore.

3-19-97.

Dear Jenny

Hi. I hope this letter finds you doing OK. I received your very nice letter, & it was really good to hear from you. You mention your wish to hear all the "Graphic" details of my crimes. And you mentioned that the last you read, I was "hunting" down a woman.

Well, to be honest, that is <u>NOT</u> true. I have <u>NEVER</u> hunted down a woman. But I guess that makes for great sensationalism in reading.

But I am willing to share with you the graphic details, although it may take several letters to do so. I really dont have an easy time talking about what all happened, especially with a stranger. But I sense from your letters you are genuinely interested in understanding this aspect of the dark side of life.

I want to tell you though Jenny that I definitely am <u>NOT</u> the same person today, that I was back then.

Today I could NEVER do anything like that. And thats a whole other story on the <u>WHY</u> behind that.

I guess the root of what caused me to act in the manner I did was simply <u>ANGER</u>. The anger didnt just happen, it built up over a long time, until it finally reached a peak at which something had to give. I was married for 10 years, I had two Sons, Michael & Jonathan who I loved deeply. In all appearances I had a good Marriage, but it slowly deteriorated.

When one day my Wife left me, & took my two Sons, & <u>VOWED</u> I would <u>NEVER</u> see them again. Well this totally devastated me, & I spent 2 years <u>fighting</u> in Court for Visitation rights to my Son's, & every time Id WIN, my Ex Wife, would pick up & move, & I wouldnt know where, & I'd have to start the whole process over again. All during this time Anger, frustration was building in me. I started drinking to try & eleviate the hurt.

I blamed it all on my Ex Wife. Till one day, I began venting my Anger out on Women. I guess this was in some way, my revenge on what I felt was done to me by my Ex Wife. Even though my hatred & anger was solely directed at HER, I vented it out on other Women. Ive had people ask me <u>WHY</u> I didnt just kill my Ex Wife. And I really dont have an answer for that except that, that would have affected my two Sons, & I loved them too much.

And to be blunt about it, a stranger was easier to kill.

However the first woman I killed, was <u>NOT</u> a stranger. She was my Wife's Sister.

The next murder was a 43 year old Mother & her 17 year old daughter.

The next two were two female hitchhikers, & the last one was a 17 year old girl, in which I was caught.

So people ask, Do I hate Women. And I can honestly say, <u>NO</u>.

Ive been here for 11 years & during this time I have come to understand <u>WHY</u> things happen. I dont carry the anger like I use to. In fact I have even forgiven my Ex Wife. In fact recently her & I have corresponded & have healed a lot of hurt & scars that were there.

I can not bring back the people who's lives I took, but if I could give my life for theres in return I gladly would.

Hatred & Anger is such destructive forces.

The first Woman I killed, was very hard. The <u>act</u> of killing is <u>NOTHING</u> like you see in the movies or read in novels. It drained every bit of life from me.

Jenny, to be completely honest, with you, what I did was so deplorable & so violent I wondered if I had a conscious.

I guess you would like to hear the details of the first one I killed. As Ive stated, she was my Wife's Sister, & her & I actually were friends after the divorce. But I had been drinking one day, & I called her up to ask if I could come over & talk. She agreed, & I went over & we talked for maybe an hour, & I was pretty loaded. And I really cant explain what all happen, maybe it was the booze I dont know. But I began seeing my Ex Wife in her, & I actually felt the Anger rise up in me, & I got up & we were standing in her kitchen, & when I got behind her, I wrapped my arm around her neck & squeezed. She tried to scream, but I held my hand over her mouth, & as she started struggling she fell, & I sort of went down on my knees with her to the floor, & squeezing her throat with my arm the way I was, she passed out. Thought I had strangled her & she was dead. I stood up over her, & then I took her by both hands & drug her into the living room, & then I sat down. There was an emptiness in me, I cant explain. I just sat there looking down at her. And all sort of thoughts were racing through my mind. I remember thinking, What have I done? & Now What Do I do with her? How can I clean this up?

And as I sat there it was like I went in a numbness & I remember thinking, Theres no turning back now, I <u>CAN</u> Never Be Normal Again.

I must have sat there for 10-15 minutes with her laying on the floor.

And then my feeling began to change, & I felt <u>POWER</u>. I felt like I was SUPER-HUMAN, I could take Lives.

And I believe what happen next, was stemming from this power I felt.

I was looking down at her, & she had her eyes closed, & her hair was sort of brushed over her face.

She was wearing a halter top & a pair of shorts. Well during the struggle with her, her halter top got pulled up above her breast, & for the first time I realized her breast was exposed, & I reached down & felt it. She didnt have big breast they were sort of flat. But when I felt her, she sort of moved & I let our a little moan, & I then realized she wasnt dead. I dont know why I didnt just

<u>FINISH</u> her off. But I took one of her sheets from her bed, tore strips from it, & then I drug her into the bedroom, & she beginning to come to, & I tied her hands to her bed post, & her feet to the other end. She is laying on her bed with one arm tied to one bed post, the other arm tied to the other, & her feet tied to the bottom.

I then took out my pocket knife, & cut off all her clothes, & took her panties and stuffed them into her mouth, & by now she is pretty conscious & staring up at me. She just had this look on her face like she couldnt believe what was happening.

I then took my pants off & I raped her. She was constantly struggling & trying to scream. I then straddled her chest, & pulled her gag out, & held her by her hair, & forced my dick into her mouth & ordered her to suck it. She tried to scream, & she was just asking Why? Why?

I dont remember what I said to her, but I can remember, thinking, "Im getting even with my Ex Wife & What She did To me."

To me I was justifying what I was doing by what was done to me. I lost all concept of reality.

Im trying to be as detailed & graphic as I can so you can maybe get a sense of what I was thinking & my interpretation of things at the time.

Well, finally I realized, I had to get out of there. And I had already convinced myself there was <u>NO</u> turning back now, & I realized I would have to kill her. But Jenny Anger at her was really raging inside of me. It was as if <u>someone</u> else had taken over <u>ME</u> & I was just on the sidelines. And I can remember thinking I wouldnt be satisfied with simply killing her, I wanted to destroy her totally & completely. And in my mind, I <u>KNEW</u> how & what I wanted to do to her. Brace yourself Jenny because from here on it gets pretty graphic & gorey.

At this point Im <u>NOT</u> looking at JoAnne (Her name) as a person, or a friend, or even a human being. I was looking at her as an <u>OBJECT</u> to be destroyed. I had absolutely <u>NO</u> feelings at this point.

I untied her from the bed post, & tied her hands behind her back, & her feet together. I put her gag back in her mouth, & I then drug her out to the living room, & then I preceded to <u>CLEAN</u> up everything so NO ONE would know I had been there.

My job at that time was Grove Supervisor. I had 1200 acres of groves I looked after. In one of the groves I had a Mobile home, & a barn. It sat right in the middle of the grove & was totally isolated, & under lock & key.

I had a truck with a tool box on back.

JoAnne had a two car garage & she lived way out in the Country. So what I did was pull my truck into her garage, & closed the garage door, then I drug her to my truck & put her in the tool box, so I could take her out to my grove.

I got some of her things to make it look as if she took off.

I then drove out to my grove where the barn was.

When I got there, I pulled her out, & drug her over to one of the barn rafters. I went & got some rope, & tied two lengths to the rafters overhead, & I then cut the ropes off her ankles, & tied one end of one rope around her ankle, AND the other end of the other rope around her other ankle, then, I hoisted her body up by her ankles, to where her head was about a foot off the ground. In other words, she was hanging upside down by her ankles, & her legs were spread apart about 6 feet.

I then pulled my pocket knife out & leaned down beside her head, & I pulled her gag out, & she started screaming & begging me not to hurt her, & she kept asking Why Was I doing This. And I was telling her she was a bitch like her Sister, & I was going to get pay-back for what her Sister did to me. She begged me to let her go.

I then stood up, & I grabbed her by her hair, & pulled her head up & I reached under her throat with my knife, & sliced open her throat, & blood poured from her, & she died, & just before she died she jerked.

I then, took & actually started at her ankles & <u>skinned</u> her just like you would a deer. I skinned her all the way down to her throat. I cut her head off. I gutted her open, & then I cut all her flesh off & cut her bones up, & I took & buried all the parts.

I confessed to her murder. In fact I confessed to all. Like I said Jenny, I did not have any emotion in me. It was as if everything in me was dead. I looked at JoAnne as a mere object.

But I can remember feeling POWERFUL. Like I was indispensable. I felt like this was my satisfaction. When JoAnne finally died, & I stood there looking at her body hanging there, I had so many emotions go thru me.

I can remember thinking I cant believe I <u>KILLED</u> her. Shes DEAD! I felt her body to see if it felt different dead, & it did.

I can remember thinking how happy I was that I <u>KILLED</u> my Ex Wife's Sister. In my mind I did it to her.

Jenny, from that point on, I remember thinking I <u>WANTED</u> to kill more now. The <u>FIRST</u> one was hard, but from here on they would be easy.

From that point on I guess you could say I <u>HUNTED</u> Women. I hunted opportunities. I rode the highways looking for hitchhikers, & I picked them up & abduct them, take them to one of my groves, rape them, sometimes torture them, then kill them. This went on for years.

And with each <u>KILL</u> they got easier, & I got more proficient. I have killed using a gun, knife, I've strangled Women, & Ive hung them.

Jenny, from the day I killed JoAnne, something happen to me. And I cant put my finger on it. It was like I no longer was in control of my thinking. All I wanted to do was vent my hatred out.

Ive abducted Women right out of their homes. Ive spent days <u>PLANNING</u> an abduction & then doing it. I was never caught. Women would come up missing & no clues. I thought I was God. I even joined the (get this) Sheriffs Dept. as a Deputy. This gave me access to so many opportunities. Well eventually I was caught, & there came a point in my life I did feel great remorse for all Ive done. Ive spent years trying to understand what happen. Ive spent <u>many</u> hours with well known Psychologist who wanted to understand along with me.

Ive spent a great deal of time with Ministers to understand the spiritual side of it. And I have changed my life. I only regret I didnt do it <u>BEFORE</u> people were hurt. I can & will go into each crime if you wish. I can share my feelings at the time.

Although after reading this letter you may not wish to write me anymore. And sad to say, it gets even more graphic than this. Anyway, I would be glad to try & give you insight into <u>WHY</u> I committed my crimes, & what I was feeling.

And now that I have open the door please if you have <u>ANY</u> specific questions you want to ask, please dont hesitate to ask. And I promise I will answer them as honestly as I can.

Do you want to know what my Victims responses were. How they reacted to what was happening? What I felt at the moment they died?

If I dont hear from you, then I'll accept you no longer wish to correspond.

I do appreciate you writing & I deeply respect your willingness to understand how a person can <u>KILL</u>. My crimes went so much further than just killing.

I might add that for the past couple years I have been working with several Law Enforcement groups who are trying to understand how a murderer thinks. Although I'm not explicit with them as I am with you, for obvious reasons. ☺

Well take care Jenny & I do hope you write back.

Sincerely
David

4-14-97

Dear Jenny

Hi. I pray this letter finds you well & in the best of spirits.

As for myself, I am doing fine. I just received your most welcomed letter.

To be honest with you, I thought after I wrote such a detailing letter to you, I probably wouldnt hear back from you. However, I cant begin to tell you how truly delighted I was when I received your letter. Thank you so much for writing back.

Jenny, I also want to thank you for sharing with the situation with yourself & the custody battle you went through for your children. Believe me, I truly understand all the emotions & feelings you experienced.

When my Ex Wife left & took my two Son's away, I felt my whole world had just ended. My emotions were in total chaos. And you are absolutely right, you do feel dead inside.

They say, hind-sight is 20-20, & thats so true. Looking back on everything now I wish so much I had handled things a lot different. I wish so much <u>NO ONE</u> had to die. There is not a day that goes by I dont regret what I did.

[I was so angry at my wife] and I believe this is why I turned my rage on other Women. In a sense, & in my mind, I WAS killing her, when I killed a Woman. I know it sounds weird, & without reason, but that's what I felt. I also believe that is why my crimes were <u>SO</u> brutal. You know how, you hear of people who get <u>SO</u> mad at someone & they <u>OVER</u> kill them. I believe this was what was going on inside me. I had SO much anger, & bitterness boiling inside of me, that I didnt just stop at killing Woman, I wanted to totally destroy her in every sense of the way.

I couldnt kill my EX Wife, & I believe there was something inside me that was so deeply connected to my Sons, that I saw if I killed her, I would in essence be killing them, if this makes any sense.

So I turned my rage on Women in general. This was the way I chose my release.

And during this period, I had NO emotions, it was like I was someone else, a robot.

I truly understand the <u>FAMILY</u> thing. I got married when I was 18 because I wanted a family. I have always been a <u>FAMILY</u> oriented person. I loved being married, having a home & children. And so when all that came crashing down on me, my World as I knew it no longer existed, & to me it was all my Ex Wife's fault.

I believe I am a much different & stronger person today. I met a Psychologist once who really helped me understand some things. Now I have never been a big fan of Psychologist, & really never had any desire to speak to one. But this particular man happen to become interested in my case, & so he came to visit me. And slowly we became friends. And I simply told him, I wanted to understand what happen. And so we approached it from this stand point. So over the years I came to understand a lot about me as a person. I even wrote a letter to my Ex Wife once & asked her forgiveness.

While I was in the County Jail I met a man who was an Evangelist, & over the course of the next few Months we became very close friends. I like to refer to him now as my mentor. We are still friends, & he really carried me through some hard times. He testified for me at my trial.

He use to tell me I spent all my life, <u>RUNNING</u> from God, & now God has me right where he wants me. And I believe this.

<u>I</u> dont like the <u>OLD</u> David. I despise him. But I can honestly say I like who I am today.

Jenny, you are the <u>FIRST</u> person who has ever wanted to understand what happen to <u>ME</u> & the reason behind my actions.

No one has ever cared enough to want to try & understand. Oh Ive had people write to me & <u>SEEM</u> concerned, & ask the usual question of "Why did you do IT." And when Id write back, I would never hear from them again.

Jenny, I have never been the type person to make excuses, & I dont make excuses for my actions. I dont believe in skirting the issues. If someone ask me about a particular thing, I would rather be blunt & honest with them than try to lie to them. Lying never gets you anywhere. I figure if a person is going to accept me, then they have to accept the truth.

So <u>YES</u>, I am <u>VERY</u> interested in writing you, & I really pray this can be the start of a long lasting friendship.

Jenny, yes, you can write a book about me if you want. For years Ive wanted to help people understand what goes on in the mind of someone who has been where Ive been. And youre right, people <u>DONT</u> understand. And a lot of that is because they just dont care to understand. I dont usually go into the Details of any of my cases. But there was something about <u>YOU</u> I felt I could trust. You seemed genuinely different from everyone else. And Jenny please feel free to ask <u>ANY</u> question you want, no matter how graphic or vivid they seem, & I promise you I will always give you an honest answer.

I dont believe its coincidence you wrote to me. You have triggered something Ive been wanting to do for years, & that is getting Society to understand.

You have no idea what it means to me to have your trust, & I promise you, I will <u>NEVER</u> betray your trust in me.

You asked why I regretted killing the 22 year old.

When I abducted her, & had her tied up, & she began begging & pleading with me to let her go, cause she had a small child. And that touched a vulnerable spot in me. But in my mind I knew I couldnt let her go, so I went ahead & tortured her & then killed her, but it was emotionally draining in me.

And as I was saying earlier it was not just enough satisfaction to just kill them, I raped, tortured & killed. And it was all driven by pure RAGE & REVENGE.

I truly wish I could bring back every single one I killed, but I cant, so I have to at least help others who may end up in the situation I did.

Maybe in some way I can help <u>SAVE</u> a life.

And would you believe this has been a prayer of mine for a very long time?

When I was arrested Jenny, I actually was relieved. I confessed to all the murders I committed. I just wanted to be free of that. I spent over a year with Detectives, showing them where all the bodies were, detailing my steps of abduction of Women.

And I even helped them to know what kind of signs to look for. I worked for almost a year with them. They could not believe I abducted so many Women right under their faces, & so they wanted to learn from me so maybe they could detect future crimes.

Jenny, something I dont tell very many people, but like I said, I trust you. I use to be a Deputy Sheriff.

So you see Ive been on <u>BOTH</u> sides of the fence. I was a Deputy for about a year maybe a little longer.

I know when I was going to trial my lawyer would tell me this didnt make sense. Because I was Not your typical serial killer.

Jenny another thing is, I will <u>NEVER</u> lie to you. What I tell you, you can check & verify if you wish. My case was in a town called Vero Beach. Fla. Believe me there arent many people in Vero who <u>DONT</u> know who I am.

Im probably the most hated man there.

You know when my Ex Wife Donna left me, & vowed never to let me see my sons, I <u>DID</u> go thru the Court system, & I finally won good <u>VISITATION</u> rights, which was all I wanted. But as soon as I won, Donna took the boys & went to West Virginia, & I went back to Court but they told me there was nothing they could do because that was out of their jurisdiction.

I was totally exhausted, emotionally, financially, & this gave way for complete rage.

Jenny I'm enclosing a photo of my two Sons. This was taken several years ago. The boy on the left is my oldest Son Michael, the one in the middle is my youngest Jonathan. The other boy is my Sister's son.

I have a photo of Michael when he is in the Army. When I dig it out I'll send it to you. I believe I sent you a photo of me, didnt I.

If you dont mind, could you send a photo of yourself, so I can put a face to your letters? I'll send it back if you wish.

Jenny, I want you to also know our communication is a two way street. If you ever Need someone to talk to, I'm a great listener, OK?

I can understand you ceasing to write serial killers because of the lies. Its sad to say, but I have met a lot of men in here who believe they have done nothing wrong, & will feed you a line of crap a mile long. I really dont care about <u>FALSE</u> people. And in a sense they live in there own sort of Prison.

The hardest thing I ever had to do in all my life, was one time one of my Victims Mother wrote me & wanted to know exactly how their daughter died. I wrote her back & told her the Sheriff dept could give her the details. But she wrote me back & told me she KNEW that, but I was the one who was there & she needed to hear it from Me. So I managed to write her a <u>BRIEF</u> note just giving the basic information cause I really didnt want to go into <u>DETAIL</u> with the Mother about how her daughter died. But she kept persisting I give all the details. So I related the whole thing to her, & was very detailed, & I figured she'd write back & tell me what an animal I was. But she wrote back & actually <u>THANKED</u> me for being so detailed & that showed her I had integrity. Can you believe that? So I wrote back & told her I would be praying for her, & I hope God would heal the hurt.

I guess why Im able to talk about my crimes is because I <u>KNOW</u> Im not that person any more.

The most profound thing about when I killed a Woman, was the utter emptiness I felt right after. I felt like I wasnt even human any more. It felt like every ounce of my emotions & feelings evaporated. It put my whole being into a sort of Numbness. But after several days or sometimes weeks, I would want to destroy again, & the whole process was repeated over & over.

Can I ask, which serial killers do you STILL write??

As I've already said, please ask any questions you wish. I will always be totally honest with you. But thats something I dont normally share unless someone tells me they WANT to hear it.

Ive been here for a number of years, & Jenny I have spent a lot of time dealing with my past. I have been very fortunate to have met some really wonderful people who have helped me understand this rage I had & why I directed it the way I did. But the one person I credit the most for changing my life is a Pastor named Fritz Bowman.

Him & I spent many hours talking. See I believed, I was to bad of a person, that God certainly didnt want anything to do with me. But Fritz helped me to come to *KNOWS* God's love for me as a child.

I truly thought I was UNSAVABLE. But God is full of grace & mercy. So I see myself <u>TODAY</u> for the man I am in God. You just dont know how much I wish I could go back in time & undo all I've done.

But I cant. However, I CAN maybe in some way help other Women & people from being a Victim.

By the way, do you have a photo of yourself or you & your family you could send? I would really appreciate this.

So Ill close this & begin another letter later. Please take care Jenny, & Im really glad our paths have crossed. Hopefully some good will come out of all the tragedies. May God bless & keep you in his care.

Sincerely
David

✧   ✧   ✧   ✧

4-23-97

Dear Jenny

Hi. I sure hope & pray this letter will find you well & in the best of spirits.

As for me, Im fine. Bet you didnt expect to hear from me again so soon did you?

Well actually I was thinking about my case, & how everything happen, & so I wanted to write you & just talk, so I hope you dont mind. To be honest in your last letter you had said something, that I have asked so many people over the years.

Jenny, I believe every person on this earth has at one time or the other wished someone dead. I use to tell or rather ask people, have they ever said to someone "Ill Kill YOU," or "I Wish YOU were dead."

Cause I believe that when you make a statement like that, you have some form of murder in your heart. So my question has always been why do most people have the restraint, & conscious to NOT let that statement manifest itself into reality, when other people like me, carries through with it?

Jenny, I honestly <u>WANTED</u> my Ex Wife dead, but I couldnt kill her. And I believe the one Main reason is, because of my two Sons. To have killed her (& Im being honest here) meant I would in a sense killed them. She was there Mother & that to me was a force I couldnt destroy.

I truly believed if we had not of had any children, I would have killed her. I felt she hurt me more than anyone could be hurt, & all I wanted was to hurt her back. And I vented all this anger, hurt, bitterness onto <u>other</u> Women.

I had so much anger in me Jenny. Its hard to explain to people what I was experiencing then. Unless you've actually experienced this yourself.

However over the years, I've come to understand the destructive force anger carries with it.

Now here is something you may find interesting. In every murder committed, I was drinking. <u>NEVER</u> once did I murder without first drinking. The Doctor I use to talk to, told me this was what gave me what is called,

"DUTCH COURAGE." He probably was right.

Im a totally different man today than I was then. But only because I wanted to <u>understand</u> what drove me to commit some of the most horrible acts you can imagine.

When I was committing my crimes Jenny, I actually <u>thrived</u> on killing. It was my release.

But I will never ever forget the total emptiness I felt when I killed the <u>FIRST</u> Victim. I was <u>SO</u> empty I couldnt move. It was as if, every emotion, every feeling in my being poured right out. And I <u>KNEW</u> at that moment, I was NO longer "human." I could never live a <u>NORMAL</u> life.

I stood there beside this Woman's body for at least 30 minutes without being able to move. It was something I will <u>NEVER</u> forget. But that was the only time that ever occurred. From that point on, killing became easier.

Yes, I did <u>stalk</u> Women. One of the experts who testified for the State said I <u>hunted</u> Women. And he is probably right. Toward the end, I went to extreme measures to abduct & kill. It was like going thru a <u>PROCESS</u>. My preferred victims were hitchhikers. But only because they were easy & convenient. <u>NOW</u> I tell people of the dangers involved of hitchhiking. There are warning signs a person can look for. Especially for girls who are hitchhiking.

This is why Jenny I really am all for you writing a book. I believe there are a <u>LOT</u> of people who Will identify with it & it will be an avenue to get a message out.

By the way, my Ex Wife & I had divorced one time before. We were divorced for about a year, then we got back together, & were married for 5 years, before our marriage ended in a traumatic way.

I really dont know <u>WHY</u> we got Re-Married. We had one child at that time, so I think a lot of it was because of our Son. By the way, my Ex Wifes name is Donna. About 6 years ago, my Cousin who I write often, wrote & told me that, Donna had called her, & asked her for my address because she wanted to start writing to me & my Cousin wouldnt give it to her. I wrote my Cousin a letter to give to Donna & in it, I asked her forgiveness for all the hurt Ive caused her. Strange huh?

Its been about 8 years since Ive had any contact with my Son Jonathan. About 2 years ago my oldest Son Mike wrote me a letter & sent me photos.

Anyway, Ill close this for now. I wanted to let you know Im still here. ☺ Please take care & I hope to hear from you real soon.

Sincerely
David

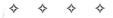

4-29-97

Dear Jenny

Hi. I sure hope & pray this letter finds you doing OK. As for myself, I am just fine. I received your most wonderful & very welcomed letter, & it was really great to hear from you. Thank you so much.

I had to smile when you said, it was 6:00 A.M when you were writing that. ☺ I do all my letter writing <u>early</u>. It is 3:53 AM right now as I write this. I just really love the peace & quiet of the very early mornings, especially in here. The only time you can have some peace & quiet. I have always been an early riser. Even when I was on the streets, I was always up before 5:00 AM. That's just how it is when you are a Country person. ☺

Thank you for the very nice comments regarding my Sons. I really am a proud father. And I do know that one day, they'll know I do love them. I have had people tell me "Well IF you really loved them you couldnt OF done what you did."

I dont even try to answer that. It may have an element of truth in it, but there is so much more behind it.

Donna (my Ex) really did all she could to try & turn my Sons against me. And I've heard this from my own oldest Son. All I can do is keep my Sons in my prayers, & just ask God to keep them in his care.

You mentioned you Wrote to Fred Waterfield. Now Jenny, he is someone I truly do feel sorry for.

By the way, him & I are First Cousins.

Did I hold a gun on him & make him do things?? ABSOLUTELY NOT!!

Jenny, he has denied everything from day one. He has totally convinced his family that he is an innocent Victim. His Mother is the nicest person you could ever meet. I have often referred to her as my second Mom.

Fred has claimed he is innocent for so long, he actually believes he is himself.

I believe with all my heart Fred is a pathological liar.

Jenny, these arent the only cases him & I are convicted of. Him & I were stalking, abducting, raping & killing for a very long time. He is as brutal & as violent as I once was.

He has raped at least 6 or 7 Women that I know of. When him & I were arrested, there were a couple of Women who came forward & identified Fred as the man who raped them.

The case that I am here on now, the Lynn Elliot & Regan Martin case, him & I <u>planned</u> to abduct a Woman that day. We sat at his shop & planned going over to the beach & just riding up & down the beach & look for a Woman alone that we could abduct. So that day, we took off on our "hunt," Then we spotted

Lynn & Regan hitchhiking, & Fred said, "Now theres a couple nice ones." It was PRE-determined that we would pick a Woman up, & if they were OK, Fred would give me a Nod, & I would pull a gun on them. This is exactly how it happen with Lynn & Regan.

A year or so before that, Fred & I abducted a girl at a gas station, & he raped her in the back seat of his car. Jenny, this is all in the records & reports. You can get anything I'm telling you right out of the files of the Indian River County Sheriff's dept. They have the evidence for all of this.

He was given two life sentences for the Murders of Byers & Lavelle.

We abducted them as they were hitchhiking. We went cruising around that night Looking for a target. We spotted Byers & Lavelle hitchhiking & picked them up, & while we were driving I pulled a gun on them, & then Fred got in the back of the Van with them, took all their clothes off, tied them up, raped one of them, & then we drove to his barn, & he told me, go get rid of them, & I drove out to a grove were I then raped them, & then killed them.

Him & I were also involved in two other murders that he Never got charged with. He actually go away with murder on them. I got two life sentences. But ONLY because I confessed. My lawyer told me if I didnt confess, they did not have any evidence to convict me. But I couldnt, it was time to change my heart, so I confessed & told them. I got 2 life sentences. Fred said he didnt know what I was talking about. So they couldnt charge him. And He raped both of the Lings & helped kill them.

Jenny, Fred I don't believe has a conscience. So I do feel sorry for him. He has all his family totally convinced he is innocent, & I am making up wild stories about him. But it really doesn't bother me, because I feel I am a better person Inside & I can live with a clear conscience. I had the State Attorney himself tell me I was much more human than Fred. Anyway, I do pray for him. And like I said you can get all the information & testimonies of people who have had contact with Fred at the Sheriff's dept.

I had my own inner motive for the things I done. But I don't know what Fred's motives were.

I have to laugh when I hear someone say how Fred says I held a gun to his head & forced him. How do you Force someone to rape, murder & all.

I really don't try to convince people of the truth. God knows my heart.

I really don't know at exactly at what point Fred & I started doing things. We grew up together, & were really like brothers. The very first thing I can remember that linked us so to speak, was one day when we were teen-agers Fred was over at my house, & he asked me if he could Rape my Sister. And I think from then on we discussed RAPE & girls & what ever. We'd always talked about doing abnormal things, but never really carried out. So when I began having troubles & anger became my force, once again Fred & I started talking & he told me that he had RAPED & killed a couple of Women, & he described every thing. And I can remember listening to him, & thinking how I'D like to Kill because of the anger in me. And so he became the catalyst so to speak. To be honest, I really don't know if in fact Fred did ever rape & kill, but at the time it really didnt matter to me. He was fueling something In me, & that's all I cared about.

I could never even think about hurting a man or boy Jenny. Woman became the object of my rage because in my mind the hurt & pain I was experiencing was caused by a Woman.

And Jenny to be totally honest with you, during this time when my rage was in full control, I <u>WANTED</u> to kill <u>EVERY</u> Woman I could. That's how intense my rage was.

I even turned my rage on my Sister-in-law, but she escaped death, simply because she didnt come home when I figured she would. Jenny, I had gone in her house, & was <u>WAITING</u> inside for her to come home, & I was going to abduct her. But she didnt come home, & I waited an hour, & finally I left. Do you know that to this day, she does <u>NOT</u> know that happen?

Yes I did mean you could write about <u>ME</u>. You are really the first person to ever want a story about Me. Most people want a story about the cases. But I'm game if you are. ☺ To be honest, you are the first person Ive wanted to open Me up to.

And as I've told you, <u>ANYTHING</u> I tell you, you can find verification in the records. I can truly promise you I will <u>NOT</u> ever lie to you. I'm simply telling you the way it is. And theres a lot of it that's not going to be pretty. And there will be times that it will be hard for Me to even talk about. Cause I can't believe I hurt so many people. But at the time I <u>WANTED</u> to hurt people. I wanted them to hurt like I hurt. Every time I killed a Woman, I always went thru a period of <u>CALM</u>, it was like I had gratified that rage in me, then it would slowly begin building up again.

Jenny, you will never see me hide behind a false perception. What you see is what you get.

I don't really have any use for people who have been convicted of a series of rapes, or murders, & then say "I'm innocent, I was framed." I mean there may be those who truly didnt do it, but for the most part, they did. In All the volumes of transcripts records, reports, you will <u>NEVER</u> read one word where I said, I <u>DIDNT</u> do it. I've owned up to what I was responsible for.

Years ago, I turned my life over to Christ & He & He Alone holds my life & future. I even told the Judge this when he sentenced me. I can't claim to be Christian & then lie. The two are contradictory to each other. And I'll get into all of this aspect of my life later on. I know we have a lot of ground to cover. I don't even know where to start. ☺

When is your birthday? I would really like to remember & send a card. This is the reason I ask. So if you dont mind, please let me know. My oldest Son was born on Dec 3rd & Jonathan May 18th. Mine is Aug 21st.

Please take care of yourself & May God bless you & the children.

Sincerely
David

5-13-97

Dear Jenny

Hi. I sure hope this finds you well & in the best of spirits. As for myself, I am doing just fine. I just received your very nice & most welcomed letter & as always it was really great to hear from you.

You mentioned you had just gotten my letter where I talked a lot about [my cousin] Fred. Did you get the letter I mailed to you just before that letter?? I mailed it around the 24th.

Thank you for telling me all you need is my honesty. You can't know how much that means to me, Jenny. And I promise you I will <u>NEVER</u> do or say something that will betray your trust in me. There may be times, it will be hard to talk about details of crimes, but I'll always tell you when that happens. <u>KNOWING</u> what I've done isn't easy. I just thank God you have believed in this enough to seek my help.

You know Jenny, <u>WOMEN</u> Need very much to hear what I have to say, Because there are a lot of Women out there who cant believe this could ever happen to them. I wasnt the ONLY one who these things were happening to. Over the years, I've tried to talk to Women (the one's who'll listen) & tell them, be careful.

People in general really do need to be aware of what's happening in peoples minds today.

You wanted to know about my years of growing up. I grew up on a small farm & we lived way out in the Country. The only playmate I had was my Sister, Wendy, who was 3 years younger than I was. We were close. Because like I said, we were each others companion in our adolescent years.

Fred & his family lived right next door to us. All of my life, Fred & I have been together. Our families were always together & we grew up more as brothers than Cousins.

I can't really pin point the exact time him & I began talking or sharing things about the "abnormal." I can remember one time when I went over to his house, & he summoned me around to the back of his house, & led me up to his window & told me to peek in through the window. When I did, his Sister was completely <u>NUDE</u>. Afterward we discussed our looking at her. I have to say, that during my teen years, I had a lot of "sexual seeds" planted in me. And what I mean by that is, I began experiencing the stimulation of sex. And Fred & I explored a <u>LOT</u> of this together as we grew up. He has 2 sisters, Connie & Debbie. Now Connie, & I were real close growing up, because we were the same age, & we were in the same classes.

Fred was really wild growing up, but I was more of the shy type & all. And I guess you can say I idolized Fred a lot. He was real popular in school, & I wasnt. He had girls crawling all over him, I didnt. I was really shy with girls. So he became my idol as we grew up. And I would have done what ever he asked me to.

He is the one who introduced me to my wife, Donna. He was one of my ushers in my wedding. So he played a big role in every major event in my life. The very first time I can remember him wanting me to do something wrong was an incident when we were about 15-16 years old. Our Mothers took us out in the woods one time to let Fred & I shoot our guns. Well at one point, Fred whispered to me to "turn the gun on our Mothers." I asked what he meant. He said, turn the gun on them & lets make them take their clothes off. Well I refused to do that, & we dropped it. But later I talked to him about it, & that was the first time we discussed actually raping a woman. Now I dont want to put all the blame on him. Cause I was beginning to experience a lot of these thoughts then also. Like I said, seeds were being planted.

Well, when me & Donna first got divorced in 1975, I can remember feeling rage then. We were divorced for about a year, & then got back together. But during that year, I changed. And I began a process of hurting. We had Michael our oldest Son then. And she tried to keep me away from him. And we fought in courts. But one day, I went to see Mike, & Donna & I talked, & we eventually got back together. And I guess it was more for the child than us, because we had done a lot of damage to each other emotionally. After we got re-married, Jonathan was born.

But during that year we were divorced, my life changed, & I began looking at my wife Donna in a hateful way. And that eventually was the breeding ground for what later would become devastation. Fred was right there with me the entire time.

He was also going through a divorce, from his Wife. And his solution was he wanted to <u>KILL</u> her. He even asked if I'd help him. I said, yes. So we planned how we'd do it. At this point, I was hurting & really just didnt care anymore. My own world had been turned upside down, & I was really resenting what Donna was doing. So yes, I was ready to strike out at wherever. And Women began the focus of my rage. Every time I struck out at a Woman, in my mind I was striking out at Donna. Well we never did go through with our plan to kill his Ex Wife. But from that point on, something happen between him & I to really seal our bond to one another.

We spent hundreds of hours discussing, how we should just take women, & do things to them. And of course the seeds in me were ready to sprout.

Our <u>FIRST</u> rape was to a girlfriend of Fred's. He came & picked me up one night, & told me of the girl we "could get" & she wouldn't tell. He said she was an old girlfriend, so we discussed it, & it was agreed that we'd pick her up, & I would pull a gun on her, & we'd force her into the back seat & rape her. Well, we picked her up, she sat in the middle, & when I figured it was safe, I pulled a gun on her, & she got terrified, & asked Fred "is he serious," & Fred said yes I think so. Well we pulled into a grove where we took all her clothes off, & took turns raping her. Then we let her go. Fred assured me she wouldn't tell no one, because she knew him. Well, she did tell someone. And the police picked me & Fred up, & questioned us for hours. But for some reason they didn't believe her story & we

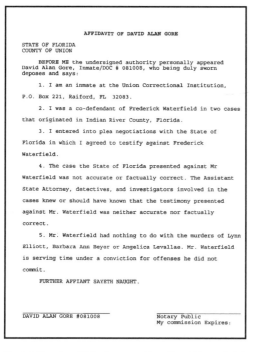

David Gore's affidavit regarding Fred Waterfield, his co-defendant and cousin.

were released. And that set a precedent for us. We thought we were invincible then. We discussed how from then on, I would always be the one to pull the gun on a girl & he would pretend he wouldn't know what's going on, so as to get the girl to trust him. And this way it would be easier to get a girl. And Jenny, this was the <u>EXACT</u> way we used to pick up Lynn Elliot & Regan Martin, for which we are in Prison for. However no one has made the connection on that & the way we used. But it was identical to how we got that girl & raped her. This is WHY Fred is saying I held a gun on him. And I'm not sure but I think he planned it this way, just for such a case as this. It was always agreed between us that I would be the "heavy" & he would act as confused as the girls were, this way, IF they did try to escape, they'd turn to him, & he could control them. And it worked many times.

Over the years, Fred & I lost contact with one another, but I had already become what I was. And I'll admit, there were many Women I got who Fred didnt have anything to do with.

I was in my own little private war. And Fred has told me that there were at least 20 women he got by himself. But I dont know. Thats just something he told me. I spent a LONG time learning how to abduct a Woman in the most proficient way I could. I devised <u>MANY</u> disguises & ruses. I then had an opportunity to get into part time Law Enforcement. So I did, & here I learned HOW crimes were investigated, what cops looked for etc. And I honed my skills to a science.

Dont get me wrong, Jenny. I'm not proud of any of this. But I had convinced myself WOMEN were the cause of my devastated life, & I declared war on Women, & I learned how to destroy them.

And for years I abducted, raped & tortured & killed Women right in my home town. And <u>NO ONE</u> ever suspected me. I took great pains in disposing of the women. Every week, there a special news bulletin on the news of a local woman who is "MISSING."

No one saw or heard anything. And Jenny, it is my belief that the reason I never came under suspicion is because I was so normal in every aspect of my life. People couldnt believe someone like me was committing such horrible crimes. I did NOT look or act like a serial killer. One of my victims was a 19 year old girl who I had known all my life. When I abducted her, & took her to my trailer she was in shock, she couldnt believe IT WAS ME.

At first she thought I was joking.

Toward the end I began focusing on members of Donna's family. She had two Sisters, & one in particular I <u>WANTED</u>. I even managed to get a key made to their home, & I use to slip in to their house while her & her husband were at work. I went through every personal item they had. I found several nude photos of her. I then began planning her abduction.

It would be easy. I'd just wait in her house & when she came in, I'd get her.

So I went & slipped into her house. I had my rope, tape, cuffs & gun, & I waited. But she never came home so I left. But IF she'd of come home, I would have gotten her.

Jenny, a lot of things I'm telling you, I have never told anyone. I'm not sure how you want to proceed with each crime. I can take them in order & tell you.

Do you want as much of the details as possible?? What I mean is, do you want me to <u>DESCRIBE</u> in Graphic detail what I did precisely to each Woman??? I will do that, if you want me to. I mean its totally up to YOU cause I don't want to scare you off or anything.

Each crime was very brutal & graphic. We are talking about me actually <u>CUTTING</u> a Womans body up & disposing of each piece. I have hung them up by their ankles & actually butchered them & skinned them.

Jenny, toward the end of my killing spree, I became <u>VERY</u> bold & aggressive in my abductions. Why I'm not sure. But it was like the more I did it, the more I thirst for it.

People have asked me how could I do such a horrible thing to someone I <u>KNEW</u>, but what they didnt understand was I had shut off all my feelings & emotions. A woman to me became simply an object. And I suppose to say I literally <u>HUNTED</u> Women would be accurate.

But you know Jenny, I had absolutely NO desire of ANY kind to hurt a young child, boy or men. In fact, I went out of my way to abduct Women who didnt have a child. That's why I was affected by the little baby. Although I abducted housewives with husbands, I didnt have any feelings toward the husband. I hunted hitchhikers a lot.

I have known Women during this time I was doing all this that I would never think of hurting in any way. I know that sounds strange, but its true. If I Liked a woman on a personal level, & I considered her a friend, she was OFF limits & I would even be protective of her. That's why people have told me none of this made sense to them. I wasnt your ordinary serial rapist killer. I really couldnt handle the hurt & pain & rejection I felt in my life at that time. It is really hard to explain the turmoil you feel, unless someone has been there. You feel totally out of control of your life. You feel <u>NO ONE </u>understands & you certainly can't talk to anyone about it. I certainly couldnt go to someone & say, "Man, I'm so angry & hurting & I'm killing Women to ease the pain." So I kept it in, & it festered. And I feel that <u>NOT</u> having a place or group where a person can seek help without being judged, is <u>SO</u> important. I know who I am, not that it makes any sense. My truthfulness will continue, despite how in so many media commendations reality has been distorted for lack of knowledge, not knowing me personally not being there, or inside of me. I have witnessed both the most horrible aspects of life, & I have witnessed the most beautiful aspects. Do I think of my crimes at night? Yes, all the time. I've seen death as close as a person could. I have nothing left to hide, & I will answer <u>ANY</u> & all questions you have, & I promise to be honest, but most people don't hear, or listen because it is too ugly. Everytime I killed a woman, I always went through a period of calm. It was like I had gratified that rage in me, then it would slowly begin to build again.

I went over to my other sister-in-law's house just to "talk" & the next thing, literally over a cup of coffee, I'm beating her over the head. I thought I'd killed her. I didnt feel bad. I felt incredibly powerful. She was laying there, on the floor, & her shirt was up over part of her breast. It excited me, sexually. And it was when I was standing over her body that she moaned. She was still alive, which really thrilled me, but at the same time I was feeling this hate for her, just because she was Donnas sister, not because there was a thing wrong with her. I took her up stairs, tied her to her bed, raped her, & then I crawled on top of her, & forced her to take my penis in her mouth; she kept crying & begging & saying "why are you doing this to me...?" I went & pulled my truck into her garage & with that privacy, I went back upstairs, untied her, & put her in the back. We drove out to the orchards where I kept a small trailer, & inside I stripped her completely naked, & tied her up by her ankles. She was pretty out of it by then. I cut her throat, & I watched her twitch until she bled to death. I couldnt stop, I was so...elated....I took my knife, & like a deer, I skinned her entire body.

I'll close this for now, & hope to hear from you again soon.

Please take care of yourself, & know I'm thinking of you, & praying for you also.

Sincerely
David

5-30-97

Dear Jenny

Hi. I sure hope this letter finds you doing OK. As for me, I am doing just fine. I just received your most wonderful, & welcomed letter & it was really good to hear from you. I am beginning to look forward to your letters very much.

So you think I should be the writer, huh? No thanks. I will leave that task up to you. ☺ You know Jenny, I have a tendency to put Me into my letters. I don't try to mash the person I am. I can't do that. If people accept me then they have to accept me for who I am. I know without a doubt a person <u>CAN</u> change, because I have. But they can't do it under their own power. You really have to allow god to Work Through & in you. And this takes a submissive will toward God.

There are very few people who know the <u>REAL</u> me, because they simply didnt or wont take the time to get to know me. They read in the paper what Other people say I am. You are the ONLY person who has ever wrote me &

said, I want to know who you are from your own words. It never has bothered me what other people said about me. Cause the fact is I have committed some pretty atrocious acts. Thats something I am not proud of at all. I wished many times I could turn back the hands of time, but I cant. And so I have to live with the knowledge of what Ive done. Ive spent years trying to make some sense of my actions. But Im happy with the David I am today.

I agree with you, I believe we both have sort of been working a greater understanding of all this. I have always entertained the idea of telling people the story of Me. But I just never had the right setting.

Thank you for your birthdate. I will put it on my calendar. My birthdate is Aug. 21st, 1953.

By the way, you said you cant send in a photo without some okay or something.

Jenny, you can send me up to 10 photos in a letter. You dont have to have any Okay or anything. There has never been a rule or anything that says this. This place allows up to 10 photos to come in a letter so please feel free to send a photo, as I would truly appreciate that. I have a whole photo Album of family photos Ive gotten over the years, so during the course of our communication I will send you some.

If I go back to court, I would very much like to call you on the phone. Thank you.

Jenny, I will share with you the <u>GRAPHICS</u> of my crimes, & all. Please keep in mind however, this isnt something thats easy for me. I have to <u>WORK</u> my way through it. There are times that I just cant believe I did some of the things I did. And so when I share details it brings the reality of my past to light. So its important to me that you know this isnt something that is easy. But I know it is for a good cause in the long run.

Im really not sure where to start.

You are correct, if Donna & I had of remarried happy, my life would have been a lot different.

Her & my two Sons were my World. And I didnt handle losing that in a positive way. When she kept my Sons from me, & vowed never to let me see them, I changed...for the worst.

But you are correct Jenny. I did have "Fantasizes" long before all this. But thats pretty much all they were. So I guess you could say there were, "Bad Seeds" planted & all that was needed was watering.

So when my World with Donna & the boys began falling, & Freddy began filling a part of my life, & the alcohol & all, the stage was set for what was to come.

And added to all of this Jenny was the fact that my sexual desire was extremely high, where as Donnas was nil. She did <u>NOT</u> like sex, & when she did, it was strictly missionary position maybe once or twice a week. So there was a lot of frustration there also. So there were a <u>LOT</u> of factors coming together that caused horrible things to happen. But you know with all this, in all the ten years Donna & I were married I <u>NEVER</u> once cheated on her. I didnt & still dont believe in being unfaithful. I was raised with high morals I guess. And it wasnt because I didnt have opportunities.

Donna had two Sisters, one was a housewife, & the other was a stewardess for United Airlines. She was a beauty. Donna was the youngest of them. Donna always resented her Sister Jo. Because she felt she had all the attention.

So when I began allowing all this frustration & all began to consume me, JO, was the <u>FIRST</u> one I targeted. In my warped sense I felt it would be OK to kill her, because Donna hated her anyway. So one day I managed to get a key made to Jos house. She lived way out in the country with NO ONE around.

So I began going into her house every chance I got, when she wasnt home. I would go in & look around. I began calculating just how I would get her. I went through every article she owned. I went through all her dresser drawers. This went on for Months. I was going thru drawers one time when I found some <u>NUDE</u> photos of her some were explicit, & some were of her taking showers, laying in bed. I never knew Who took them. But seeing these <u>NUDE</u> photos fueled my desire for her. I knew all I had to do was hide somewhere in her house, & wait for when she came home. I carefully orchestrated my plan. I used Donna to find out when she would be home etc. The day came, & I slipped into her house, with a gun, knife, some rope, duct tape. And I waited. But she NEVER came home when she was suppose to, so I got impatient & left. I really dont know if she realizes to this day, how close she came to being one of my Victims. If she would have came home, theres no doubt I would have got her.

It would be a few weeks later when my next opportunity would come to abduct a Woman, & this time it would happen. This would be my <u>FIRST</u> killing. And from that point on, I would become a monster so to speak. Getting the <u>FIRST</u> killing over, the rest would become easier & easier.

Actually the day I abducted the two Oriental Women, I wasnt <u>LOOKING</u> for a Victim. They just happen to be a set of circumstance that presented the opportunity.

It was a normal day, I was working, making my rounds to the Citrus groves, it was probably around 2:30 or 3:00. I was heading west on route 60 heading toward my grove, when I saw a school bus drop a young girl off & as I passed, I noticed she was walking down a dirt road which was very secluded, & there wasnt but one house at the end, so I know this was where she had to be going. She was a <u>VERY</u> nice young girl. <u>VERY</u> pretty.

Now during this time Jenny, I was a Reserve Deputy for the Indian River County Sheriffs dept. I carried an I.D. & a badge.

Also during this time, I carried in my truck rope, handcuffs, duct tape, handgun. I kept these things with me all the time. So I made a U-turn & pulled down the dirt road where this young girl was walking. I pulled up along side her & showed her my Deputy I.D. badge & told her I was a "Detective" with the Sheriffs dept., & I was investigating some burglaries in the area, could I ask her some questions. She said, yes, but she had to ask her <u>MOTHER</u>, which threw me for a second, cause I hadn't counted on a mother. I was committed, though, so I told her, okay, get in & I'll drive you up to your house & talk to your mother.

Now before I pulled up alongside of her, I had tucked my handgun into my pants & my hand-cuffs into my pocket.

So she gets in, & we drive up to her house, & we get out & walk just inside her house where her Mother meets us. The girl tells her Mother who I am & what I want. Now in my mind. I'm thinking on just when I will make my move & pull my gun on them. But first I have to size everything up. So I ask the mother if I could speak to her husband. She tells me he JUST LEFT for work. Perfect I thought. So now I realize I have the mother & daughter alone & they are both standing side by side listening to me. Then I reach & pull my gun & point it at them, & I tell them, "dont move, I am placing you both under arrest, I have to take you down to the Sheriffs Office."

Now they are 100% convinced I am a DETECTIVE.

They have no reaction when I pull the gun on them. They just act somewhat confused, so I take my handcuffs out, & I cuff their hand to one another, & I order them to walk out to my truck, which they do, I make them get in. They <u>BELIEVE</u> I am taking them to the Sheriffs. We leave & I start heading toward one of my groves close by, & they both try to talk in their language & I tell them to be quiet. When we pull into the grove, they dont say anything. I pull down into some trees where no one can see us, & I park & I put the gun to the Mothers' head, & tell her, NOW, lets see what you have & I reach & pull up her blouse & when I do this the realization hits them that I am <u>NOT</u> a cop, & I'm going to do something bad. When I pull the Mothers' blouse up over her titties, she isnt wearing a bra, so her titties are exposed, & she begins begging me NOT to hurt her daughter, she tells me to DO HER. Please, leave my daughter alone. The daughter is just sitting there sort of in shock. I squeeze the mothers titties & put the gun to her daughters head. I tell the mother to do what I say, or I'll kill your daughter. She starts saying, PLEASE, yes, I'll do what you say, please dont hurt my daughter.

The mother was 43 years old, & not a bad looking woman. She had a nice figure. Her hair was in a frizzy style.

Her daughter was 17 years old & everything was perfect on her. She had the real long straight coal black hair & an hour glass body. She was the one I was focusing on, however, the mother got caught up in it. And I had to get the Mother also.

So I wanted to get them out of my truck so I could have more room to do what I wanted with them. I made them get out, & lay down on the ground face down. Then I got rope, tied the Mothers feet together & then the daughters feet. I then uncuffed them & tied their hands behind their backs. I then rolled the Mother over, & took out my pocket knife, & began cutting all her clothes off, turned to her daughter, I haven't messed with the daughter yet. In my own mind, I'm <u>SAVING</u> her. The mother is constantly begging me <u>NOT</u> to hurt her daughter. I have all her clothes off, & what really surprised me was the Mother didnt have <u>ANY</u> pubic hairs. And she didnt shave them, they just weren't there. I began rubbing her pussy, & felt a string protruding from her hole, & I pulled it & I pulled a TAMPON she had in her out. It was bloody from her period, so I took the tampon & forced open the daughters' mouth & shoved it in. And the mother screamed, NO leave her Lone. I then took the mother & sat her up beside my truck so she could watch, & I then focused my attentions on her daughter. I began cutting off her clothes, & the Mother became really belligerent, yelling at me & all, when I had all the daughters clothes cut off, I viewed her body. She was flat chested. She just had nipples where her titties were. She had the softest body, & she had the perfect slit for a pussy. And she really had <u>THIN</u> pubic hairs, maybe a dozen total. She was also a virgin. I then pulled down my pants, & exposed my dick to her, & the mother really was yelling, screaming, & just being <u>LOUD</u>, & she was so loud I was afraid even out there someone would hear her, I walked over & ordered her to shut up, & even slapped her, but she was out of control, & what I did next was more or less a reaction. I grabbed her by the hair, & pulled her down to the ground, face down, & she was kicking & hysterical so I put my knee on her back, grabbed her by her hair, to hold her head, & put the barrel of my gun to the back of her head & shot her, & killed her instantly. I rolled her over, put the barrel right between her eyes & shot her again to make sure she was dead. I put my knee in her head. She was kicking. I put the gun next to her head & shot her. In the back of the head. I think she died instantly. I went & did it again, just to be sure, between her eyes. This was to make sure she was dead, I guess.

I looked over at the daughter & she was like paralyzed with shock. She just was staring blankly. I cut the ropes lose from the Mother, grabbed her arm, & pulled her lifeless body over next to the daughters. I rolled her over on her stomach, & then got straddled on her back & pulled her head up by her hair, &

took my knife & sliced her throat open so she would bleed & I'll explain the purpose of this later. Even though she was dead, the cutting of her throat had a purpose.

When I did this Jenny, I stood up, & looked down at the dead Mother, & every bit of emotion drained out of me. I was paralyzed with this emptiness.

All of a sudden I realized that I had just done something that separated me from the human race, & it was something that could <u>NEVER</u> be undone. I realized that from that point on, I could <u>NEVER</u> be like Normal people.

I must have stood there in this state for 20 minutes. I have never felt an emptiness of self like I did right then & I will <u>NEVER</u> forget that feeling. It was like I <u>CROSSED</u> over into a realm I could never come back from. I literally could not move or function Jenny, that's how much I was affected.

But there after about 20 minutes, it was like I began getting some feeling back. I kept looking at the dead Mother asking myself, what have I just done. She's dead, I can't undo that. Then there came a point when I said to myself I might as well go forward with this cause I can <u>NEVER</u> go back. And when this realization set in, it was like I began to function. And I then bent down beside the daughter which all that time just laid there in shock. I Began sucking on her nipples, I stuck a finger up into her pussy, but I could NOT get a hard-on to rape her. What I had just experienced took that out of me I guess. I tried, but I could not get hard, even though I <u>WANTED</u> this girl. The desire & thirst to destroy her was still in me. I then wanted to get rid of the body of the Mother, & I wanted to <u>KEEP</u> the daughter alive until at some point I could rape her. I took the panties I'd cut off her & stuffed them into her mouth & put strips of duct tape over her mouth. I then set all the tools out of the big tool box I had on the back of my truck & I managed to put her into the tool box, & close & lock the lid. I drug the mother over to a spot, & the first thing I did was cut her head off. I put her head in a plastic garbage bag, tied it, & set it in the truck. Then I cut both of her titties off, & put them in a bag, & put them in the truck with the head. I split open her chest down to her pussy, & removed all her intestines & stomach. Then I cut her liver, heart & lungs out. I cut her hands off, then her arms, I cut her feet off, & then her legs at her knees & then I dug holes & buried all her body parts.

Then I got in my truck & headed to my house. Now Donna & me were still married at this time, but she had gone out of town with her Mother. We were having a LOT of problems, & were right on the verge of divorce. When I got to my house I pulled around back & up to the back door. I could get the daughter out & into my house with no one seeing me. I drug her into my bedroom, & I put her up on my bed. I then went around & closed all the curtains in my house & put towels up where there might be the chance of someone looking in. I then got the bag with her mothers' head in it, & brought it & the bag with her breasts in & put them in the kitchen sink. I tipped the daughter next spread eagle on my bed, I tied each hand to each bed post, & her ankles I tied to each bed post at the foot of the bed. We had a Polaroid camera in the closet, so I got it & took several pictures of her.

I sat down & began rubbing her body, & stroking her hair, & fingering her pussy. I pinched her nipple & she winced at that. She still would not say a word. She acted more traumatized. I still wasnt able to get a hard-on, so I left her like that, & went into the kitchen, took the mothers head out of the bag & set it up on the counter. I got a couple knifes, & took the head & literally cut the scalp of hair off, & then I cut her ears off. I then cut her tongue out, & cut off her lips.

I put her hair, & took it into the bedroom & held her Mothers scalp up & let the daughter see it, & she just stared at it with a blank look. I put the scalp in a zip lock bag.

I have been told that the reason I cut the head up so much is this was my way of releasing my anger out in a destructive way.

I then put everything in a bag to be buried later. I took the breast I had cut off & just played with them, looked at them.

I then went in the living room, sat down & drank a beer, & I just sat there recuperating so to speak for probably 2 or 3 hours. During this time I was completely naked & I would play with my dick trying to get some sort of stimulation up. And after a hour or so, I started getting my stimulation back, & actually got really hard, so then I went in the bedroom, got a jar of Vaseline & smeared a gob over the head of my dick, & climbed up between her legs, & I began trying to insert the head into her pussy. Now I'm sort of **BIG** & she was so small & tight, but I managed to get the head started in, & then I just began forcing it in & ramming the head in & out & it was so tight. She winced from it hurting & was letting out moans of pain & tears were coming from her eyes, & I didnt really last long. She had begun to bleed from her being a virgin, & it was really slick with the blood & Vaseline smeared over the shaft. And so I cum immediately, & it filled her up.

I kept her tied up most of the night to my bed, & I fucked her several more times. At one point I forced my dick into her mouth & tried to get her to suck, but she wouldn't.

On into the morning, I knew I had to get rid of her & clean up. So I took a broom from my closet & used the handle & inserted it into her butt hole, & ass fucked her with the handle, & then I shoved it up into her pussy & fucked her with the handle & at one point I left the handle protruding from her pussy & took a photo of it.

I then got straddle her chest & wrapped my hands around her neck & I just squeezed hard & strangled her to death. It took several LONG minutes to kill her. She kicked against her ropes, & her eyes bulged out, & when she went limp, I tied a rope tightly around her neck. Then cut her loose, & grabbed her by one of her ankles & drug her body off my bed across the floor into my bathroom, where I put her body in my bathtub & I cut her throat so her blood could drain into the bathtub. I cut her head off, & cut her up the exact same way as I did her Mother. I got a bunch of garbage bags & put all her body parts in them, & took out & put into the tool box on my truck & then spent a couple hours cleaning the house up from ANY sign of what went on. I took all the parts out to one of my groves & buried them.

That day the husband call the Police & reported his Wife & daughter missing. And it was all on the news & all.

That was the first kill so to speak. And from that point on, it was like I kept going forward, & my aggression got worse. I began LEARNING how to abduct Women & get them unseen. I had now found a RELEASE for everything that had been building up inside me all this time. I would now turn my hate, bitterness on Women. I would use Women to VENT all my frustration on. I would literally hunt for opportunities to abduct & rape & kill. This would be my outlet.

And as time went on, & I actually got away with killing the Mother & daughter, that only bolstered my courage. I set out to perfect the abducting of Women.

In one of my groves I had a trailer & I turned this into my lair when I would bring my victims to destroy them. This trailer had a double bed in it, in which I attached eye holes at each corner so I could tie a girl, with her legs spread & bent backward up over there head to give me deep unobstructed penetration into her pussy.

I had a closet & dresser drawer where I kept an assortment of TOOLS I would use on a girl. One item was a rubber dildo I had purchased thru an underground source. This dildo was 18 inches long, & 2 3/4 inches in diameter. It was shaped exactly like a dick. This would become the "TOOL" I'd literally inflect as much pain on a girl I could. I would hurt them like I was hurting. It was during this time Donna left me, took our sons & vowed never to let me see them. This only fueled my hate. It became my conviction to abduct & kill. This would be the avenue I used to ease the hurt I was experiencing.

When Donna divorced me, I focused my attention on HER family.

I lived in sort of a zombie state during this time, I just existed. And always under my thoughts was the fact I had killed two Women & had gotten away. The knowledge that I could actually KILL was a reality to me. It make me dangerous. It was no longer something I <u>WONDERED</u> if I could actually do, or wonder what it would be like. I now knew it would be no trouble for me to <u>KILL</u> a Woman. All I had to focus on was being able to <u>GET</u> her without getting caught.

So this was the area & learned, "How to abduct a Woman." I studied different ideas of disguises. I determined that <u>HITCHHIKERS</u> would be the best & safest victims. All I had to do was drive around until I found a girl by herself hitchhiking. I fixed my truck so once a girl go inside the door handle would <u>NOT</u> work so she could jump out. This was one area where I would get Victims. Another area was on the beach since I lived on the beach. Up & down the coast was many <u>PRIVATE</u> beaches, that were totally secluded. During the week days when the husband would go to work, Wives would take off & go to the beach for a couple hours, by themselves. They liked going to these secluded beaches away form people. And these secluded beaches became one of my favorite hunting grounds. I would simply drive up & down, pulling into these secluded beaches, & if I saw a car parked there, I would step up to the dune & see <u>WHO</u> was on the beach & if it was a Woman by herself, I would plan her abduction. What I would do was I'd either disable her car by flattening one of her tires, or opening her hood & doing something to the engine where it wouldn't start. Then I'd pull down away from the beach where she was at, & watch her through binoculars. When I saw her gather her things & start to leave, I'd give her a few minutes to get to her car & realize her predictament, then I would come driving up, as if to go to the beach, & I'd notice her predictament & offer to help, & they would always ask me to help. Then It was just a matter of waiting for the moment to pull my gun on her, force her into my car & take off with her.

Another disguise I used was driving around until I found a Woman at home alone, & approaching her door with a number of ruse's that would cause her to open her door to me. Once she did I would pull my gun on her & abduct her.

Sometimes I would inter mix these throughout the day. I'd drive the beaches then into country areas, then along the highway to look for hitchhikers. 99% of my hunting was done during work hours during the week. When a person is in the state of mind I was in Jenny, you feel like it's the , "Other" persons fault that causes you to these despicable things. In my case, what Donna was doing to me caused me to do what I am, therefore in my mind I was justifying my actions. Therefore to plan out an abduction with precision all was in my mind justified. I saw what was being done to me just as equally wrong as what I was doing. & You really lose a sense of reality. You live in your own little world, with & us against them, attitude.

I created my own World, & I became totally obsessed with abducting

Woman, taking them to my "Lair" & destroying them. I thought about this every waking moment, I couldnt go anywhere, where I didnt <u>LOOK</u> for an opportunity to strike. I would go to bed at night reviewing thoughts thru my mind of possible targets I could grab. Or I would see a Woman during the course of the day, & at night I'd lay in bed forming a Plan to abduct her.

It came to the point I was consumed with this & it controlled Me. I'd go out to the groves early & get the crew started on their daily jobs, & I'd put a man in charge & by 9:00 AM I would take off on my hunt for a Victim. I'd hunt till 4:00 or 5:00, go back to the grove to knock everyone off for the day then I'd go home. If during the course of the day I did abduct a woman, I took her to my "Lair" & "Do" her, & by that evening she was dead & disposed of. For practically day in & day out this was my existence. It came to the point that <u>EVERY</u> Woman I met or came across was a <u>POTENTIAL</u> target for me. This included members of family, etc. I was totally possessed by this.

Jenny, I'm giving you a LOT of my past, <u>BEFORE</u> I changed, & I'm trying to give it to you as events happened. I will go into what changed my life when I reach that point. This way you can pretty Well follow my life as it happened.

When Donna left & took our Sons, Life as I knew it pretty much ended. I was hurting emotionally more than you can imagine, & I had NO release for it, except........

I <u>NEVER</u> targeted children, I didnt see kids as a <u>SOURCE</u> of why I was hurting. Children always held that soft spot in my heart, & probably because of my own sons. I focused my aggression on just Women in general.

All thru my life I had these sexual tendencies, & they were always enhanced when ever I was around Freddy which was a <u>LOT</u>. We spent hours upon hours talking about how it would be to rape a girl, & we'd fantasize together. So when I say these fantasizes were in me before this is what I meant.

When Freddy & I were teen-agers, we raped or attempted to rape his two Sisters. One was the same age as me her name was Connie. The other was several years younger & her name was Debbie. Freddy told my to take Debbie into another bedroom & keep her there while he "FUCKED" Connie, will I heard Connie saying NO Freddy what are you doing, <u>STOP</u> it. And I could tell he was forcing her. I held Debbie & tried to slide my hand down into her pants, & feel her, & she would keep pushing me hand away.

Then Freddy & Connie came out of the bedroom & Connie was really crying & holding her stomach. She kept asking Freddy WHY Freddy? They both left & for some reason they <u>NEVER</u> told anyone what we did. Freddy said he didnt penetrate Connie, I dont know. But today they get along fine. I guess they have forgotten the incident.

So there were <u>EARLY</u> seeds being planted in both me & Freddy.

So I guess if you add fuel to already smoldering embers a fire erupts.

Right now, I'm studying a process that has to do with Generational Curses in the spiritual realm. You see this all thru the Bible & God has spoken of this on many occasions. Anyway, this is food for thought, for later on. ☺

When I was finally arrested, I was at life's end. I heard the State was going to seek the death penalty on me, & I was actually relieved & glad. I knew this pain would be over. The day I was arrested, I had every intention of walking out of my house & dropping my hands which would force the cops that were surrounding my house to shoot me. I had made my mind up, & I called out & said I was coming out, & all the Police took positions & began aiming & cocking these guns at the door. As I came out with my hands, raised, I <u>TRIED</u> to drop my hands, but I couldnt. Jenny, I <u>FELT</u> someone holding my wrist, & I thought it was a Cop who had come up behind me, but when I looked around no one was there, & I couldnt pull my hands down, I <u>FELT</u> the pressure from "SOMEONE" holding my hands up so I couldnt drop them. Just as the cops rushed & took hold of me, I felt this pressure let go. For Months I never thought about that incident. It was only much later that I came to believe that on that day, there was an <u>ANGEL</u> behind me holding my hands.

You see just two days before this I had come to a spiritual crisis in my life, & I got down on my knees beside my bed, & <u>BEGGED</u> God for help. I couldnt take it any more. I had no where else to turn to.

So the "ANGEL" that prevented me from dropping my hands was just the first of many events to come that transformed my life. Although I didnt know it, God was answering my prayer. The next event that took place was several days after my arrest, they had a couple of Chaplain coming in to show a film called "God's Prison Gang" & they asked if I wanted to attend. I thought this was a good way to get out of my cell for a little while so I went. There were about 40 men in the room, & they began showing the film, & it was dark, & one of the evangelist started walking back through everyone, & I watched him. He walked up to me, leaned down & asked if he could tell me something. I said, sure. He said, "God just spoke to me, & told me to tell you he has you here for a purpose."

This blew my mind. I said thank you & he walked off. I couldnt believe it. I asked myself, <u>WHY</u> could God tell **ME** this, out of all the men here, why did he single <u>me</u> out. If he (God) knew what I'd done he wouldn't say that. Well that began a conviction in my heart, & a spiritual journey for me. Finally one day I called this Evangelist up & asked him <u>Why</u> did he tell <u>me</u> that. He said he'd come talk to me. He came & we met in a room & he began telling me how God had spoken to him about me, & that God had a plan for my life, but first he had to bring me to a point where I would have no one to look to but <u>GOD</u>.

Well this began a real conviction in me & I began crying & I asked him how could I do right, surely God couldnt want me after what I've done.

Then Jenny, he placed his hand on my head & began praying, & Jenny, I felt this warm ooze come over me. I felt just like someone poured oil over me, & I FELT something happen to me, & I asked God to forgive me for everything I'd done, & asked him to take control of my life, & tears flowed down my face, & Jenny when it was over, I WAS a new person. I felt like someone had lifted 2,000 pounds off my shoulders. I got back to my cell & I couldnt get enough of the Bible. I read constantly. I told everyone who would listen what happen to me. That began my spiritual walk with God that continues to this day. I have grown in SO many areas over the years. I still write to that evangelist & over the years we have become as close as brothers. He has been my mentor so to speak. I truly thank God for him.

One of my favorite scripture verses is II Corinthians 5:17. I don't dwell on the past, & when I do talk about it, it is only so people can under stand what was going on in my life back then. I have regretted my actions immensely.

I know I jumped ahead on this, but I wanted to give you an overall perspective on everything. So much has happened in my life. I lot of bad, a lot of good.

Please take care of yourself, & I hope to hear from you real soon. May God truly bless you. You are very much in my thoughts.

Always
David

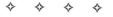

6-24-97

Dear Jenny

Hi. I sure hope & pray this letter finds you well & in the very best of spirits. As for myself, I am doing really good. I received your most wonderful letter & as always it was really good to hear from you. Your letters are really great. And I do look forward to them.

Yes, I would have to say that Donna & myself did have some sexual problems, along with others. And the pain of rejection is something that is really hard. That was a time in my life that I seemed to have no control over.

I saw advertisements for the movie Con-Air, & it seemed quite exciting.

You know Jenny you said something in your letter that really hits to the core as to why a serial killer can KEEP killing. Because they look & seem SO normal. And this is the portrait they want people to see.

When I was abducting & killing, I could change to fit into any circumstance. The FIRST goal of a serial killer is to, get his or her intended victim to drop their guard, & be caught unaware. This is why the "COP" disguise was so effective. When I approached a Woman as a cop, They just assumed they were safe, because I was a cop. They would let me right into their house, & once I was inside, they had no chance. The majority of my Victims I got were right inside their home.

This is why I am so adamant now to <u>WARN</u> people to not trust even someone they think is a cop. If a man comes to your door & says he's a cop, DO <u>NOT</u> let him in. Tell him you wish to call the Police station for verification. A REAL cop, will not have a problem with this. If someone would have told me that, I would have got away as quickly as possible. People can't be trusted like they use to. We live in such a violent World. And then there are the disguise of Repairmen & such. You see these are disguises of <u>NORMAL</u> people.

The main goal of a serial killer is to <u>NOT</u> bring attention to himself. To FIT-IN.

You were asking about how you maybe should feel more frightened. You know Jenny, you should feel frightened, but not so much from the men in prison. But just of every day people around you. These are serial killers who are still walking our streets.

But it's who I tell people I write, the best Defense is plain ole Common Sense. Don't put yourself in a situation where you could be hurt. If you walk out to your car at night in some shopping center, <u>KNOW</u> who's around you. Look at the cars parked around your car, is there anyone sitting in them. If so, just keep your eye on them. I dont know what sort of serial killers you have been in contact with, but I will be the first to admit, these are killers who I would <u>NEVER</u> want to see out on the streets.

Most people don't think They could ever be abducted or raped. I dont mean anything by this, but when I was out & I was abducting Women. I pretty much could get who ever I wanted. It may take me several attempts. If I saw a Woman I wanted, I just waited for the perfect opportunity. I abducted a Dental assistant one time right out of her office in the middle of the day in a crowded shopping center. I saw her, wanted her, so I set up a plan to grab her, & I got her. I watched her for several days, & at 12:00 Noon Every day, the Dentist would leave for lunch, & the assistant would go to a deli near by, & she would always return about 15 minutes till 1:00. The Dentist came back at 1:30 just like clock work. So I simply waited until she came back. Walked in under the pretense I needed some dental work done, pulled a gun on her, made her walk arm & arm outside to my car parked right in front of the door, & took off with her. What I'm trying to express, is Serial killers dont just strike in dark alleys or on secluded streets. I spend a <u>LOT</u> of time now days clueing people in on the kinds of dangers there are. If I can keep one person from being a Victim, that's great.

Well Jenny, let me close this for now, so I can get it into the mail today. I'll start you another letter. So please take care of yourself, & May God Bless You.

Always
David

✧ ✧ ✧ ✧

7-10-97

Dear Jenny,

While a lot of people will cry & scream how they didnt do anything wrong, I have never done that: I've faced my demons, actions, & I am certainly not proud of anything, but maybe something CAN be learned from this. There was a time when I liked hurting women — people ask the same question, "if you hated Donna so much for moving why not just kill her?" Yet, in my own reasoning, I couldnt, because she was my children's mother, & I couldnt take her away when they would be needing her, so I channeled that hate everywhere but where it belonged. I once killed a mother, I didnt know it until the abduction was a done deal. She pleaded with me, but she'd already seen me. She begged that I would just let her go after I had raped her & tortured her some, because she had a baby to go home to. If I would have known, I never would have taken her to start with. Yes, I would have to say that Donna & myself did have some sexual problems, along with others, the pain of rejection is something that is really hard. I seemed to have NO control over it. You said something in your last letter that hit to the core, about why a serial killer can <u>KEEP</u> killing because they look & seem so normal — this is the portrait they want people to see; when I was abducting & killing, I could change to fit into any circumstance. The <u>FIRST</u> goal of the serial killer is to catch his intended victim off guard. This is why the COP disguise was so affective. I am <u>SO</u> adamant now to WARN people to not trust even someone they think is a cop. If a man come to your door & says he's a cop, call — a <u>REAL</u> cop will not have a problem with this, & then there are the disguises of repairmen & such. These are disguises of <u>NORMAL</u> people. The main goal of a serial killer is to not bring attention to himself, but to FIT IN. Jenny, you should feel frightened, but not so much from the men in prison, but just of everyday people around you, still walking our streets, & the best <u>DEFENSE</u> is common sense. Dont put yourself in a situation where you could be hurt. I dont know what serial killers you have in your book, but there are those who I would <u>NEVER</u> want to see on the streets!

Sincerely, David

7-21-97

Dear Jenny,

Hi. I sure hope this letter will find you well & in the best of spirits. As for myself, I am doing fine. Please forgive me for the delay in responding, I had to wait until I could get a couple stamps. My mom normally sends me postage stamps, however, my Dad went into the hospital for major surgery a couple weeks ago, & it has really taken a toll on them financially. So for right now, I really have to be conservative with my stamps.

Things here are pretty much the same. It has been unbearably hot. And these cells are <u>NOT</u> Air Conditioned, which is contrary to what much of society believes.

Thank you for your nice comment as to me being a teacher. Telling people about that I caused the death of a person is not easy. But I know that through what I've gone through, I may be of help to someone else. You asked about actual facts about me & Fred. I'll go through my legal work, & I have a lot of papers with all my actual charges, Fred's charges etc. And I can send those to you.

You know Jenny, I am free from the past in the sense I dont have that demon in me that caused me to abduct & kill. But when I was out & doing these things, its what I lived for. Every thing I did, focused on my "NEXT" victim. You get to a point where it literally consumes your life. I looked for potential victims where ever I went. Many times I would be just simply driving up town & I'd pass a car on the road with a woman by herself in it, & I'd turn & follow her to see where she went. And if she drove to some place secluded, she became a target.

Serial killers will <u>ALWAYS</u> be on the look-out for a victim. A lot of times they will display the actions by stalking, or following a girl in a car, or driving up & down streets. You know, Jenny, I hear so much about Serial Killers, & the reason they kill is for the POWER they feel. But to be completely honest, I NEVER once felt that type of power. I didnt kill to feel any power. I'll be honest, I killed in order to destroy women. I mutilated their bodies so much.

It was more of a destruction thing. I was hurting, & I felt the reason for my hurt was a woman so women became the object of my rage. And I was meticulous. I would actually <u>STUDY</u> ways to abduct women. I just believe the different reasons & why of serial killers vary from one to another. But I believe the <u>BASE</u> & <u>ROOT</u> cause they kill is <u>ANGER</u>. And they turn that anger on other people. Anger is a very destructive force. I was doing what I did, then I began the process of dealing with it, & getting rid of what was going on in me. And I really believe there is only <u>ONE</u> way a person can truly be released & that is through GOD. God is the only way. I've written to a lot of people who have had the exact kind of anger & rage in them, & they would vent it out in different ways. I also believe another strong motive I had for abducting women was sexual. And I dont mean sexual in the NORMAL sense. The very first thing I would do once I had control of a woman was to get her clothes off. I would NOT just KILL a woman. I mean, I wouldn't just see one & shoot her & then leave her. To me that was a waste. I <u>HAD</u> to get them in a way I could <u>HAVE</u> their body & could do things to it. I had a friend ask me to <u>KILL</u> his sister once. He wanted to get rid of her so he could have all of his family inheritance. She was in her 20's. And I thought this was the easiest one I'd ever get. He was going to actually bring her to my house, so I could kill her. He wasnt able to actually kill her himself. So I agreed to do it. I told him once he brought her to the house, I would grab her, tie her up, & then he would leave. But he decided not to do it. But those were the opportunities I looked for.

Well Jenny, let me close this & get it in the mail to you. I'll get together some legal papers with dates & all on them & send to you.

Please take care of yourself, & know you are in my thoughts & prayers.

God Bless You
David

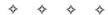

the desire & thirst to destroy her was still
in me. I then wanted to get rid of
the body of the Mother, & I wanted to
keep the daughter alive until at some point
I could rape her. So I took the
panties I'd cut off her & stuffed them into
her mouth & put strips of duct tape
over her mouth. I then set all the
tools out of the big tool box I had on
the back of my truck & I managed to
put her into this tool box, & close & lock
the led. Then I drug the Mother over
to a spot, & the first thing I did was
cut her head off. I put her head in a
plastic garbage bag, tied it, & set it
in the truck. I then cut both of her
titties off, & put them in a bag, & put
in the truck with the head. I then split
her open from her chest down to her pussy,
& removed all her intestine & stomach.
I then cut her liver, heart & lungs out.
I cut her hands off, then her arms, I
cut her feet off, & then her legs at her knees
& then I dug holes & buried all her body
parts.
       I then got in my truck & headed to

A page from one of David Gore's letters.

Jeff Libby

W hat a strange guy, Jeff Libby. Most people who have been accused of murder either insist they are innocent or they admit their guilt. Jeff Libby, on the other hand, claims responsibility for crimes that he has never been accused of and for which there is no evidence indicating that they even occurred. And not only does Libby claim to be a killer, he claims to be a serial killer.

The only murder that Libby has been convicted of, and to which he readily admits, is that of his grandfather, who he drowned in a bathtub 25 years ago. Libby says he killed his grandfather because he was a selfish, arrogant and abusive drunk. If, as others claim, Libby hoped to collect on his grandfather's life insurance policy, he killed him in vain for he never saw a penny. Libby says the reason he was never convicted of the other murders he lays claim to is because he was so careful and methodical that he never left a clue and no one was ever able to catch him. Libby proudly claims that he raped, tortured and killed 12 prostitutes — slit their throats, tied them to trees and went on his way.

Libby says that he started hating women after he witnessed his favorite uncle's death in the electric chair. Apparently, Libby focused all of his anger on a woman he didn't even know and with whom he had no personal involvement — the "sadistic female warden" who pulled the switch on his favorite uncle. Apparently, he believed that this warden was responsible for the execution and from that moment on, he decided that it was his calling in life to get back at all women (although whether he actually killed is unknown).

As soon as Libby discovered that I was corresponding with Harvy Carignan, he became interested — obsessed is a better word — in one thing only: establishing, through me, a relationship with Carignan. Libby claimed that he needed desperately to correspond with Carignan because he wanted to share his feelings about murdering young girls with someone who could understand where he was coming from and who enjoyed this activity as much as he did. Furthermore, he said he would only discuss the details of his crimes with me if I could persuade Carignan to respond to him. But it was Libby's hammering obsession with getting Carignan to discuss only one particular crime — his involvement in the death of a young girl named Kathy Sue Miller — that made it increasingly clear to me that Libby had an ulterior motive. I find it hard to believe that Libby didn't realize how pitifully transparent his pleadings were. It was so obvious that he wasn't as interested as he claimed in discussing the fine art of murder with Carignan as he was in trying to coax an admission of guilt out of him for the death of "the Miller girl." Although Carignan refused to correspond with him, Libby claims in his last letter to me that he did in fact "accomplish his purpose."

He also added cryptically that everything he had written in his letters to me was "false and fictionalized." Despite this statement, because lies and deception come so easily to Libby, perhaps his boasts are true — that he really is "just a classic serial killer" who "loves the high" he gets from killing. Whatever the case may be, Jeff Libby is serving a life sentence at Mansfield State Prison in Maine for murdering his grandfather.

The Libby Letters

Dear Jenny,

    I'm in reciept of your typewritten letter, which I got in the mail on 3-21-97. I just returned from a court hearing yesterday and so I am writing to you today. I assume that Harvey [Carignan] sent my letter to you and that this is how you have become aware of me and my crimes. I have no problem corrosponding with you, but I would like for Harvey to reply to the letter I sent to him. The reason I wrote Harvey is because I think we both have alot in common. I'm particularly interested about that 15 year old girl Kathy Miller Harvey wasted, because of the 13 year old I spoke of in my letter to Harvey. I say that because I have more to tell Harvey about what happened to the 13 year old who by the way was a prostitute. Tell Harvey to write me right away. I've known other prisoners to send their letters to people on the street, who in turn send them to other prisoners, but thats between you and Harvey. You could even read my letter to Harvey over the phone. If you choose to do this, thats up to you. I am fascinated about Harvey and this Miller girl and that nearly 20 years has passed and the law can't trace the killer. My case is simular in that so many years has passed in the murders I am suspected of, including the 13 year old girl. Its a rush knowing that the law can't close in for the bust in my cases, they never will figure it out. This is what I want to know from Harvey, (How he feels about never being caught for the killing of the Miller girl). I'm just a classic serial killer, I love the high it gives me. I have a deep passion for hot sexy sassy woman. I'm not going to really open up to you in my letters until I hear from Harvey. I did alot of murder for hire jobs, for people who had money also. The woman I wasted were really into sex and loved money as did I. There were moments during some of the murders that threw me on such a high at times, that I became addicted to all the morbid acts involved. Anyway, I sit here in my world of concrete and steele, empty of passion, compassion, friendship, love and privacy, relishing the taste of freedom each passing day. Your question to me about the tourture I inflicted upon my victims is one that calls for a very long and detailed answer and I am willing to comply with your request and to

dignify your question with an answer, but I first must hear from Harvey. I can
tell you however, that I did all my killing at night, and I convinced all my
victims to have sex voluntarily first before I engaged in forceful acts, which
would ultimately result in their demise, but there was alot that happened in
between the time I became forceful and brutal and the time my victims died.
There was much, much more that transpired than just cutting their throats and
tying my victims to trees, in fact I will tell you that in 3 of the murders, I
partially disected my victims in a way, if told to you in vivid detail, would
make your stomach turn. Other kinds of torture took place during sex acts,
(E.C.T.). Like I said, I want to tell you every detail, because it would be healthy
for me to disclose my inner feelings about my victims but I first must recieve a
reply to my letter, from Harvey, so if you would, get this message to him right
away, so we can corrospond in horrifying detail about my past acts. If you
would, send a picture of yourself and $15.00 for stamps so I can write you two
or three times a week. As I mention in the beggining of this letter, I just got
back from court. I had to go to probate court, because some of my relatives are
contesting my great grandmothers will, due to the fact that she left me a
substantial amount of money. Due to probate proceedings, it could take another
7 months before I see a penny. Any funds you send me I will of coarse
reimburse you for. I hope this can be the start of a long healthy relationship and
will look forward to your next letter. For now, peace & love,

Yours
Jeff

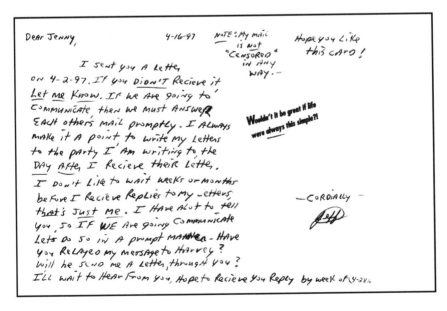

Dear Jenny,

Sorry I could not respond to your latest letter, but we had an incident last week. An inmate made a homemade shank out of his "pen" so they locked us down for a week and took away our pens. We just got them back 2 hours ago and so here I am responding to your letter. You mentioned "honesty" in your letter. Well, I may be alot of things, but I do not lie. I see no point in lying because deception does not appeal to me. I did not mention the family member I killed, because you never asked. I killed my grandfather, he was a despicable man, he was a gambler, spendthrift alcoholic who abused his wife and his grand children, who was careless in his person and his friendships, selfish and arrogant. I drowned him in his bathtub, then took his body out of the bathtub stripped and layed him face up in the tub. You would not believe some of the nightmares that occurred when he was alive. I will talk about this in more detail in my future letters. Did you tell Harvey to write me about that Karen Miller? I have alot of things to tell you about the 13 year old I killed, that perhaps was my worse crime but I must hear from Harvey first before I tell you the horrible details of her death at my hands. I have reoccurring nightmares of what happened that night in a secluded wooded area. I did not think, that as a human being I was capable of such an act. You told me that if I did not hear from Harvey, that I was to let you know. I have not heard from him. Make sure to send him a copy of my letters or tell him the contents of my letters to you. I want to tell you how it felt to take all those womans lives and why I wanted to, but as I told you I have to feel comfortable in doing this and so, again, I ask you to tell Harvey to write me telling me how he felt taking Karen Millers life. I am anxious to see, if he felt the same way about killing that 15 year old as I did killing the 13 year old. So be sure to tell Harvey to include these details in his letter to me, then I will open up to you and tell you everything, but I must hear from Harvey first to know in my mind that all three of us can communicate openly and freely about our feelings. I hope you understand this. Now, what I want to tell you in this letter is chilling, but it has alot to do as to why I set out on a killing spree although its not 100% of the reason why I set out to kill these woman and the 13 yr old. A few years after my sister Leann died from an overdose of speed, my uncle was arrested for her death because he had confessed to selling her the drug that killed her. I knew it was all a mistake that it was my sisters choice to do drugs, my uncle was not at fault for her death, but a court did not see it this way, they convicted him of first degree murder because of aggrivating circumstances, and they gave him the death penalty. I loved my uncle dearly, we were close, and I certainly did not want to see him executed. He lost all of his appeals. Before a handful of witnesses, myself included, my uncle was executed in the electric chair right before my eyes. I remember sitting in one of the witness boxes with my brother. We were completely seperated from any sounds or smells in the death chamber. My uncle was escorted into the death chamber, fully clothed, and shaved on his head. He made a final statement which was read off by the "female" warden a sadistic looking bitch known for her romatic affairs with some of the guards. She was a fucking hor in my mind. Anyway sitting there, looking though the glass partition into the death chamber, they secured his head, chest, arms and legs with leather straps, then a leatherette cap containing an electrode was placed tightly on his head. Other electrodes were affixed to his legs and calfs. Sponges dampened in a solution, saline solution were inserted between the electrodes and his skin. A black hood was then dropped over his head hiding his face. The prison guards then left the chamber. When this "female" warden pulled the switch sending all that voltage through my uncles body, I saw his hands turn red, then white and I saw the cords of his neck stand out like steele bands. The force of the electric current was so powerful that his eyeballs popped out on his cheeks. I saw this as they lifted the hood off his head after he was dead. My uncle deficated, urinated, and vomited blood and drool during the execution. I could not help but see my uncles gray face and blue lips as doctors lifted the hood to check his eyeballs which were sitting on his cheeks. When the doctor announced through the microphone that my uncle was dead, I remember storming out of the witness chamber in a furious manner. I wanted to kill the female warden that took my uncles life. Who the fuck was she to pull the switch, to kill my uncle? Well, anyway, 2 years later, I went on my killing spree. Although I loved hot sexy and sassy women, I now wanted it both ways, which was, to have sex, then to kill these woman while they begged for their lives, just like my uncle did when the "female" warden pulled the switch that would terminate his life, but there was also more reasons why I killed these woman, but I will reserve those details until I hear from Harvey. If you can, please send me a few dollars for mail money. Pursue Harvey, tell him to write. Will expect to hear from you week of 5/26.

Yours,
Jeff

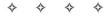

[Jeff Libby asked me to mail the following letter to Harvy Carignan.]

```
Harvey (What's up?)

     Saw your profile the other night. Pretty radical man! I'm serving
six (6) life sentences. I went on a killing spree in 1988, killed 12
women and a drug dealer, but so far, they have  only nailed me for (6)
murders. I expect they might try to charge  me with (2) more murders
soon. Maine doesn,  have the death penalty so I'm not too worried about
it,(Know what I mean?). I tortured my victims and made them beg for
life.I had a lot of sexual fantasies and fulfilled them all through my
victims. I picked up prostitutes mostly, and treated themlike the hors
they were before I cut their fucking throat. I tied my victims to trees
after I killed them. Most of the dead women were found a couple days or
so after I tied them up to a tree. I had no fucking mercy for my
victims. I saw that scumbag detective talking about you, saying you
deserved to die and that he wanted to drive a stake through your
heart. Hey, fuck that pig. I hate pig ass cops. I killed  two mother
fucking chicks in Connecticut in 1987, met them at a local bar. I got a
real rush killing those two because they put up a real struggle. They
went out with me to smoke a couple joints in a secluded wooded
area. After, we had sex and drank some booze. I asked them to go for a
walk with me. I used a tire iron to bash their heads in, then tied them
up to a tree. There was a lot of press on their murders, but it is still
ruled unsolved. I don't fuck  with to many people,I'm very selective
about who I associate with, can't stand to be around a lot of people. I
thought I would write you because I can definitely relate to your
situation. I know what it's like to exist in this world of concrete and
steel,which is empty of passion,love, friendship, and privacy. I'm (58)
years old, will be fifty-nine next month. I'm tatooed from head to
toe. I used to run with the Outlaw Motorcycle Gang up and down lthe east
coast. Sold a lot of drugs in the Florida Everglades.I miss all the
action. Anyway, I think we might have a lot of shit in common. Serving
time in Alcatraz must have been a rush. I did a couple of murder for
hire jobs, but I always did them with someone else. I remember reading
about that  (15) year old girl, Karen Miller, who waskilled in
```

Seattle.She must have been a slut. Did she put up a struggle? Did you
get some of that tight pussy before you killed her ass? I hope so, I
would have. To me, if a girl looks older than her age, she is eligible
for my list. How did you kill that bitch anyway? Think she knew you were
going to waste her? Bet she had a sweet little ass.I had a 13 year old
give me oral sex before. It was the best experience of my life. Well,
listen, when I hear from you I'll write you back. Tell you some wild
shit. Hope we can write to each other,getsboring sitting around all
day. My great grandmother died six months ago.Left me a lot of money. If
you need a few bucks, just let me know in your letter. Stay strong
Dude.

                          Later,

                          s/Jeff

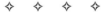

*[The following letter was written to me by Harvy Carignan in response to Jeff
Libby's letter (above) to him.]*

Dear Jenny,

Jeff Libby is a study unto himself! I suppose I could write concerned he is
human egesta. His spoliating defers whatever possibilities there were for my
writing to him. I am amused. He is idiotically making assumptions, the most
egregious of which is that I am not sure whether or not I was with Kathy Miller:
I was not with her, not ever, and I talked with her only twice over the telephone.
His second mistake is believing that I would ever so denigrate myself to a
lowness from which I could correspond with him and on his level. He is a liar
of no little magnitude and such a stool pigeon he is lucky to be alive. He is the
most hated person in Thomaston. He pretends to have committed crimes, and
asks others to exchange notes about their crimes with him. He confesses to non-
existent murders; then, when someone is gullible enough to tell him anything,
he goes to the police, offers to testify for a time cut off of his sentence, a first
degree murder conviction for killing his grandfather in a bathtub for the
insurance money. Him suggesting that you and he must influence me to admit
having murdered Kathy Miller is nothing short of hilarious and him failing to

exercise prudent judgment or to display common sense. He is beyond silliness and what he is doing far surpasses ludicrousness. He is enamored with the idea that the SERIAL KILLER documentary was true — and it was less true than what Ann Rule, that bucolic witch, wrote! — Even an idiot such as he should discern its claims as absurd and incongruous as to be laughable. His lugubriousness magnifies his ludicrousness and exaggeration to where I find it more and more easy to doubt his sanity. Enough about what I could write about that cretin. Just let me say I pity him and he is mistaken, so misled. Now he is being misused. The letter's not so silent desperation convinces me that it was not he himself who wrote it. It is obviously the work of one or another kind of police person. Jeff Libby is too stupid to be so subtle or to portray such a sublime scheme as you and he getting me to confess a crime. What I wonder is where whoever wrote the letter got the idea that I am not sure about whether or not I was with that young lady. I am sure I was not with her, not ever. Never was I any closer to her than the distance between my telephone and the one she used to call me. Use his letters if you will, but I suggest you write it is evident a police person is involved with him in this exploration for what they deem truth! What an imbecilic show of unconcern the writer has of our joint intelligence! If only they knew what I have to fall back upon. When the Seattle news media and Police Department were "coming down" on me hard and heavy I decided I needed an attorney who would come to the county jail night or day, weekend or holiday, if I was arrested. I never was. The first lawyers I went to had done some legal work for Miller's mother and to represent me would have constituted a conflict of interest. The second lawyer refused emphatically to touch the case as it being "too political". The third made me submit to a lie detector test before he would represent me. The person who gave the test was an ex-police officer for the Seattle Police Department. He assured me after three four-hour sessions that there was "no way you could have committed this murder".

✧   ✧   ✧   ✧

6-4-97

Dear Jenny,

Got your letter on (5-23-97), it sent me into such a rage that I hit my cell wall several times with my fists, I busted 3 knuckles. A guard caught me punching my cell wall, and they put me on observation watch, I just came off and was brought back to my cell 20 minutes ago. What made me furious about your letter was the second line in where you say ("He denies guilt about the Miller girl.") I've been wanting to tell someone for years what I did to the 13 year old, but it had to be someone I could relate too, I thought that person would be Harvey, and then ultimately you, but I'm not so sure anymore. Harvey seems to be my class of people, but for whatever reason, he wants to deny guilt about the Miller girl. I thought me you and Harvey were going to be "honest" with each other. Do you realize what all three of us can accomplish if we are honest with each other? Tell Harvey that I was counting on his honesty to get me through my nightmarish haunting from the 13 year old I killed. She haunts me all the time, and you and Harvey can never know exactly why she haunts me until I tell you and Harvey. I need this clensing process, I need to get all this off my chest, but I've got to feel Harvey is being honest. By denying guilt in killing the Miller girl, makes me feel I can't relate to Harvey. If only he would be honest and open up to me about the Miller girl, so I could feel his rage, his fantasy, his desire to kill as he did, then I would open up to you and Harvey, the line of communication would be open with no limit. You and Harvey would be able to extract things inside me that are so deep inside me, that what you discovered would probably wake you up at night in nightmares. Tell Harvey to write me, he has not written. I need to hear from him, not just you, so me and Harvey can open right up to each other and so I can open up to you and give you what you need. Believe me Jenny, you have no idea how badly I want to open up about the 13 year old girl, what I did to her physically and sexually is beyond imagination, but I guess what I am trying to say is that I need to hear another serial killers same experience such as Harvey killing the Miller girl. I have to feel what he felt during the killing, this will trigger me to open up to you as you want. Sometimes human beings cannot put down on paper exactly what they mean to say, sometimes it needs to be communicated by verbal translation, so if you would, send me your phone number, so I can call you in July. We are on this fucking stupid computerized phone system and I have to submit the new numbers I want to add to my phone request slip by June 24, 1997, so I can call you in July, so send me your phone number, so I can feel included in your life and please send me a small picture of yourself so I can write to you and know in my mind the face I am communicating with, and finally, I wasn't kidding when I asked you to send me a few dollars so I can write you often.

We have to get this issue with Harvey resolved before we go any further. I know and he knows and I'm sure you know he wasted the Miller girl, stress it upon him that I want us all (me, you and Harvey) to be a team, sort of like a mini mafia where only we know what goes on in each others heads, but in order to do this and to accomplish this, me and Harvey need to dig deep inside ourselfs and turn out all the truth, all the rage and horrid vivid details of our crimes. After all Jenny, thats what you want, and you should be as upset at Harvey as I am for not telling the truth about the Miller girl, once Harvey admits to killing the Miller girl as I have admitted to killing the 13 yr old girl, then we can move foward, then I will feel like we are sort of like family, divulging and disclosing our inner most secrets to each other, and as I said, this is what you want. People need to feel they are dealing with people who are sincere, honest and true when they release their deepest secret. This 13 year old girl I killed brutally is mine, just as I know in my heart that Harveys deepest secret is killing the Miller girl.

I hope you understand where I am coming from and I hope you will not give up on me for telling you what is in my heart. Please stay on Harvey to write me, and discuss the Miller girl with him and tell him to include the Miller girl in his letter.

Yours,
Jeff

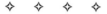

6-25-97

Dear Jen,

Yes, I am in alot of mental pain but I am doing fine. I read your letter several times and what caught my eye is where you say ("He still believes he isn't involved"). Jen, either he did it or he did not do it, there is no in between. I think this is the start of Harvey trying and wanting to open up about this Miller girl, and so, I feel we have to help him open up. I think he took a big step, in telling you ("honestly") that the Miller girl called the garage where he was working, the same day she disappeared, and that he went to pick her up that same day. Can't you see, Jenny? We are half way there, with having Harvey, tell you that much. Just between me and you Jenny, do you really think for a minute, that Harvey, (a serial killer), went to pick up the Miller girl the very same day she disappeared, for any other reason, than to rape and kill her to forfill his fantasy? Don't you find it odd, that this Miller girl was with Harvey on the same day she was killed? (I want you to ask Harvey if the Miller girls boyfriend actually saw Miller get into the car with Harvey). Whatever pressure Harvey is under, we must help him release that pressure and to open up about this murder. (I also want you to ask Harvey if he killed her "AGAIN"). I know you do not want to pressure Harvey or to press him, but there is no other way. We have to make him feel that he can open up to us, that all three of us are out to accomplish one thing, that being the "truth," so we can start communicating our deepest most buried secrets about each other. There must be a bond between us, so I can start telling you and Harvey about the 13 year old girl I killed and about other things you want to know, but first, we must pursue Harvey, you cannot settle for Harvey's answers about this Miller girl, you have to make it clear to him that before we go any further, we must resolve this.

When you say in your letter ("perhaps Mr. Carignan feels too much pressure to speak of something he is committed not to speak of"), thats exactly what I am talking about, thats just the kind of thing me and Harvey must communicate with you, things that we are not, have not been committed to talking about (i.e.) the Miller girl, the 13 year old I killed. We must be able to freely discuss these kinds of things, before we can accomplish what you want, ("the truth about everything we have done"). Talk to Harvey, send him a copy or discuss this letter, make sure you get answers to the two questions I asked you to ask him. If me or Harvey have reason why we are not comfortable or are in denial of something we did, we have to let that go, and begin the process telling our deepest secret. As I said in a previous letter, the 13 year old I killed is my deepest secret, just like I know the Miller girl is with Harvey. We have to get everything out on the table before we start to delve into ourselfs about other things.

I have every intention of telling you everything you and Harvey want to know, I need Harveys willingness to open up about the Miller murder before I can feel like we are bonded. Please send me a $10.00 postal money order. I even ran out of pen ink. I am allright, and will look foward to your next letter. I'm feeling closer + closer to you with each letter I recieve. I hope you will make it a top priority to pursue Harvey, be firm with him, sometimes thats what it takes to get a person to open up. (Send me picture of yourself and your new address you plan to move too).

Peace + Love
Jeff

7-16-97

Dear Jenny,

Got your letter Monday 7-14-97. I hope the things he will tell you will be about the Miller girl. Once we have Harvey open up about the Miller girl I will open up and tell you everything. I've already explained this to you in my previous letters, so I will not waste ink. Let this letter reflect for the record that I am giving you my full permission to incorporate any and all of my letters as you deem appropriate, into any publication of your choice, which may include any book you may decide to publish and/or write. I think you have a terrific goal in that you aim to paint us serial killers as human beings. Be sure to send me the money order and your photo right away. Also be sure to send me a copy of Harvey's letter to you, or all the contents of your conversation with him over the phone in your letter to me. I've got to get ready to go see the doctor to get an xray of my knuckles. Hope to recieve your letter by next week. By the way, your last letter to me, which is the letter I am responding to, made me feel a little better and more secure about our relationship, now only if Harvey opens up about the Miller girl we will have that special bond I talked about between the three of us.

Your Friend
Jeff

✧ ✧ ✧ ✧

DeAR JeNNy, 2-13-98

In Reciept of your most Recent Letter. I thought it Appropriate to inForm you At this time that the inFormation I provided to you in my Letters was "FALSe" And I "FictioNALized" my Letters to you For the sole ReAsoN oF Extracting inCriminating inFormation on the "Miller" Murder. I Do Not wish to be in your book. Things Are being pursued through the WAShingtoN AttorNey GenerALs oFFice in connection to your Letters to me And your stated converSAtions with HArvey cAirigan Regarding the Miller Murder. I HAve Accomplished my purpose For this mAtter And things will now be in HANds oF WAshington AuthoritieS. Further, I Am FowArding A copy oF this Letter to the WAshingtoN AttorNey GenerAL For the Record. Any Further corrospondence you mAiL to me will ALso be turned over to Authorities. pLeAse ReFrAin From writing to me.

— SincereLy —
Jeff Lbty

(C.C.) WAshington (AG)
Files

Douglas Clark

ouglas Daniel Clark vehemently denies that he is the maniac responsible for the vicious murders of six pretty young prostitutes who worked on Los Angeles' infamous Sunset Strip. Clark's ex-lover, Carol Bundy, says he's the killer and she gave him up to the police. Bundy also confessed that she had just killed her lover, Jack Murray — butchered is a better word — she shot him twice, stabbed him 22 times, sliced off his buttocks and then chopped off his head. Despite the fact that Bundy might not have been the most solid witness, her testimony sent Clark straight to death row.

Not only does Doug Clark say he is innocent, he says that Carol Bundy ("a sadistic lesbian serial killer") and her now dead lover, Jack Murray ("S&M freak pedophile crime partner") were the killers. Clark admits to having had a relationship with Bundy, but says it was just a casual one — that they were never lovers, just occasional sex partners. Carol Bundy says he's lying. She says that when she first met Clark, she thought his bizarre and violent desires were only fantasies, but as he

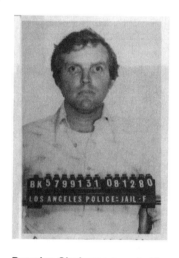

Douglas Clark was arrested in 1980 and charged with child molestation until detectives could conclusively link him to the Sunset Strip murders.

slowly began to involve her (she has said she was only a "mesmerized victim" of Clark's herself) she realized they were very real indeed. She says that she would help him find prostitutes for three-way sex and that she once delivered her 11-year-old babysitter to him for his enjoyment and hers. Their three-way "relationship" with the child went on for three months. Carol also reported that she would sometimes coerce prostitutes into their station wagon, where Doug would be waiting. He would get the girl to perform oral sex on him and, just as he was climaxing, Clark would shoot the girl in the head.

Whether it was Carol Bundy and Doug Clark, or Doug Clark alone who did the killing, the murders were brutal and ugly. On June 23rd, stepsisters Gina Marano and Cynthia Chandler were raped and shot to death. A short time later, Exxie Wilson and Karen Jones, prostitutes who had come west from Little Rock, Arkansas, were killed by a .25-caliber revolver and raped both before and after death. Exxie Wilson had been decapitated. Her head was discovered three days later in a wooden chest in a Studio City alley — washed, carefully made up and frozen. Bundy and Clark both say that the other wanted to keep the head as a trophy. And while Bundy insists that she was not involved in any of the murders, she once told a magazine reporter: "We had a lot of fun with her [head]. Where I had my fun was with the makeup. I was making her over like a big Barbie doll.... And then he wasn't happy with the way I had done her eye — her eyelid kept folding funny, y'know, because she was still half frozen." On June 30th, the body of Marnette Comer, a 17-year-old prostitute, was found in the San Fernando Valley. Her stomach had been slit open and she had been shot three times with a .25-caliber revolver, the same gun that had been used to kill the other women. One last body that has never been identified was discovered just before Clark was arrested. Though the gun used in these murders was found in Clark's possession, he claims that it did not belong to him. In fact, it had been purchased by Carol Bundy.

On March 15, 1983, Douglas Clark was sentenced to death for his role in the murders of six women and the attempted murder of Charlene Ackermann. The most damaging testimony came from Carol Bundy. He now sits on Death Row in San Quentin Prison. (Carol Bundy got 52 years to life for killing Murray and for participating in the killing of the last unidentified victim.)

Clark insists that he was framed by Carol Bundy and because of a series of incompetent lawyers, he has not been able to prove his innocence. He ended up writing his own court petition for a new trial, but it was summarily dismissed and denied. He says that he will continue searching for a lawyer who will prove his innocence.

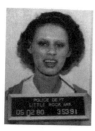 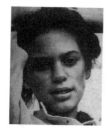 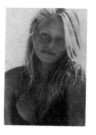 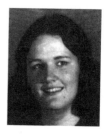

Sunset Strip murder victims (from left to right): Exxie Wilson, whose body was found in a Sizzler parking lot — her head was found later, frozen, washed and freshly made up; 15-year-old Gina Marano, whose body was discovered on an on-ramp to the Ventura Freeway; Cynthia Chandler, Gina's 16-year-old stepsister, of whom Clark says: "The only victim I knew and Carol *hated* her"; Karen Jones, who became a prostitute to support her little boy.

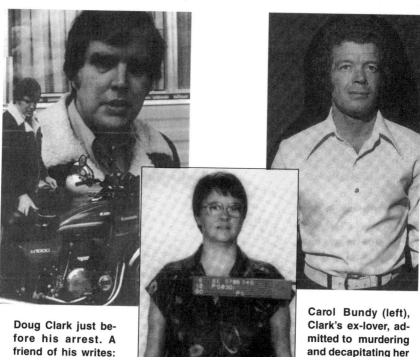

Doug Clark just before his arrest. A friend of his writes: "Danny has many friends from all over the world who are cheering for him to get a new trial."

Carol Bundy (left), Clark's ex-lover, admitted to murdering and decapitating her boyfriend, Jack Murray (above). She insists that Clark is the Sunset Strip Killer.

The Clark Letters

— december 31 — [1996]

Jenny,

Thanks for your interest — although misplaced in me and the case. Sorry to disappoint you — the vast mountains of evidence (alibis, proof of Carol Bundy copycat of Ted Bundy, her S & M lover & victim Jack and even DNA — not accepted in U.S. courts in 1980 — all will free me, in the pending retrial.)

We can now prove 1) I could NOT be [Carol Bundy's] partner, and, 2) <u>who was</u> and even <u>WHY</u> & HOW she became a sadistic lesbian serial killer

So — Thanks for your interest — but as "they all say," I didn't do it — so — look for a lovely condemned serial killer to write to, in <u>someone else</u>. <u>You</u> sound interesting, to <u>me</u> — married, nearly 30, parent — attractive...sounds to me you may be looking for vicarious thrills — I'm always interested in a sexy 'playmate' — any age, race, or even 'size' — but I don't 'play' at what you seem interested in. Sorry!

D.

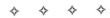

March 13 1997

— Jenny —

I really wish we'd met when I had the time & energy to enjoy & entertain you. Your last letters hint at a fun friendship — but with this fucked up stupid pack of assholes delaying incoming mail an extra 2 weeks, usually, it's not likely we'd have much of a conversation.

You don't pay much attention to detail — Carol [Bundy] and her <u>proved</u> S&M freak pedophile <u>crime partner</u> [Jack Murray] (with an 11 year old in his van, <u>FACT</u>) were the killers [of the women I am accused of killing]. She was NAILED LYING, denying [having] any Ted Bundy knowledge (proved by her letters, even). She denied being even FRIENDS with Jack [Murray], in 1980 — we proved she was into 3 ways, KIDDIESEX, 'SWING,' SM, etc, up to Aug 4, when she rimmed Murray's asshole and blew his brains out... She <u>also</u> tried to cover up the fact that for several 'events' (at least 6 murders) I had alibis for — from "DA" witnesses

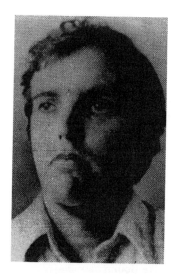

Doug Clark was found guilty of six counts of first degree murder and was sentenced to die in the gas chamber. He insists that he's innocent.

I don't have time or energy to spend discussing it — and I want to make this clear — you sound like an interesting person — anyone would be glad to have such a quirky funny (WRY) pal...I wish we'd met under other, better, conditions. I do have real friends of your "gender." (most men, some <u>women</u>, can't befriend the other gender.)

I have no problem with "honesty" — or "brain picking" — but I'm stretched so far & wide — I'm trying to groom a Swedish pen pal and my first pen pal to be SISTERS — they are like TWINS — love to travel the globe — same outlook on love, life, sex, future...adventure! These two mean so much to me — (you may think its weird!) — I helped a female (21) lifer to fall in love with another gal — 'IGNORING' gender — because they FIT, (except for gender!) It is odd — okay — but why not help people enjoy love & life, if I can? (Why do they listen to me? No idea!)

<u>5' 10</u>" — add <u>heels</u> — hair — yum!! I just imagined being under your desk, tasting you, as you type on your PC — So? I like the scent & taste of a naturally healthy, sexy woman...I'm a "slut" — so what? (Religious/moral repression is considered a mark of "value" in this fucked up country...)

As to the "facts" — you can buy the <u>next</u> book, in 2001, and find out I'm not bullshitting — as for now, I don't care enough about it to bother telling <u>anyone</u> (I don't really know well) what is <u>proved</u> — gotta go. I'm <u>broke</u> — if we write, send stamps?

Doug

✧   ✧   ✧   ✧

— AUGUST 5, 1997 —

Jenny —

The U.S. DIST COURT just fired my (useless) attorney. "Fred" could have, <u>should</u> have filed a 20 page MO-SU-JU (motion for summary judgment) 30 days after being appointed (<u>1992</u>). He <u>refused</u>...I did it — court refused to accept it <u>except</u> from counsel. I'd have been <u>freed</u> by now, if the stupid son of a bitch didn't go for the "long term" (bucks) rather than a "quick WIN". Here I sit...

So I'm busy as hell — but wanted to write to chat. I really hate this time of year, extra much when the day/date lines up to 1980 — as of next Monday, the 11th, it's 17 years of this — and the "GUMMIT" is dragging its feet — They know they'll lose the appeal, and retrial — so <u>delay</u> is the name of the game. They took TEN YEARS to do what would have usually taken THREE...tops. I yelled — I filed my record corrections in 3 months, the lawyers (4) redid it (exactly the same) in 4 YEARS...the court refused to accept mine.

I'm pissed off...oh well. Life sucks!

You got problems, you have dreams that you gave up on? I <u>want</u> to hear...talk to me about <u>whatever</u> interests you. Okay? And I'll share <u>me</u>. Why not? What "secrets" matter? I really wish you'd been there, to watch the mail with Veronica Compton...you know about her — (& Bianchi)...do you know that coke snorting bisexual submissive chick she (nearly) had sex with? What an old story — but also, how <u>odd</u> it hit a tiny place like Bellingham [Washington]. There's a crooked cop there, "Nolte" — truly <u>STUPID</u> and <u>crooked</u> — a bad mix...he will be in the crossfire — an LA cop reports Nolte faked an interview — a pack of <u>lies</u> — and Los Angeles cops and DA went nuts over it...used it...and it exploded in their faces... Also, 3 Sacramento cops blew the lid off 2 LA cops on fabricated evidence and perjury...It's always <u>best</u> when we get cops ratting off other cops!!

Summer... I'd love a good <u>swim</u>. Lazy, cool water, relaxed... Do you like to sit back, eyes closed, get a really good firm expert foot massage? I've only met one woman who knew how to give & get them. Our poor <u>feet</u> are beat up, smashed, battered — and never appreciated as having as many "feelings" as <u>hands</u>..., a good <u>patient</u> foot massage can really change a person's day — alter the 'path' — hookers love a good foot massage (and french session) after a hard day (or nite). I dated a waitress who worked streets at night — double-sore feet! Debbie...she is <u>cool</u> ("D & E" cups!).

So, when do I get to "pose" you? Hands & knees, big <u>smile</u> — flirty eyes? no? (okay, "school marm" will do!) (I even prefer bra & pants to 'nudes' — I kind of prefer the elegance of lingerie!)

gads, I'm horny, I guess. Sorry. Usually I sublimate it into "work" —

be good — write soon — remember, it takes 2+ weeks to get to me — 2 days to get to <u>you</u> ...TIME WARP! Thinking of knowing you —

"KINDRED"
Douglas

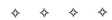

— August 17, 1997 —

Hi Jenny!

You're sweet to have sent the $15 — but as I (hope) I warned you — they seized it — and $1.70 of money I'd slipped in "under the wire." It's fairly silly, really — see, 1) any funds I receive OVER $10.00 in "any month" is "seized" at 40%, and all medical, copy service, legal postage. I had $5.00 medical hold (skin cancer spot on my hand — can't get it cut off — have to use a cigar, out on yard, to burn & kill all the cells...a friend'll do it — I don't like doing the burn — we use a "foil" cover to avert ashes in the hole...) I had $1.30 + postage owed — $5 medical (for the visit where an alcoholic reject from the real world said it's only a rash...) and "40%" waiting to pounce. So please — never ever send $ here! Stamps, yes, money NO.

I need to get my time clear, so I can discuss all that Veronica, Ted, Van, Carol stuff. That'll be fascinating but I got a new lawyer and things are amazingly confused — (he's written 3 times he says — I got ZERO...?!)

Talk to me — I do listen...would you like me to call? (collect only, all they allow). So be well — peaceful too — Send me what you feel you want me to know — I'd like to admire, enjoy, adore ya. Trust me not to be cruel — you'll be glad you did.

Douglas.

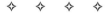

— Sept 2 97 —

Jenny —

Just to say, Thinking of you — and after a miserable week of lockdown & shakedowns, finally getting out for sun & air, and it RAINS. Ha!

A lesbian (butch) friend went to the "freak" ball in L.A. Sent pix of herself in "drag" — with TWO half naked chicks — now — this gal's doing something right??? ☺ I mean, as a "man" she scored better than most men do! Ha! I love it...sent me some fun pix of her vacation —

Listen — you're married — no? so — try this — open a can of sliced peaches — bathe slow and sexy — and...let those little slippery devilish "tongues" raise your mood — and his, too — done (gently) he'll be astonished — you'll be (hopefully) dessert!

Just my horny side surfacing now & then — I'll bet you're delicious! X!

Douglas

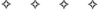

— September 8 — (Monday)

Hi! Been up to my ears in work — sweat, too — it's suddenly HOT, here. I'm OK — new lawyer is coming up here for 8 - 2 PM, Tuesday & Wednesday — taped meetings. No more B.S. from lawyers on "welfare". He sounds energetic — fairly skilled. That's a <u>good</u> mix.

So, I'm <u>OK</u> in legal factors — <u>don't</u> try to stir the pot, yet — let's give this new guy a chance to prove himself.

Which lawyer did you contact? Maxwell (BURP!) Keith is (drunk) disbarred — <u>legal bar</u>, (not just cocktail bars!) He's <u>scum</u>. Never interviewed <u>one single</u> key witness (of over 100). He told a judge he'd talked with over 100 — he clarified later, "I mean, I read their story or report." Gads... The DA closing argument conceded I was with his witness "CISSY" — the entire weekend, 9 PM Saturday (May 31) to 4 AM Monday (off to work), (June 2.) met at C/W bar, with her pals — even wrote her that 1st week's "rent check" ($30.00) naked in the bed...all <u>april</u>. Max in closing argument argued against all that — claimed I was guilty, inspite of proof I <u>couldn't</u> be... Lawyers like max keith are morally <u>obscene</u>.

Check this action out...The DA's BOUGHT Charlene Williams' stories — gave her an <u>easy deal</u> — she's now OUT — look up People vs. Gerald GALLEGO, in Nevada & Calif. She was the one <u>fully</u> into it — leading in the murders & tortures — she's <u>free</u>...Gads! Justice at work. See — in that era, (pre-'90) the macho stud male police forces couldn't imagine a lil ol' <u>woman</u> doing any sadistic sex murder, unless "forced to" by a male. They INSTANTLY gave women deals. Well, Cynthia? Charlene? Williams (his common law wife) proved 'em wrong — so did Cameron (?) Hooker's wife — she was in on a murder, then, keeping a "sex slave" for <u>seven years</u>. Remember that one? She was let go — the VICTIM proved the wife was a full partner, but DA let her walk. Oh well. <u>Carol's</u> [Bundy] going to get her story proved false — <u>bank on it!</u>

how about a <u>photo</u>? anything? I like <u>you</u> — relax and <u>be</u> yourself.

Great! bye for now pal. if your husband buys "playboy" — don't toss 'em out — clip a few pix for your lusty ol' brother-in-jail? (<u>not X rated</u>) Cool! X!

D!

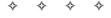

— January 30 1998 —

Jenny —

I had no idea the horrors you were immersed in [i.e., because of the kind of people you correspond with]. <u>Listen</u>, you do need to find some "center" — someone NOT in this "mess" — to anchor yourself back in reality — these ted bundy types are something you may think you can match wits with — but the others — the <u>really</u> depraved ones, comparatively speaking — the <u>Ed Gein's</u>, Kempers — you need to stay by the exit — sunlight & fresh air.

All's well here. I'm okay — case is going <u>fine</u>, at long last.

a quick note — I have never "owned" either gun [that was used to kill the women I am accused of killing], and all witnesses & DA/COPS agree — they were <u>Carol's.</u> All witnesses say

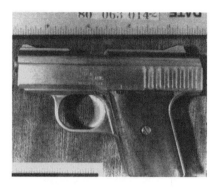

A) <u>doug</u> had <u>CHROME</u> gun
AND/OR
B) <u>carol</u> had the <u>NICKEL</u> one.

Chrome was the MALFUNCTIONING one Carol gave me, then repossessed when <u>I</u> gave it to Joey. That's all

Doug Clark's nickel Raven linked him to the Sunset Strip murder victims.

uncontroverted. Okay! I frankly admitted, "at one time I had access to each or both guns." But <u>carol</u> admits one was <u>her's</u>, one was for "doug" — and — she had both, <u>OFTEN</u>, "HID them" in her locker at work. (<u>on tape.</u>)

Then — too — she ADMITS:

Aug. 4 1980 she had both, in her makeup bag, with 2 small EXCEDRIN bottles, 6 bullets <u>in each</u>...<u>2 guns, 2 bottles, full "load" in each</u> in her makeup bag — NO PRINTS on shells, bottles, guns, magazines... She admits on AUG 9 she gave guns to me, saying "get rid of them where no one'll find them." No conjecture, fact. She had them — thrust them at me within an <u>hour</u> of the cops finding her lover's corpse she killed with one of those guns. NO doubt, no debate, fact. Okay? If you hear otherwise, say so — it's proved false!

— Here's a question —

What happens to JUSTICE when 8 veteran cops realize (suddenly) their stupidity let 5 people DIE — after they should have arrested 2 killers? And, blaming the guy <u>carol</u> accused CURES their career woes? You're aware, I know it.

be good — get away from this vile depravity — it sickens the soul of anyone who has to view it.

D.

Just got an article about Paul & Karla Bernardo, in Canada (from AUSTRALIA) someone sent it re: "WOMEN" — They all whine HE MADE ME. hey — some <u>men</u> do 'it' some <u>women</u> do 'it' <u>FRY 'EM ALL</u>

- February 11 -

Jenny -

I'll assume you're sincere in your
letter - and say that I don't think
"psycho" is at all appropriate as a
way to define ya -

Relax, okay? It seems to me
you feel like your thoughts push
you outside of any possible
friendship with someone who doesn't
always agree with you... as I said,
relax.

You could have 20 tattoos, a
double mastectomy and purple hair -
hang by your feet in a casket
at night and dream of really
unusual things - so? So what?

I only want to hear from you
if you decide it's a valuable
and fullfilling event for both of
us. Be yourself - I'll be me...

I won't write for you - but I'll talk with you...

My interests won't be as exciting for you, since the retrial is about to occur, and prove Carol Bundy & Jack copied Ted Bundy, in these crimes. That'll reduce your interest in me, I guess. So? If you get bored, say so - it's not a mine!

I'd like to see you - (polaroid film isn't allowed) - do you like cats or dogs? Are you fit? like to daydream?

let me know if you want to be you - I'll be me... could be FUN!

D.

Lawrence Bittaker

From the moment of his arrest in 1981, Lawrence Bittaker has insisted that he didn't kill the five women whose murders eventually landed him on death row and Roy Norris, his partner in crime, in prison for life. Severely undermining Bittaker's staunch denial of guilt is the fact that Norris openly admitted that the two of them did indeed kill the women in question. Following their arrests, each man gave a completely different account of what had actually happened and today they still claim that the other is lying.

While the two men first met in the mid-1970s when they were both imprisoned at the California Men's Colony East, it wasn't until after their release that they came up with the plan to abduct and kill young girls. Some accounts say that their goal was to kill a girl whose age matched each teenage year — a 13 year old, a 14 year old and up through 19, but I don't know whether this is true or not.

Once they had their plan in place, Bittaker bought a van, customized it to facilitate easy abduction and christened it "The Murder Mac." Apparently, they had no trouble abducting victims; they lured girls into their van by flirting with them and promising them drugs and when neither of these did the trick, they simply used physical force.

Their first victim was 16-year-old Cynthia Schaeffer, who they abducted from Redondo Beach, California, on June 24, 1979. After raping and torturing her for hours, Bittaker wrapped a wire coat hanger around her neck and twisted it so tightly with a pair of pliers that he crushed her windpipe, strangling her to death.

Less than a month later, on July 8, they kidnapped their second victim, 18-year-old Andrea Hall. Before strangling her to death, Bittaker took a photograph of her begging for her life and then drove an ice pick into her head, through the ear and into her brain. (Later, when Bittaker was in prison for these crimes, other inmates would refer to him as "Pliers Bittaker" and "Ice Picker Bittaker." Some accounts say that Bittaker himself used these monikers when he would sign autographs; apparently, he must have liked something about these references to his favorite tools of torture.)

In early September of the same year, Bittaker and Norris picked up 13-year-old Leah Lamp and her 16-year-old friend, Jackie Gillam, while they were hitchhiking along the Pacific Coast Highway. After terrorizing and torturing Gillam for more than 24 long hours, Bittaker strangled her to death. Lamp, who probably witnessed her friend's torture and murder, must have thought a miracle had occurred when Bittaker told her he was going to let her go. But he was just kidding; instead, he killed her with a deft sledgehammer blow to the head. The two men then tossed the girls' bodies over a cliff.

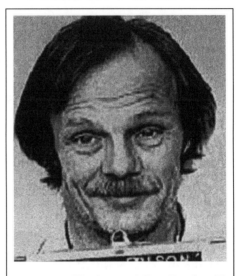

Less than two months later, on Halloween night, Bittaker and Norris abducted Shirley Lynette Ledford from a gas station. They raped her over and over again and then bludgeoned her with a sledgehammer, specifically, bone-crushing blows to her elbow — a sadistic act if there ever was one. Bittaker and Norris are perhaps best known for the bizarre fact that they tape-recorded

Lawrence Bittaker and Roy Norris will always be remembered for the fact that they tape-recorded their last murder, preserving forever Shirley Ledford's blood curdling screams for mercy as they raped and tortured her. Bittaker claims that they "asked" Ledford to scream, that she was only "acting."

this particular murder. I have listened to the tape of Shirley Ledford screaming for mercy and begging her torturers to just get it over with and kill her — and it is chilling beyond words.

In late November, an old prison acquaintance of Norris' tipped off the police about the murders. When the two were arrested, Bittaker denied involvement, but Norris caved in easily, confessing that they were both responsible for the murders. Norris also led police to the "Murder Mac" and to some of the victims' bodies. One skeleton still had Bittaker's ice pick protruding from the skull. In the "Murder Mac" police found photographs of over 500 smiling young girls, 19 of whom were currently missing. Police eventually thought that Bittaker and Norris were responsible for as many as 40 murders, although in the end, they were only charged with five.

To this day, Bittaker maintains that he is innocent, that he was framed, and that there has been a legal conspiracy against him from the beginning. During his trial for the five murders, the jury was not impressed with Bittaker's defense; they found him guilty of the five murders and on February 1, 1981, he was sentenced to die in the gas chamber. Bittaker has appealed his death sentence several times, but with no success. His death warrant has been signed once, but on July 9, 1991, he was granted a stay of execution. Now 58 years old, Lawrence Bittaker remains on death row in San Quentin Prison, hoping his death warrant won't be signed again, at least not in the near future.

The Bittaker Letters

December 30, 1996

Dear Jenny,

Hopefully you will receive this; if not, it's your own fault for writing your return address so illegibly.

As to your question [about the crimes I was convicted of], I am sorry to say that you have been greatly misled; I have always denied committing the crimes. If you have read the usual sensationalistic blurbs about the case, it is easy to believe that I confessed to a variety of people. However, that is not the case, and the people making those claims were either my business partner (trying to avoid the gas chamber with the only bargaining power available to him: someone else to lay the blame on), or various jail inmates (seeking a quicker release from jail, or future forgiveness for some yet undone crimes).

I don't mind if you don't believe my disclaimer; you surely believe in the "system" and that it doesn't convict the innocent. How naive!

Or you assume that I had a trial, and the jury decided on the evidence. Again, how naive and ignorant.

But then the media never cared to report much of anything I said, or find out that (like you) 'my' attorney also believed I was guilty (before he even heard my side, or did any investigations), and failed to investigate and present a defense. In effect, there was no trial, and I might as well have pled guilty.

I have been trying for the past 15 years to get someone, anyone, to listen to me, but the 'system' seems composed only of those who believe in my guilt, and who will do nothing to determine the true facts. But then the 'system' is set up to make the trial the 'main event,' and all that comes after is pushing papers around, and which are then reviewed by 'packed' courts (of conservatives) hardly likely to give a "convicted killer" a fair hearing. They weren't elected or appointed to do that: just affirm such sentences and speed executions.

I don't even have (as a practical matter) any attorney at the moment, as I became tired of their incompetence, routine lies, even stealing from me, and ceased communicating with them 8 months ago. I suppose they're necessary, but I learned long ago why there are so many bad jokes about them.

254

In any event, it is a long and rather complex story, and I have repeated it too many times to do so again to you, especially as it requires about 200 pages to do so.

I will answer specific and pointed questions, as long as you provide the postage. I have no family and my income is quite limited, so I can't afford to even pay the postage for idle inquiries from strangers.

L. Bittaker

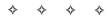

Jan. 21, 1997

Jenny;

Now to see if I can figure out what you are saying; some of your comments are rather unclear.

I can only assume that you based most of your comments on the alleged "torture tape" of the girl Ledford. Unfortunately, I am not in the best position to explain its content. The cops originally gave my trial atty a poor copy of it, and when he pointed this out, they gave him another poor copy (which he didn't realize was poor). He also didn't have the tape subjected to any examination by anyone, and I only heard a clear copy once (perhaps twice, although I don't remember it), at the trial. So there was no real effort made to determine what was on the tape, or what it meant.

The media reports make it sound like there is no question of what is happening on the tape, while that is actually not the case. It is difficult to hear what she is saying on it, as the screams (mostly done at our request; i.e. scripted) cause one to prejudge the rest of it. While I have a transcript of it, and the jury was given a copy, that doesn't demonstrate her very inconsistent (with torture) tone of voice she uses. For someone allegedly being hurt, she is not crying, or giving any other sign of being hurt; merely the screams. So something doesn't make sense.

Because I had been drinking all evening, and smoking grass, I simply can't remember everything that happened, or why I said certain things on the tape. I have tried for years to get my attys to give me a copy, so I could erase the screams on it, and we could then listen to the rest and try to understand it, but they refuse, or to do that themselves. So it is very hard to 'defend' such tape, when I have no access to it, and can't demonstrate my claims.

And despite the extraordinary claims made by certain witnesses, that is the only tape that every existed, with that sort of content. But I can't prove that others didn't exist: one can't disprove something that never existed!

Anyway, the short story on that subject.

Since I don't know what 'information' you are relying on, I can't adequately respond to your (implicit) accusations. If you have specific questions, ask them. I don't expect you to believe my answers as it is impossible for anyone to prove most of the 'facts' in my case, one way or the other. It's mostly a matter of "he said, she (or he) said." Who you believe is mostly based on bias, and the almost total failure of 'my' atty to demonstrate that the other witnesses are liars, while nothing I said can be demonstrated as a falsehood.

A trial is supposed to be where both sides put on their evidence, and the jury decides who is telling the truth, and thus what the 'facts' are. Well, that didn't happen in my case, and thus the jury didn't learn that most of the witnesses against me could reliably be proved to lie about various things, with no motive except to 'frame' me for the crimes. So I don't blame them for their verdict: I blame my totally unethical and incompetent atty for abandoning me as a client, and the cops/prosecutor for allowing various people to testify, when they had to know that they were lying.

So yes, I'm "pissed" to say the least!

So Norris, who pled guilty to 5 murders, and misc. other crimes, (effectively) received life without parole, while the state intends to execute me, and I'm still waiting for my "day in court"!

And whatever happened is not simply the "past." I daily have to live with such events, attempting to correct matters, or at least living with the results of such events.

But the legal system is not set up to really rectify 'mistakes,' but to make it difficult for anyone to obtain a new trial, once they have been convicted.

Given such screwed up legal 'system,' while I may eventually obtain a new trial, it will probably be useless, because by now evidence helpful to me has been lost, and previous events make it very difficult to determine the truth. Witnesses who lied back then, have to continue such lies, even if they don't want to, because to now tell the truth gets them in trouble. Some lied back then to get out of trouble, and because they thought me guilty, but no matter how false their past claims, we're all stuck with them, so there can never be a "fair" trial after the cops and prosecutors start pressuring a witness to say certain things, or put a suspect in certain circumstances that will cause negative things to happen.

It goes without saying that if I catch you in a lie, I will probably cease writing, and I expect the same reaction from you. If there is one thing I "hate," it's liars.

For what it is worth, I've spent much of my life in prison for (rather minor) property offenses (mostly because I didn't care if I was in or out). And those results were based in part due to my admission of guilt; if I did something wrong, I accepted the punishment. So I am not someone with a record of denying guilt or accepting blame.

Why do you mention sending drawings? I don't care how well you draw; unless you send interesting letters, I will not continue to write.

Given your repeat comments, I assume you live only with your children. No mention of a job??

Anyway, you don't say much else that I can respond to, so I will get this off. Hope you are doing OK. Take care.

Larry

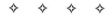

February 1, 1997

Jen;

Will try again; are you writing any others on the row here? No surprise that most [of the inmates you write to] say they are innocent. I would prefer not to even have to say it, as most probably don't care to believe that. But simply discussing that I didn't get a fair trial, isn't enough for most people.

Guess I'll remain less "respectable" to you, if a confession is necessary to be otherwise. And it's not so much a matter of waiting to get screwed; no waiting is necessary. Got another dose of that on Monday, during a telephone interview for the Leeza Gibbons show. So what else is new.

I'd be interested to learn what book printed a transcript of the Ledford tape; haven't heard about that yet. Am sure curious about whether they copied the 'official' version used at the trial, or some other.

Your suggestion that [Ledford] spoke as she did, from knowing she was going to die, is a rather unusual one. I'd say few people would be able to adopt such an attitude, unless they had been told that was going to happen, which supposedly didn't happen with her.

And again, even if she was that gutsy, that doesn't explain her cool/neutral response in the midst of the alleged gross physical mistreatment. Something just doesn't compute there. But as long as you only look for explanations that follow your presumption, they most likely won't fit.

No, I'm not a "bullshit" type person. Fun and joking is OK in their place, but the case is hardly the place for that. Also, we haven't developed a relationship on that level, so it would be out of place. As for writing just a chatty letter, of frivolous chit-chat, I'm really not into that sort of thing, absent special circumstances.

(My letters are also terse and grammar sometimes clumsy, because I type it directly into the memory, and print it without editing. I'd prefer to do otherwise, but the supply of ribbons is limited. Also, I get tired of typing, as I've been at the keyboard about 6 hours already today, doing legal things.)

I can't say I'm familiar with your marital problems; have never been married outside. Wanted to be, but my goofy 'life style' and experiences conspired against it. Sure kids are extraordinary, but so is a flower or bug. That doesn't equate to 'there must be a God'. Lack of logic there, although the proposition is attractive. Why do people also need to find some 'higher power' to explain their lack of knowledge?

I don't really know or propose to guess why my trial atty did as he did. Maybe he was just the lazy sort, who didn't like to do the necessary work. Maybe he figured the evidence looked so bad, by only chance to live longer was for him to screw everything up, so I would eventually get a new trial. (Curiously, my subsequent attys couldn't believe that might be the case.)

I can merely speculate, but have no real data to make a judgment on. I knew 3 of the other 4 victims, having met them under similar circumstances, for similar reasons. And yes, they would all seem to be logically connected, which is a factor that is hard to explain away.

I can largely destroy the credibility of Roy, and some other important witnesses in the case, but the tape and the apparent pattern of it all, are more difficult.

Woops; am really getting senile. Just remembered that the tape transcript was in Alone With the Devil. And it does read almost as "bad" as it sounds on hearing it. But Marman adds his own editorializing, which is merely speculation.

And in a sense I do accept responsibility for the deaths. I should have known about Norris, and not created opportunities where he could have done what he did. As I told someone just last night, a witness who had nothing good to say about me, says Norris drove to my place very late on that night with the last victim, and wouldn't let her near the van. He then went into my room for a few minutes. Almost nothing that witness said was the truth (she made up some outrageous and bizarre claims), but that was one of the few truthful things.

Actually, I had gone home early, and Roy was still out in the van with Ledford. Roy essentially denied that such a meeting happened, and I can't think of why it would have happened, or in that manner, if we had both been in the van at that point, with Ledford as a prisoner.

As for who I "really" am, I wouldn't know how to being to answer that, or even understand what it means.

Anyway, enough for now. Take care.

L. Bittaker

March 13, 1997

Hi Jenny,

Another short missive from you, eh?
You ever write a long letter to anyone?
I meant to ask: that's an odd apartment (?) address, or
is it some type of box at a convenience address?
Again, I'm not really "bitter," just frustrated. And no
reason to 'fear' my letters, as I don't 'go off' on people (except
in a sarcastic way).
Yeah, I acknowledge being preoccupied with my legal situation,
but then my very life depends on it, so that's to be expected.
The Leeza show just screwed me. They invited me to comment
on my (alleged) "broken cookie" law suit, and then set me up
for the kill, by having my prosecutor on the show to make me
out the very devil. So from the general subject of prisoner
law suits, it changed into why should scummy killers on death
row have any rights? *(and me in particular.)*
Not that I got to say much I'm sure; probably just the usual
5-second sound bit, but I haven't heard what was actually broadcast
yet.

I wouldn't have minded that so much, as the producer offered
to take some photos in her area, that I need in my case. She
also asked for one of my cards, which I sent. But now she's denied
offering to take the photos, and hasn't had even the courtesy
to send a note of thanks for the cards, or replaced the stamps.
So they used me up one side, and down the other.
So what has been your "obsession, rage" "for so many years"??
My case??
I just compared the court exhibit (tape transcript), and
it differs here and there from Markman's 'quote' in his book.
He has her saying "ouch" in one of the earlier lines, and the
transcript says "ough." He also characterizes the sounds as
"slaps" and that I "struck" her, while the transcript merely
describes them as "sound." (Just noticed that he has me beating
on her elbow, when in fact Roy admitted that.)
But of course merely reading such words is largely ineffective
in proving things either way; only hearing the actual tone of
her voice would reliably indicate the true conditions. But as
yet, my attys have refused to do anything about that.
I do have room for humor and witticisms in my life, but
sometimes they get rare. Indeed, the other night I was fingering
my extension cord, and considering ending it all. But have mostly
come out of that black mood.
And I find it harder to make funnies in letters, while I
do so pretty easily in the flow of a conversation.
Am not sure who I 'really' am. Was raised by adoptive parents,
who were less than affectionate. Nice, but I often describe
the relationship as not much different than being the family
pet.
I didn't mind school that much, but it was often boring

```
(too easy).
        And your question made me reflect: I probably never have
loved anyone in the usual meaning. Of course that has been my
greatest desire for a long time, but it just never seemed to
happen.
        Sorry to hear about your bad family life. I wish you could
get things together now.
        Curious that you should mention SLO; got a letter from a
new pen pal tonight, who lives in that area.
        Yeah, I know that area, having done 3 terms in the Men's
Colony there.
        Am a bit surprised that I didn't become an alcoholic or
drug addict. I seemed to steal when younger to compensate for
the poor family life (replacing love with material things?).
But I seem to fear heavy drugs and avoid them, although I've
been less careful with alcohol. So I know it can be a seductive
escape.
        Seems like I asked you my last, as to whether you wrote
others, and where. I answer all your questions; why not equality?
        And unless your letters improve (seems I said that also),
I won't be writing much longer.
        WHY are you writing??
        Thanks for the sketch and stamp. WIsh I could draw as well.
        Take care.



        L. Bittaker
```

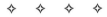

July 18, 1997

Jenny,

Any reason I should be "crazy" about you?

Obviously I have a lot to say, and am "intelligent." So what else is new? Hearing that does not bother me in any way, as I am hardly unique.

Would it do any good to object to the publication of my letters? It seems obvious, despite your "research," that you have yet to understand the facts.

Yes, had I been wealthy, I would have received a trial that was much more fair. But that doesn't end the question: my particular case was not so much affected by wealth (and thus the quality of my representation) but by the operation of the 'conviction machine' established by the authorities, with the approval of the courts.

Money could not have competed with the favors the district attorney could offer. It couldn't have purchased the dismissal of charges against various they use (and abuse) that power to achieve the ends they see fit. Yes, a good attorney and thorough investigative efforts could have damaged the credibility of most of the witnesses against me (to a greater or lesser extent, limited primarily by the particular claims they made), and I might have been acquitted on that basis.

Objectively, that wouldn't mean I was innocent, but...only two people really know, and you either make your own judgment (usually based on emotion), or simply accept the jury verdict.

As to having my letters read by "people who may make a difference," there are only a few of those: the judges who will decide my federal habeas corpus petition, and — to a much lesser extent — my present counsel. No one else really matters, or can make a difference, and those judges certainly don't care what I have to say.

If you think anyone else can "make a difference," you understand the 'system' even less than you think. The 'game' is in progress, and nothing matters except the events of the trial, now carved in stone. Nothing can change the claims of the jailhouse informants, whose testimony was purchased by the highest bidder. Nothing can change the faulty memories of those who believed I am guilty, and whose recollections were shaped by those beliefs. It is too late to secure certain evidence that would have demonstrated the various lies and mistakes; that evidence is gone forever, and I cannot now even prove it once existed. It is too late to go back and start over.

Take care.
L. Bittaker

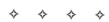

August 24, 1997

Jenny;

My problem is trusting people too easily; a character flaw I guess. Surely not a survival characteristic.

I question your judgment of me, based on our limited correspondence.

I'm sure it would be easy for all but the most selfcentered or sociopathic in here, to write a few letters giving someone a positive impression of their character. But, to each their own I guess.

As for your request to "continue our relation," that is not reasonable for two reasons: (1) your referenced belief, and (2) the fact that there has never really been a relationship. How could there be when your 'letters' were usually just a few sentences?

Again, to each their own. But since that isn't my thing, I'll pass.

I wish the best for you all. Take care.

Larry

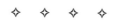

Bill Suff

A fortune teller once told Bill Suff that someone put a black spell on him. It's the only explanation Suff can come up with for why "darkness" has followed him for most of his adult life. The way he looks at it is this: How else could he, a completely innocent man, be suspected of as many as 26 brutal sex murders, wrongfully accused of 20 murders — and have been solidly convicted of first degree murder of 12 women?

Bill Suff's troubles began back in Texas when he was arrested for beating his two-month-old daughter to death. Although he claims that he was asleep when his daughter was killed and that his wife was responsible, official reports say that Suff was home alone with his infant daughter and young son when the baby was mercilessly battered to death. Despite his claims of innocence, he was found guilty and sentenced to 70 years in prison. Released on parole after only ten years, Suff headed west to California to make a fresh start.

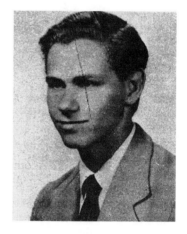

Bill Suff's 1968 Perry High School yearbook photo. Five years later, he would be arrested for the murder of his baby daughter.

In 1984, Suff settled in southern California near Los Angeles. Over the next six years, Riverside County, California, became the scene of a series of extremely violent sex murders of as many as 26 young women who had been raped, strangled, stabbed near the heart and mutilated, sometimes with their breasts sliced off. The bodies were found all over Riverside County, many of them near Lake Elsinore, often positioned by their killer to expose the fact that they were prostitutes and drug users — their legs were pulled apart to show their genitals and their arms stretched out to show their needle marks. It was clear that the killer thought these girls were nothing but trash and he wanted to tell the world.

By April 1991, it was evident that a serial killer was at work and a special task force was established to find him. As the months wore on and more and more girls were killed, police slowly began accumulating evidence. They had distinctive tire prints, shoe prints and hair fibers that were found near the bodies of several victims. By August 1991, they had a description of the man: white male, 5'10", brown hair, medium build, slight mustache, metal frame glasses, driving a late model, blue over gray, Chevolet Astro van with gray-blue carpeting. But still the killer eluded them, month after month.

In January 1992, police stopped William Lester Suff for a traffic violation in the red-light district of Riverside. Upon realizing that Suff looked exactly like the man they were after, the officer called in a license check and discovered that Suff was in violation of his Texas parole. When police searched his van, they found some items that

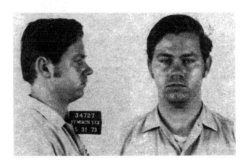

Bill Suff in 1973 after he was arrested for the beating death of his two-month-old daughter, Dijianét. She had 13 broken ribs, a broken arm, human bite marks on her forehead and stomach, a cigarette burn on her foot and was bruised from head to toe. Even though Suff claims his ex-wife killed her, he was convicted of the crime.

sparked their interest: a bloody kitchen knife, rope, a policeman's uniform and what appeared to be a big stain of blood. Suff was indignant when he was promptly handcuffed and arrested.

Apparently, people that knew Suff were shocked to hear that their odd but sweet and helpful friend, a mild-mannered stock clerk, had been charged with the Lake Elsinore murders, as they were now called.They didn't think he was the kind of person who would look down on prostitutes, let alone kill them. Even the detective in charge of the investigation at first didn't consider Suff a likely suspect. After all, here was a man staunchly, vehemently opposed to drugs and alcohol (friends testified that Suff was so "moral," he couldn't be in the same room when people were drinking alcohol), who was also known to be hardworking and a regular churchgoer.

Nevertheless, Suff was brought to trial in 1995 and although he was suspected of killing as many as 26 women, in the end, he was charged with only 19. He was found guilty of first degree murder in 12 of the cases (the jury could not agree on a verdict on one case and there was not enough evidence to tie him to the other six cases). It took the jury less than ten minutes to decide his fate: death. They felt that if William Lester Suff didn't deserve the death penalty, then who did?

Suff himself says he is flabbergasted and outraged about the whole thing, that his conviction is a sham, that he was framed. He has explanations for most of the evidence used to convict him. For example, he says he has nothing against prostitutes, that he often employed their services and even considered some of them to be real friends; that the hair, blood and semen used to connect him to the murders was planted in his van; that the "blood" in his van was actually Dr. Pepper that his wife had spilled.

According to Suff, the real killer is still out there and he's being railroaded for crimes he did not commit. He is hoping authorities will realize their dreadful mistake and set him free. Investigators involved in Suff's case believe that the evidence against him is overwhelming and there is no question in their minds that they have the right man.

Today, Bill Suff sits on death row in San Quentin prison. Things don't look so good for him. It appears that his own lawyers have lost interest in his case and will not even return his calls. Neither will any of his friends, and with the exception of a recent truce with his mother and one of his sisters, none of his relatives want anything to do with him.

If only he had paid the fortune teller the $20 worth of sugar and coffee she wanted to remove the black spell...

The Suff Letters

Hello Ms. Furio,

May I call you Jenny? Please call me Bill. I do not care to answer to either of the appellations of William or Mr. Suff. All of my life I've been called either Bill or Lee (sometimes Billy) and prefer to be called that. Whenever someone calls me Mr. Suff, I tend to look behind me to see if my father is there. To me, he is Mr. Suff, not me. And my birth certificate says my name is Bill, not William. Only the legal system and a glitch when I was in the Air Force changed my name to William. So, if you decide to continue our correspondence (or anything more in the future), please call me Bill.

I usually don't write back to people who have written unsolicited letters to me (unless they have gone into some great detail concerning themselves and the reason for their letter). To date, there are only three people to whom I have decided to write back to and have continued a corresponding relationship with them. You are the first lady that I have decided to answer. I'm not saying that you're the first lady to write to me nor the only one to whom I am writing. Others have written, but for one reason or another, I didn't write back to them. I cannot give you a clear answer as to why I have decided to write back to you. One reason is the intense hope that I can convince you that the court (jurors) made a mistake and that all of the little tidbits written about me are in gross error and outright lies.

Needless to say. I cannot go into great detail regarding my case. My appellate case depends on keeping too much from being found out regarding my defense and the proof we have to show that I am actually innocent (wrongly convicted). So, please understand my reluctance in discussing legal matters. I don't even discuss matters of my defense or my case with my attorneys when we are talking on the phone (even though our conversations are **supposed** to be case. This much I can tell you: What you have read was a one-sided report coming from the prosecution and police investigators that worked on the case that was **waged** against me. But we have proof the prosecution lied, left out evidence that would clear me, and misquoted evidence to the jurors and the

266

public. We also have real and circumstantial evidence that misleading information was leaked to the news media and relayed to the public. (Just one instance: My family, my ex-wife and her family, my co-workers at my job-site, and the public were told that I had confessed to the killings. In actuality, I had not confessed to anything other than to being in the area where one of the bodies was found!) And, we have proof now that evidence was planted in my apartment, at my job-site, and in my van. As I said, the reports about me were awfully one-sided.

You also say that you understand that I have a really nice side. To say the least, that is a gross understatement. All of my life it has been my belief that women should be protected and respected, almost as much as children. Along with that, I've always believed in the following credo for my life: "Be happy, try not to hurt other people, and hope to fall in love someday." The first has happened more often than not. The second has been a constant in my life. And the third has happened a few times. I lost Bonnie because I didn't show her exactly how much I actually loved her. Cathy was killed in an automobile accident the evening after she said she was moving in with me. Florence, well....that's a whole different case...she's married. But I have a great deal of love that I can give to the right girl, if I can only find her.

A little more about me: I never was a party-goer. I preferred to spend quality time with the girl I was currently with. I didn't ever really drink, either. When I did, I drank Vodka Screwdrivers, and then only on my birthday, New Years Eve and the 4th of July. Alcohol and drugs never were a part of my life. Talking about church, I was a member of my church's choir and was the puppeteer for our Vacation Bible School's mascot. I really love nature. I've raised all kinds of birds: Chickens, ducks, quail, pheasants, canaries and finches. I also raised fish (both fresh water and marine), dogs, cats, and even a rabbit. I've taken trips to Zion National Park in Southwest Utah, to Sequoia National Park and the Grand Canyon to enjoy the surrounding beauty. Like I said, I love nature.

Your comments about my guilt of killing **anyone** distresses me. The reason is because I know that I am innocent and so do the people who **really** <u>know</u> me and have stuck beside me throughout this entire mess. The person (or persons) who actually killed the women I am charged with killing knows I'm innocent, also. To a lesser degree, the police and the prosecution knows that someone else is responsible for those murders, too. But they had a scapegoat in me and decided to clear their books by manufacturing my guilt. So, I'm sorry that you believe in all of the things the news media reported, prompted by the police and the prosecution. It really hurts me that people believe I could do something that terrible.

As for schooling, I graduated from High School and College, obtaining both my Associate's Degree and my Bachelor's Degree in the combined fields of Sociology/Psychology. I also amassed about 2,000 hours/credits in computer sciences (specializing in the Apple computer field). But all in all, I'm a private person, comfortable with being alone, but preferring the company of other people....I'm a 'people person'.

Like you, God has blessed me with the inability to hate. I don't hate anybody. However, the prosecutor and the police scare me. It scares me that they can create evidence to the degree that they can find **anyone** guilty. **Nobody** should have that much or kind of power. And the fact that our justice system is a lie saddens me very much. The legal system says that a person is supposed to be presumed innocent until found guilty. In actuality, the person is presumed guilty until, not just **thought** innocent, but proven innocent. With the help of the news media and our flawed legal system's laws, the prosecution is allowed to successfully convict the charged person by having the first and last words ever heard by the jurors and the public, therefore making it nearly impossible for the charged person to get a fair trial. And the defense doesn't help much by forcing a virtual gag-order on the client and refusing to give away any hint of a defense to be heard by the public before the trial starts. Therefore, the accused is placed at a disadvantage long before they get a chance to publicly proclaim their innocence. Much as was shown by my case.

Sincerely,
Bill L. Suff

P.S. — Please forgive me for not signing this letter. I'm still gun-shy (of autograph/souvenir seekers.)

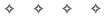

24 May 1997

Hello Jenny,

I received your letter yesterday and thought I'd better answer it right away. I don't recall whether or not I told you in my first letter, but I do a lot of writing: Two novels (currently in progress), three short-stories (completed) and a cookbook containing recipes I created myself (currently standing at 39 recipes and growing as I recall more of the recipes I created). I have also penned a few poems (though none have been written in the past few years) and even drew a few cartoons when I was a lot younger. I don't draw anymore, though. I think it's partly because I've lost interest in drawing. But also, I think the motorcycle accident I was in destroyed the minor ability I had in the drawing field. But then, there's a lot of my youth that I can no longer recall because of that accident. It did some big time damage to my body and my mind.

Thank you for the compliment (I think). I've never read anything by Nabokov (I suppose you're talking about Vladimir V. Nabokov, the Russian-born, American novelist and poet -- see, I do know a few things). I **have** been described before as being eloquent in my writing and speaking, but this is the first time anyone said that my writing was perverse, or that it contained great insight. I've never thought of myself in those terms. What exactly brought you to that conclusion?

I'm glad to hear that you don't believe **everything** you read and hear (and I hope that doesn't apply to what I have to say to you). After all the bad things and derogatory remarks that were made about me, it's refreshing to hear that someone out there might have some doubts as to the veracity of what the police told the media and the media reported to the public. But I **can** tell you this much, there are certain members of the media that are beginning to doubt what they were told by the police. They are now beginning to seriously question the guilty verdict in my case. Did you hear that some guy was arrested in Chicago for killing prostitutes? He has given them a written confession and claims that he also killed prostitutes in Riverside County and a girl in San Diego County. My attorney and investigator have been paying real close attention to that case. They are wondering just how many of the killings he did in Riverside that I took the fall for. Riverside cops are **NOT** talking! My attorney says they are ducking and avoiding all questions regarding my being blamed for the deaths of prostitutes in Riverside.

You asked me why men kill. I wish I could give you an answer to that question, but unfortunately, I can't. There are only a couple of people I know who admit to killing someone, thereby ending up here. But I don't feel comfortable talking about their cases. I don't talk about my case to other people and I don't care to learn anything about anyone else's case. So, insights as to why someone would want to kill someone else -- I can't afford to discuss those reasons or rationalizations in this format. If I were to do so, the Attorney General could possibly get hold of those comments and twist them to use against me in my appeal. I don't know if you are aware of it, but every one of the letters generated from here are closely examined and xeroxed for possible use against us in our appeals. Therefore, it behooves me to **not** discuss particulars about my case or others, so please have the courtesy not to ask.

You asked me what life was like for me in here, in regard to special privileges, bad food, rape...etc. And no, you probably haven't been watching too much Hard Copy. Those things have been going on here or in other prison units. I've talked to a few of the people those things have happened to. But me? Well, I don't think I'm getting any special privileges. At least, no more than others on the Row are entitled to: I have a TV, this typewriter (of course), and a watch. But only because my attorney cared enough to send me money to buy them. No one else has cared enough to send me anything, not even a letter or a stamp, let alone money, not even my blood-relatives. I go out to the exercise yard for a little sun and fresh air Monday through Fridays from 7 a.m. until 1 p.m. We shower and have access to a razor three times a week (Monday, Thursday and Saturday for me). On Condemned Row, we are confined to single man cells. We only come into contact with each other when on the exercise yard, at religious services or in the visiting room. I've been assigned to the protective custody exercise yard (tell you more on that), and the church is segregated as to which yard the inmates are assigned to. The visiting room is the only place inmates come into contact with inmates from other yards. So rape or any other kind of violence doesn't really factor into what privileges I'm entitled to. The PC yard is off-limits to any kind of violence by mutual agreement of the inmates. So is the church and the visiting room area. So I think that I have very little to fear in those areas. However, I'm still in jeopardy here. It seems a contract has been put out on me from someone in Riverside County [Prison]. I've suspected it for some time now, but it was confirmed last week... Once on the yard and again when I was talking to my attorney.

Whenever a condemned row inmate needs to go to the unit hospital, the clinics or to the main visiting room for a legal visit, we are escorted by one or two officers past the main-line inmates. During an escort to the hospital or clinic, we are escorted by two officers, a chain around our waist and our hands handcuffed to our sides at that chain. When going to a legal visit, we are escorted by a single officer and we have our hand 'cuffed behind our backs. No real way to defend ourselves in case of an attack. Last week I had to go to the clinic to have blood drawn for diabetes testing. I informed the escorts about the contract on me before we left the building I'm housed in. The escort said for me not to worry, nothing would happen. On the way to the clinic, we passed a large group of main-line inmates (about 100). We had only passed a few of them when we heard someone shout, "There he is, that's him. That's Suff!!" Nobody made any movement in our direction, but there were two inmates pointing at me. It shook me up some. You see, all it would take is for 10 or 15 inmates, en masse, to attack me and any escort with me. One inmate to take me out while the rest kept the escort(s) busy. That really bothers me. Foremost, because the escort(s) might get hurt. Then there's the possibility that I might be killed. Now, dying doesn't bother me, however, the **manner** of my death does! I cannot tolerate pain at any level. What really bothers me about my prospective death is dying for something I didn't do! All of my life, if I did something wrong, I've always accepted my punishment without question. But when I get blamed for something

I didn't do, I have to protest...loudly and passionately. And in that lies the reason why I am protesting my conviction and death sentence so vigorously.

I'd like to know more about your family. Since I don't seem to have a family anymore, I'd like to hear about the families of other people I write to.

Well, I guess I better close this letter here. Write back when you can.

Sincerely,
Bill Suff

✧   ✧   ✧   ✧

21 July 1997

Hello Jenny,

I received your letter last Friday, the 18th, and thought I'd better answer it right away. I can't go into any great detail about how the evidence was planted against me, so let it be enough that much of the trace evidence that was presented in order to implicate me didn't exist until <u>AFTER</u> I was taken into custody. For instance, head hair and pubic hair was claimed to have been found on some of the victims. However, when I was taken into custody, the police took massive amounts of hair samples from me twice. Then the sheriff's

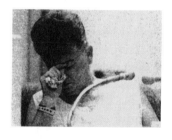

Suff's mother testifying at Bill's trial. Recently, she and her daughter have appeared on the "Leeza Gibbons Show" and "Geraldo" discussing Bill and his crimes. *Photo courtesy of The Californian.*

deputies took a third sampling of hair from me. All three times, it was head hair, arm hair, chest hair and pubic hair that they took. My question is: why did they need <u>that</u> <u>much</u> hair? If they had as much hair from the victims as they claimed to have, all they would have needed from me would be a comparison sample: Just a few hairs from each of the above mentioned sites. Right?! DNA? That's easy to manipulate. I've done an awful lot of reading up on how DNA tests are performed and it can be manipulated to prove anything you want it to prove! And as for the major evidence that was conveniently "found" in areas connected to me. The majority of it wasn't found until a <u>third</u> search! A search over areas that had already been searched twice before. So what does all this suggest to you? Doesn't it make <u>you</u> wonder?!

About my family: A mother, a father, three brothers and three sisters. My father is in Michigan somewhere and hasn't had anything to do with me since 1966, when he left my mother and five kids for some other woman. None of my brothers and two sisters won't even write a letter to me, let alone accept a phone call from me. My mother and baby sister (half-sister, actually) have just lately begun to accept my calls, but cannot send money nor any quarterly packages because they say they can't afford it. Yet they can afford to live in Las Vegas and pay phone bills that amount to a couple hundred dollars a month. No, I don't call but twice a month. My sister makes a lot of long-distance phone calls back east. Also, my mother and sister have been making the rounds to the various talk-shows. They <u>say</u> that they are attempting to help me and prove my innocence.

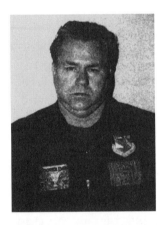

Suff was charged with the brutal murders of 19 women. He claims he is innocent of the crimes. "The police had a scapegoat in me and decided to clear their books by manufacturing my guilt." Clearly, Suff's jury, who decided on the death penalty after only 10 minutes of deliberation, did not believe him.

However, I saw them on the Leeza Gibbons Show in 1995 and the Geraldo Rivera Show last month. It didn't sound like they were helping me at all. In fact, they hurt me rather badly and really ticked off my CAP attorney. My CAP attorney said that she doesn't want me to have anything to do with those shows and has asked my mother and sister to stop appearing on these shows, also. But I've got a strange feeling that they're going to keep right on doing it. That's the way they are. Especially if the show offers them some money!

Yes, there <u>is</u> a disparity between what the media and police have been saying about me and what my friends said about me. There is a dichotomy there and that is what I've been saying all along. The person (or persons) that committed those crimes is <u>not</u> me! The problem is, the person(s) who did the crimes, seems to have moved on to other areas...like Chicago. Did you hear about the guy that was arrested up there? He's given the police there a written confession that includes a statement saying that he committed a lot of the crimes that I was accused of! Plus, he has red hair and the pathologist reports said that a lot of red hair was found on many of the victims I was charged with! I don't have red hair!

Yes, I admit to using the services of prostitutes. But I didn't have a "thing" about it. I was with them only on the spur of the moment. I never went out "looking" for them. I never "planned" on going to a prostitute, it just happened. And yes, like your friend in Minnesota, I was charged with so many cases and suspected of so many more in order to clear the books. I was picked out as a very convenient scapegoat. They built up their case with manufactured and planted evidence. Then they pointed their collective finger at me and said "there he is, go get him!" And yes, I do believe in conspiracy theories. Riverside

County, California is full of them.

Tell you what...if you send me a couple of dollars worth of stamps to cover the postage, I'll send you a copy of my short story "Tranquility Garden." The main character, Lee, is loosely based on me, including my own characteristics and morals. And the place, tranquility garden, actually exists. Not exactly as described in the story, but it does exist. Also, if you're interested, I'll make the same offer to you that I've made to a couple other people: For fifteen dollars (a postal money order), I'll send you an autographed copy of my cookbook, including my award winning Sweet Chili recipe. And yes, I will send you a photo of me (as soon as I have the money to buy a photo ducat) with the return of one of you in exchange. Trouble is, I don't have any money right now to get the photo ducats (coupons) that I have to have in order to get a photo taken of me. That's one of the reasons why I'm offering my cookbook for sale. Eventually I may do the same with my stories that I'm writing.

Jenny, what do you mean by wanting to write <u>about</u> me? In what media? What exactly do you want to write? You are wrong on one count, though. I <u>don't</u> want to die. At least, not for something I didn't do. I'm not afraid of death and I will embrace it when it comes. But I'm not **looking** to die either. I know what happens when we die and it doesn't scare me. But, like I said, I'm not hunting it.

You said I have an important message and that people could learn from me. What do you think that message would be and what could people learn from me? I've been told this before by the police. They wanted me to confess to everything they were claiming I had done. I'm not about to confess to something I didn't do. No matter <u>what</u> supposed evidence they claim to have. I know where that supposed evidence came from and how it came into being. And those few people who <u>really</u> know me are standing up for me and protesting the guilty verdict the jury passed down on me.

Sincerely Yours,
Bill S

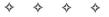

Saturday — 2:00 AM
23 August 1997

Dear Jenny,

How are you doing? I'm well enough, considering. I got your letter yesterday (Friday) afternoon.

You mentioned that after re-reading my letters, you found that I didn't mention anything regarding anyone I ever laid a hand on. Maybe that's because

I never laid a hand on anyone in anger or malice. Huh?! I've always treated people the way I wanted to be treated. I've always accepted people for who I learned they are from personal experience, never from what I heard or read about them. I guess that's one of the reasons why I get along with people in here. I don't care what they did or didn't do that put them in here. How they treat me is how I treat them. If they are gossip-mongers or can't be trusted, I have nothing to do with them. I give myself no reason to trust them. And there are about a half-dozen people that fit into that category, one of them is my brother, a couple are guards here. Everyone who <u>really</u> knows me know that I'm a caring and sensitive man. I fall in love very easily and out of love very difficultly. I cannot hurt what or who I love; not willingly or otherwise!

You are right about the difficulty I have trusting anyone. I trusted my family, my lawyers, my friends and my wife. For the most part, they've all turned their backs on me and/or betrayed me. At least, that's the way I feel. Lately, over the past couple years my depression has grown and so has my paranoia. Recently my paranoia was justified. I found out that two members of my family were going to be on the Geraldo Rivera Show. I was told that the show was going to be about how I was unjustly prosecuted and erroneously given a guilty verdict. I tried to find out <u>when</u> the show was going to air. I wanted to see if my family was going to present a worthwhile defense of me. I finally got the number in New York for one of the show producers. I called her, talked for awhile and she was very sympathetic toward me. She said she didn't have a confirmed date for the airing of the show as yet, but that if I could call her back the next week, she'd probably know then. So a week went by, the show was taped on a Tuesday. I tried to get in touch with the family members who were on the show, to no avail. I was wanting to know how the show went. On the Friday after the show was taped, I placed a return call to the show's producer. Instead of her, I was patched directly to Geraldo, himself. I said that I hadn't called to talk to him, that I just wanted to know when the show was going to air. He said he just wanted to ask me some follow-up questions and then proceeded to lambaste me, spouting of moral outrage with every question. He said that blood, women's clothes were found in my van...a lie. He said that I had confessed to the crimes, another lie. He never gave me an opportunity to properly respond to his accusations, so I finally hung up. A week later, the show aired and portions of our conversation was aired, also. Trouble is, they spliced everything together to get the effect he wanted and then made believe that I had called in right at the time the show was being aired. Making it seem as if the show was live! I was never informed that I was being taped, was never told about the tone the show was going to take, and never told that Geraldo was going to re-prosecute me. I only found out when the show was on, when someone else here yelled to me that I was on the show! Everything I was told, about how the show was going to support me, about how evidence was going to be given that would show I was framed, and about how the police and D.A. broke the law to prosecute me; it was all a front. Geraldo wanted to have a show that would back up the prosecution of what the public viewed as a heinous, illiterate monster! He didn't want anything to do with presenting the truth about me or showing that there might have been massive misconduct by the law and the D.A.'s office in their efforts to prosecute me, wrongly! In light of all this, can you really blame me for being paranoid and wary of trusting others?

Sorry, I didn't mean to get off on that negative tone, but I wanted to show you the lengths others have gone to make me appear as something I am not now, nor have I ever been. It almost has gotten me to the point that I'm even afraid to trust those who are truly attempting to help me and have my best interests at heart. So, I hope you'll forgive any initial skepticism I may have shown, or that you may have read in the words of my previous letters. Alright? Now, back to your letter.

Of course, my trial was nothing more than a mockery of justice. The trial didn't determine my innocence or guilt. That was determined long before a jury was chosen. Anymore, almost any big decision is made by our supposedly "unbiased" news media.

In my case, the media took every unsubstantiated rumor, every lie "leaked" by the police and printed or broadcasted them as fact. That's where Geraldo got those outrageous accusations that bloody clothing was found in my possession or that there was a confession. In reality? Yes, there was a few items of feminine clothing in my van...belonging to my wife. The police thought there was blood sprayed across a seat in my van...it was Dr. Pepper that my wife had spilled. And as I've already said, there was never any kind of confession. The police sergeant in charge claimed that in order to attract the news media into giving negative information about me. (The police sergeant has since been fired for criminal acts that she committed!!) After that "leak," she began "leaking" half-truths and other outright lies. The news media then proceeded to run away with their "feeding frenzy" of reporting everything and anything that would make me appear in a negative way. None of my accomplishments, good deeds or benevolent acts were reported. Nobody heard or read anything good about me before or during my trial. So it wasn't surprising that I was found guilty, or wound up with a death sentence. It was decreed by the news media. There's an old saying that people generally apply to fighting a war. However, that saying is more aptly used when it's applied to criminal trials (or elections). The saying... "Control a nation's news reporting agencies, and you control the nation!" It's proven all the time, when you actually sit down and give it some serious thought. And I dare anyone to prove me wrong in that statement!

You said that it's hard to believe how many people (men) in prison would have possibly not wound up in prison if they'd had some place to go or someone to talk to; that they might have gotten families or good jobs. Well, I don't know if you're aware of what my living conditions were like before I was pinned with this rap or not, but I was fairly well off. I had a good wife, a daughter, a terrific job and friends that liked me and valued our friendship. I didn't have a lot of money, but I didn't need a lot of money. I always had my bills paid, tithed to my church and was able to donate to the needy. I didn't have a lot of possessions, but I had enough to keep me occupied. Whenever one of my friends needed help, I was the first to volunteer my assistance. Whenever someone needed something and it didn't run me short and I had it to spare, it was theirs. That's how I was before I was arrested, that's the way I still am and that's one of the reasons I get along with anyone I meet. Does that sound like someone who might have committed the crimes they blame me for?

You are correct in the point you made about my not being allowed to speak for myself. My trial attorney (the lead attorney) would not allow me to testify in my own defense. The only time I was allowed to speak was after everything was over, when I was allowed to give my final statement. Then I was just scoffed at. Hopefully, what you are doing will give me a voice that so far has been completely ignored or silenced. Also, if your desire is to be featured on the "Headliners" with Geraldo (or whomever he has hosting it), I hope you are very skeptical of his promises or statements as to how the program will develop. Remember what he did to me and my family!

Going to sign off here. Take care and write back soon.

Best Wishes
Bill S.

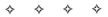

23 September 1997

Dear Jenny,

I just got your letter a few minutes ago and decided to write back immediately and try to get this out tonight. I'm not feeling very good right now. I went out to the yard today and on my way back in after being out there all morning, my knee gave out and I began to fall. Luckily, there was an officer nearby and she grabbed me, kept me from falling and held me up until I could get my leg under me again. My left knee is swollen some now and it hurts quite a bit. I've taken a couple pain tablets (Ibuprofen) and hope they take effect soon. If I can bring the pain down to a tolerable level, I can use self-hypnosis to get rid of the remaining pain. I'm glad I learned how to perform self-hypnosis all those many years ago. It helps me at many points in my life.

I was re-reading some of your past letters and located one that I did not answer as yet. Somehow I missed it. So I'm going to answer this one first and then answer the one I missed.

Yes, I <u>do</u> have a rather dysfunctional family. None of my 3 brothers will write me, send stamps, money or even a greeting card. In my family, I'm the eldest, then there's Bob (2 years younger), Don (3 yrs younger), Ken (5 years younger than me), then my sisters — Roberta (9 years younger), Deena (my daughter by marriage, sister by adoption — a story in it's own right), and Bernice (my half-sister and the youngest). Bob is a mechanic in Vegas lived with my mom until just recently. Don also lives in Vegas and is the trouble maker in the family. He has caused endless problems for just about every other member of our family. Since my arrest and conviction, he claims that I am reason he lost his wife, job and was forced out of our home town. In all honesty, my problems, and the overdone publicity might have contributed to some of his problems, but they were not the cause. Don's wife, Leah, left him because he was arrested, tried and placed on probation for molesting (sexually) her younger sister. He was employed as a disc jockey for a teen night club. He lost his job because the nightclub was closed down. The kids began to loiter in a famous inn that was across the street and began causing problems for staff and patrons, so the police and city government closed the nightclub down. And forced out of town? People began to find out that he had been convicted and served time for raping a prostitute in the early 80's (or late 70's) and also found out about his crime regarding Leah's young sister. Nobody would employ him nor rent him an apartment. Every girl he became friendly with would break up with him after discovering he had lied to them regarding his losses. Now, though he is still married to Leah, he is living with a black girl whom is employed as a guard at a Prison near Las Vegas. Whether or not she knows the truth regarding his troubles with the law, I'm not aware. As I've said already, he will not contact me in any way, shape or manner. I only know what's been happening from what my attorney finds out from my sister, Bernice. Ken still lives in Riverside County. He works as a construction worker, has his contracter's license and works nearly everyday. He lives with his common law wife and 5 children, each child's name begins with a "K". Roberta lives in Las Vegas, is married with 4 children. She had a daycare service operating out of her home. I heard she says the parents stopped using her service when they heard she was related to me. Now she works as a secretary in an office building in Vegas. Deena is in the Army, living somewhere in North Carolina. She's married and has a son. She won't let me know where she lives because she doesn't want any negative publicity associated with her family. I don't blame her, but I miss her. Bernice lives in Vegas with my mother. She's attending a nursing school and plans on becoming an R.N. She still believes in me, but doesn't write much and prefers I not call but once a month. I've got no problem with that, I don't want to run my mother's phone bill up, seeing as I can no longer help her with her bills. I've been limiting my phone calls to my civil attorney, my CAP attorney and to one of my trial attorneys. Trouble is, they're out of their office more often then they're in. Since I can only call my mother and Bernice once a month or so to get updates on them, I get real lonesome to hear the voice of someone that isn't a prisoner. A couple that I used to know before I was arrested used to write me in the county jail before I came here and would let me call them collect when I felt lonesome. But they won't accept my calls now and don't write anymore. None of my old friends that I have phone numbers for will accept my calls, either. Anyway, you now know more about my family than you probably wanted to know. Right?!

If you ever consider appearing on Geraldo — My best advice is: Don't!!! He verbally attacks anyone defending prisoners, especially death row prisoners, or fighting for prisoner's rights. His people told us that he was going to come down on the way the police and prosecutor <u>persecuted</u> me and my family, and as an attorney, would realize how the police planted and fabricated the evidence in my case. When my mother, sister and civil attorney got on the show, and when he got me on the phone after the show was taped, he immediately jumped in with both feet, spouting off righteous indignity, that we would dare say the law and the courts could have made mistakes or even committed criminal acts themselves. If you don't have hard, factual and tangible evidence to back up your comments, Geraldo won't give you a chance to get your points across. He takes what the cops and prosecutors say as gospel truth, but everyone else is a liar. He was told that the police found bloody, women's clothing in my van. Untrue! The clothes they found belonged to my wife. What they found that they <u>thought</u> was dried blood, was actually spilled Dr. Pepper. When the truth regarding those two subjects was discovered, it was conveniently kept from the press so they wouldn't print a retraction about me.

Regarding prostitutes: I did <u>not</u> use the sexual services of prostitutes while I was married, nor while I had a steady girlfriend. Between '89 and '90 I did; but before '89, I was with Bonnie and <u>never</u> cheated on her. After I married Cheryl, I again had no reason to obtain sex outside of my relationship with her. <u>However,</u> I did visit with <u>one</u> prostitute but <u>not</u> for sex. We had become friends and I promised her that if she ever needed any help, to call me...or if I saw her on the streets, I would stop and if I could, I would help her out with some cash.

Her name (street name) was Michelle, but after I was arrested, no one could find her. I never told Cheryl about Michelle, because she wouldn't have understood. Cheryl's mother surely wouldn't have understood. Trouble is, without Michelle, none of what I say can be proven. Also, without Michelle none of what the prosecution said can be <u>disproven</u>! The only connection to prostitutes they can make after I was married is the evidence they <u>manufactured</u> that <u>looks</u> like I was with those who were murdered. However, someone has come to my attorneys who says they have proof that DNA evidence collected from me <u>AFTER</u> I was arrested was added to some of the cases, saying that it was collected <u>from the bodies</u>! This person also says that proof exists that tire and shoe tracks used against me in all of the cases did not come from the murder scenes! Again, that information cannot be used to clear me until my attorneys bring it up at my appeal.

My past record? I guess you're talking about Texas and my daughter, Dijianét Jawn (Dee-Sha-nay Shawn). I can't really tell you a lot about that case, except that my first wife (Teryl) and I were both tried by the same prosecutor,

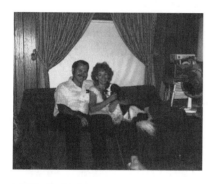

Bill Suff with his ex-girlfriend, Bonnie, prior to the Riverside convictions. Suff says she is the love of his life.

the same judge, jury and evidence. After the trial was over, two jurors told the attorneys Teryl and I had, that they could not decide who was guilty, so they found both of us guilty. The only factual evidence that was presented against me was the fact that I was home at the time D.J. was inflicted with the fatal injury. However, so was Teryl. But there was more against her. The morning of the afternoon I found D.J., Teryl was getting ready for work when two ladies she worked with came to the door to pick her up. Usually, Teryl would open the door and let them in to wait. That morning, she only cracked the door open and made them wait on the front porch in the cold. Those two ladies testified that they could see into the bedroom and saw me asleep in bed. Teryl said that when she left that morning, she yelled at me as she walked out the door to wake me up. The two ladies testified that they saw I was still asleep and that Teryl said not one word to me! Also, when I called her at work telling her something was wrong and she should come right home, she said "What's wrong with the baby?" One thing that never came out at the trial was her deciding she did not want Deena, her first daughter (more on that later). She told me and her mother that she didn't want a daughter! That's why she gave Deena up for adoption so my mother could have her (hence, my daughter by marriage — sister by adoption). When D.J. came along, Teryl was very upset and wouldn't have anything to do with her caretaking. I had to do everything: I changed D.J.'s diapers, fed her, bathed her, and played with her (what little play you can do with a 3 month old). After D.J. was born was when Teryl began to have another affair. This time with one of her co-workers. And then you should see another inconsistancy, when you look at what I did before D.J. died... I was in the Air Force working as a medical corpsman in the base hospital on the pediatrics ward. Six days a week, I took care of children from newborns up to 16-year-olds. I've always loved children and was very happy when Deena, Billy Jr., and D.J. were all born. I lost Deena because I was in the Air Force in Texas and because Teryl decided to give her up because she had <u>supposedly</u> been raped, thereby giving her an unwanted daughter. I had nothing to say in the matter, because I wasn't the father! That's what Teryl and my mother told me over the phone (I was in Fort Worth, Texas — they were here in California). By the time I came home on emergency leave, the adoption was already done and over with. So you can imagine how hurt I was when I found D.J. dead. The first daughter I had was taken from me by Teryl's and my mother's choice. My second daughter was taken from me (I can only guess) by Teryl's insistance that she not have a daughter (her own words)! My son was taken from me by the courts because I was in jail. That's three children I've lost. Because of this current case, the state took my 4th child from me, another daughter. Everything in my life that I've desired, has been taken from me. So you can see how I can get so discouraged and depressed? The Texas case took more than 10 years of my life from me for something I didn't do. And now because of the Texas case, a bunch of cops and a prosecutor picked me as a good prospect to place the blame for a bunch of killings. They saw me as an ex-felon on parole that no one would miss. So why not blame me, let me take the fall, clear their books and make the public happy? Make everyone believe they caught their killer, while the real killer (or killers) moved on to other areas...just like the Green River Killer did.

My friendships? I had many friends, more female friends than male friends, and they all knew that if they needed help, I was the <u>first</u> person they could come to. I helped my friends to move; I babysat for my friends; when they needed to go somewhere, I took them there. One friend had to go to court regarding her daughter. I took off work all day so I could sit with her in court to give her moral support. She finally got her daughter back, but I don't think my being there helped that much. One apartment complex I lived in was at the base of a mountain range that catches fire every other summer or so. One summer I was there and a fire was going right down the mountains toward us. The police came around asking that everyone leave for their own protection. I wouldn't leave. I had a neighbor take my birds with her and I stayed on top of the roof of the complex with a water hose. Hot and firey embers were coming down on the roof and I stayed there, putting them out with the hose. Everyone else left, but I stayed on. A couple other roofs in the area wound up with burned holes in their tops, but not ours. I protected my place and my friends places. That's the kind of person I am.

Death Threats! I got my first one three days after I was locked up. The second night I was in the jail, the TV News broadcasted that I had been arrested and had given the cops a confession. The next day, the area newspapers picked up the story. As I told you before, it was a lie put out by the cops. However, you know how people are when they see something on the news or in a newspaper...if it's there, it must be true. So that next day I was on my way to the showers and several inmates in their cells told me that they were going to kill me and save the state the cost. That's continued ever since. All based on that one news report.

Conditions here at San Quentin are fair enough. I'm treated civilly by the guards. The meals are decent and for the most part filling. I get to take a shower and shave three times a week (not as often as I'd like) and am able to go out to the exercise yard seven days a week, though I usually stay in on Saturday and Sunday to rest and catch up on my sleep. But Monday through Friday I'm usually out on the exercise yard (from 7 am to 1 pm) and playing dominoes, pinochle, Uno or just walking around the yard talking to some of the other guys assigned to my yard. Not quite what the prosecutor from my case claimed about me on Geraldo ("Suff is so afraid of being shanked, he never leaves his cell!"), then showed a picture that was taken of me on the yard!

Anyway, the last chance I have to send this out tonight is only a couple of minutes away, so I'm going to end this here. I'll write more when I hear from you again. Take care and write soon.

Love & Wishes,
Bill S

16 November 1997

Dear Jenny,

I hope you are well and surviving all of the cold and wet weather. I received your letter of 10/18 this past Friday (11/14). I'm definitely not giving up. One man that is on my exercise yard and lives just a few cells down from me, just found out from his attorney that he's got a reversal and the D.A. has decided not to re-file on his case. I can't tell you his name or what his case is about because I promised him I wouldn't talk to anyone about him. That's a promise I intend on keeping. Besides, I don't talk about my own case and there's no way I'd talk about someone else's. Anyway, besides him, there are two other guys that I know who got their cases reversed also and are getting results. It gives me hope and that's why I'm not giving up. Regarding that man in Illinois that you mentioned who finally got his hearing on DNA...because of bureaucracy and red tape, not to mention slow moving appellate attorneys and judges, that guy lost 20 years of his life. When you're an innocent person in prison and the public believes you are guilty, you wind up losing **many** years out of your life (and sometimes they **lose** their life). And it's all because of lies, misinterpretation of evidence and mistakes made by jurors who don't understand all of the court's instructions. And, of course, some of the mistakes made by the jurors are because the prosecution will lie to them, saying the evidence points out one thing, when actually it says something else. (For instance, the DNA evidence that was presented against me was supposed to prove that I was the killer. Actually, all it really proved is that, if it **was** my DNA, maybe it was there because I had had sex with them sometime **before** they had been killed by the real killer. Curious thing, the victims who supposedly had DNA evidence matched to me were girls who had been killed during the time period after Bonnie and I broke up and before I met Cheryl. However, I still maintain that a lot of the DNA evidence that was presented didn't exist before I was arrested and they collected it from me, then applied it to the cases they were trying to clear up! After all, the police were under a lot of pressure to solve those murders. They had to find someone they could pin it all on.) And when the defense tries to correct those mistakes, human nature takes over. That human nature wants to believe the worst in all instances. They **want** to believe that the accused is guilty. If a poll had been taken before my trial, it would have come back 95% in favor of a guilty verdict and a sentence to death! How do I know that? From the way the news media talked about me and the results of the voir dire questionnaires the juror pool filled out before my trial. Of all the questionnaires I examined (about 50 of the 400 plus), only 3 or 4 of them were really impartial and unsure of my guilt or innocence. Only one of those jurors were finally picked, and that juror only served as an alternate juror. He never even got a vote in the decision. The others were excused by the prosecution as being undesirable jurors. The entire jury was stacked with people who believed I was guilty before my trial even started. But now I'm getting into sensitive territory here. So on to other subjects.

Regarding Michelle, the girl I was seeing, even after I got married. I think I first started visiting with her (accepting her generous offers) about 3 or 4 months after Bonnie (did I tell you about her?) and I broke up for the last time. Michelle was a very pretty mexican girl (about 5'4", 100 lbs., dark brown hair and eyes, a cute tattoo of Pegasus on her left hip and a rose above her right breast) and in her early 20's. Whether or not she used any form of drugs, I never found out. I had asked her to leave the Riverside area and move in with me after a couple of months of "seeing" her and getting to know her. But she refused my request, saying that she already had a boyfriend and wouldn't answer any of my questions about him or even if he knew how she spent her evenings. However, when I got engaged to Cheryl (about six months later), Michelle became extremely upset with me. She wouldn't even talk to me the next few times I saw her on the street. Finally, she began talking to me again, though she was still slightly miffed because I would no longer accept her offers. I'd like to think that she came to respect me for my steadfast faithfulness to Cheryl. At first, she couldn't understand why I was offering her help (financially and materially), but wouldn't go to bed with her. However, she finally came to see that I truly liked her and only had her welfare in mind. Of course, I never told Cheryl about Michelle, she wouldn't have understood. Besides, being a complete mama's girl, she was always telling her mother everything that happened in our lives. Her mother would have blown my relationship with Michelle all out of proportion. Her mother didn't much care for me because I was 21 years older than Cheryl and only 2 years younger than her. Also, I believe she tried to hit on me a couple times. She was always brushing up against me, touching me and leaning over me while resting one of her breasts on my shoulder. Once she even tried to get me to drink with her during a card game and became perturbed when I wouldn't (I don't really care for liquor or wine). But I never caught on to what she was trying to do (I never claimed to be that smart -- remind me to tell you about Virginia Baldwin at March AFB). It wasn't until I realized that her husband worked some very odd hours and that she'd had two affairs already that I added it up. After that, I was hesitant about going to visit Cheryl's family and then tried to stay out of her mother's way. Cheryl's father liked me, however, and her younger brother and sisters absolutely loved me. Her older brother didn't care for me at first, but came to like me after he got to know me better. Anyway, back to Michelle. I described her to my attorneys and investigators, telling them that she could testify as to what type of person I was and probably even give me an alibi for the time periods/days that I was supposed to have committed one or two of the murders. But my investigators couldn't find her. Therefore, an alibi that might have cleared me, was never brought out. Anyway, I told you all of this just to let you know a little more about my relationship with Michelle.

Regarding Geraldo...again! I've watched a lot of his programs both before and after the fiasco he pulled on me. Did you, by any chance, catch any of his programs regarding the Jonbenet Ramsey case or the British au pair case? He is absolutely convinced of their guilt and calling for a conviction in both cases. He wants to see both of the Ramsey's convicted of the murder of their daughter, Jonbenet. And he's outraged that the British nanny was sentenced to time served and released. He led off that program with the statement:

"You've all heard about the British au pair being released from jail with a time-served sentence. First of all, I believe she is as guilty as can be of killing that poor baby and deserves the maximum punishment!"

He doesn't want to hear any kind of extenuating evidence or anything that might prove the girl innocent. He's got his mind made up that she's guilty and nothing will change his mind. That human nature that I mentioned earlier in this letter? Geraldo Rivera carries that human nature to it's farthest extent. If someone is just suspected of wrong doing, Geraldo's positive that that person is guilty of that crime and probable more! You can't deal with a person who thinks like that. He's a radical of the worst type. He's worse than any criminal prosecutor! Please, don't have anything to do with him. He'll tear you apart and preach the worst kind of filth and slime about whomever you're trying to help. Me or anyone else. It's a no win situation.

I just got a letter from one of my attorneys the other day. He told me that my mother and baby sister have left the west coast. They were living in Las Vegas, Nevada. My attorney said that they have once again been run out of another town. That makes the fifth town they've had to leave now. This time they moved to the east coast and now live in North Carolina somewhere. He said they were receiving a lot of crank and obscene calls on their answering machine and that their apartment windows had been broken several times. The apartment complex they were living in served them with eviction papers because of the broken windows and obscenities painted on the apartment walls. He didn't say anything about how he found out that information or exactly where in North Carolina they moved too; no address, no phone number. I was hoping that I'd finally get through to them and get them to come here for a face-to-face meeting. Guess that won't be happening now.

Well, I guess that's about all I've got to write about for now. I've covered all of the subjects that you mentioned in your letter and got into another one or two. I'll be sitting here, patiently awaiting your next letter. Take care of yourself and your children. Write when you get a chance. Wishing you love and happiness, as always...

Your friend,
Bill L. Suff

Dear Jenny,

I just got your letter this afternoon (I made out all my Christmas Cards late last night). Your letter was a little hard to read (You evidently wrote it quickly), but I was able to work my way through it. To be perfectly honest with you, though, I really don't know how to respond to it. You seem to be unsure **what** I am...in your words "utterly evil, in denial or innocent." Of course, not knowing me before, I can see why [you] might be skeptical about my claims of innocence. I wish you could talk to the people who do believe in me and know that I am innocent. A husband and wife couple I've known since the mid-80's when I worked for the husband (Dave and Florence).

Since your last letter, I've found out just how much my civil attorney, Brian Lane, lied to me in order to write his book about me. He told me how much he believed that I had been railroaded, framed and convicted on false evidence. Then he turned around and tore me apart in his book. All this **after** he told me that witnesses had come forward explaining how the prosecutor in my case mis-represented evidence that was said to have been found at murder scenes, when actually it was found nowhere **near** the scenes. Tire and shoe prints, body hairs, etc. Because of him and one of my trial attorneys, I'm becoming very paranoid of everyone! My own family proclaimed over the phone and in person that they believed my statements of innocence. But then they went on Geraldo Rivera's and Leeza Gibbons' shows and say that I must be guilty because of all the evidence that was produced against me! Throughout this entire mess, only two people have stood steadfastly by my side: Florence and Dave. They **know** how the police have been framing people for various crimes. They were witness to specific threats made against prostitutes and street people. Florence was also approached by a prostitute requesting money so she could get out of town because she had just seen two men beat another prostitute to death. She knew those two men to be police officers on the town's police force and that they knew her! However, all of this evidence was not allowed because it was decreed to be hear-say evidence (no matter <u>how</u> true it might be)! But I'm getting off the track. Back to your letter...

I know how just about everyone in prison hollers at the top of their lungs that they are innocent. Some of them might actually be innocent. In my case, I **am** innocent!!! But because of everything the news media, the police and the prosecutor in my case claim, no one believes me (except Florence and Dave, of course). As I think I've already said in a previous letter, the public tends to believe that the police and the prosecutors are infallible; and that if the news media reports it, it <u>must</u> be the truth. But the public in general doesn't read of the retractions that are printed on page 22-C! The newspapers have never, in my memory, come right out on the front page with an apology for mistakes made in previous newspaper editions. And the television and radio news broadcasts never admit to an error in their reporting, either. Can you recall that kind of admission ever being presented to the public right up front? I can't and neither can anyone else I've talked to. Admitting mistakes is bad for business. You can't make any money if you let the public know that you make mistakes in your reporting of the news. Also, the news media can't come right out and say that the police are making a mistake when all they get is one side of the story...the prosecutor's story. The defense can't afford to reveal the defendant's side because then it allows the prosecution to fabricate some evidence that negates everything the defense is trying to prove. So in that instance, the defendant can't get fair treatment by the press.

Well, I think I've gone off on this tangent long enough. Besides, I want this to go out with your Christmas card tonight. Be careful in all you do and have a very joyous holiday season. Wishing you a very Merry Christmas and a prosperous New Year. As always...

Warmest Wishes To You,
Bill S

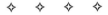

23 February, 1998

Dear Jenny,

I got your letter of 31 January this past Friday (the 20th). It was very nice to have gotten another one from you after such a long time of not hearing from you. I was beginning to think that you were going to do the same thing that Brian Lane did to me. He got what he could from me so he could write his book and then he wrote me off. What he couldn't get from me, he made up or lied about. So many of the people who began writing to me when this nightmare started have thrown me away just like the state and my family has done. Needless to say, your letter brightened my day considerably. And, with all of this gloomy weather lately, I needed a lift from somewhere. So, thank you for writing back to me at last.

If I remember correctly, some time ago I promised to send you a photograph of me as soon as I was able to get one taken. Well, enclosed you should have found a recent photo of me (yes, I know, I'm beginning to put on some weight). I got pictures taken the same day I got your letter (last Friday). Ergo, you get the one I promised to send you. Hope it doesn't scare your kids. I know that I'm not among the best looking of guys. In fact, I think I'm rather on the homely side. Oh well.

Since I haven't been going out to the yard, I haven't had much of an opportunity to talk to Doug Clark lately. I do see him every few days, though, when he passes by my cell heading for the showers. He's a dozen or so cells further down the tier from me.

Jenny, if I have any say in the matter, I hope to remain friends with you for as long as you want to be my friend. I have so few friends (and I've lost so many of the ones I had before this nightmare started), that I cherish every one I do find. Other than you, I've only got two other people that I can honestly name as a friend. One in Riverside (that I hear from every few months) and one in Tampa, Florida (who writes a little more often).

You know, it's strange that you mentioned the odd circumstances of the darkness that has followed me throughout my adult life (from Texas to Riverside). There is an eerie explanation for it, the only one I've been able to come up with. Back in '87 I went to see a fortune teller/palm reader at a local flea market with a friend. This fortune teller/palm reader read my palm and had some **very** interesting things to say. Then she read her Tarot cards and said that I was in trouble. She told me that my "aura" was being attacked because someone had placed a black spell on me. She said that it had been placed on me by someone I had once known whom had hurt me and caused a death in my family. She said that she could remove the "curse," but that it would cost me about $20.00 in coffee and sugar. I was willing to pay it, but when I went back the next weekend, she wasn't there anymore. That left me with no other option except to watch my step and be very careful in my day to day travels. I did some long and deep thinking, though. The only person I could possibly think of that fit the two statements she had pointed out was my first wife. Teryl had hurt me several times by having affairs with other men. Then she killed our daughter, Dijianét (pronounced Dee-szhuh-nay), and left me to face the punishment that she actually deserved. Also, Teryl believed in the "black arts" and was in the habit of practicing with the Tarot. I don't know how much credence **you** place in those beliefs, but **I've** come to believe in them from personal experience. I've seen things happen that had no other explanation. Yes, it was gut-wrenching to me when I found Dijianét dead. I cried so hard that my throat and chest hurt. I still remember it vividly. And that intense pain was brought back to me when, during my trial, the prosecutor brought the whole thing up in front of the jury. Do I believe Teryl killed Dijianét? Yes!!! There is really no other answer that can be derived when the actual clues are examined. I still remember the off-hand things she said when her first daughter (Deena) was born, things she said during our marriage and off-hand comments she made after I found Dijianét in her crib. What would it make me feel toward women in general? Nothing in particular, certainly not any kind of anger. What did I feel about Teryl? I just wished that she could have faced the punishment she deserved for what she did. Actually, if I had been the type of person that the police, the prosecutor and newscasts said I was, I would never have gone after someone who had nothing to do with Dijianét's murder. I don't believe the innocent should suffer for the crimes of the guilty. Neither should everyone pay for the actions of one or two people.

As for your other personal question ("I **seem** charming, like I had a variety of "choices" among women. Why pay? Excitement?") No, not excitement. I was looking for love. I was looking for a lady that would love me as much as I could love her. It didn't matter to me that she might be a prostitute, as long as

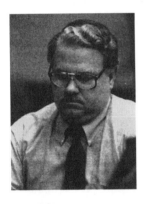

she was willing to change for me. But I think I told you that I had more or less proposed to two different prostitutes at one time or another. I was willing to overlook their past. I just asked them to change before becoming my girlfriend. They didn't want to be my girlfriend though, so I went on with my search. And as I've told you, when I found the girl who decided to marry me, I quit using the services of prostitutes. But as for your question as to why I visited with them...I am quite a bit on the shy side and find it difficult to approach women who don't start up a conversation with me first or is introduced to me by another person. I've always needed to feel wanted, even if I had to pay for it. And one of those girls did become a good friend of mine. I think I told you about Michelle, didn't I? Trouble is, the police were able to use the fact that I had visited with prostitutes against me. And they blew the

Bill Suff during his trial. He says he was devastated when he was found guilty of 13 counts of first degree murder. *Photo courtesy of The Californian.*

relationship I had with them all out of proportion, making up their "facts" to suit their own perverted theories. But now I'm getting too far into my case again. Sorry about that.

Well, Jenny, I think I'd better close out this letter here. Until my next letter to you, take care of yourself and your children, stay healthy, warm and dry and write back when you can.

Love and best wishes to you,
Bill S.

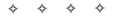

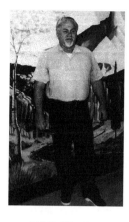

Bill Suff today.

26 April 1998

Hello Jenny,

   I happily received your latest letter this past Friday (the 24th). I haven't received any mail from **anyone** in such a long time that I was rather startled when the officer stopped in front of my cell with the mail-cart. Strange, I also got a letter from some lady in Dublin, Ireland. I'm still trying to figure out how she got my name and CDC number. I don't mind the letter, though. Being Irish myself, I'm always interested in hearing from another countryman (or woman). I **was** writing to one guy from Dundalk, Ireland for a short while just after I first arrived here. But I quit writing to him because he was so persistent in asking me about pertinent details regarding my case. He kept asking me specific questions as to how the crimes were committed. I couldn't answer them because I didn't commit the crimes and don't know the answers. Other questions, I wouldn't answer because they might be detrimental to my appeal. I **can** not and **will** not answer any kind of question that may be harmful to my appeal.

   Easter. Well...it was very much like Thanksgiving, Christmas and New Year's for me: Just another day. No, I didn't see anyone. There's no one that will come to visit with me. So, I spent the day in my cell, working on my Fantasy-Fiction novel ("A Whisper From The Dark"). I did get the phone at 1:00 pm on Easter day, though. I tried to call the three people whom I have phone numbers for. Unfortunately, one was refused and the other two didn't pick up the receiver to answer my call. I was really lonesome that day and wanted to hear the voice of someone who knew me and was at least a little sympathetic toward me. However, I had to spend the day with only my memories. So I just tried to escape from the loneliness I felt by immersing myself in the TV programs I was watching.

   I'm glad to hear that you and your family are all feeling well. Glad you were able to visit with your folks on Easter. I'll bet the kids had a blast. Grandparents do tend to spoil their grand-kids rotten. I know all about that. My mother fawned over my daughter whenever I took her down to Salton Sea for a visit. Like you, I wasn't rich, but I had enough money to pay my bills and afford a few extras. That's all I needed. Like now, I have a TV, a typewriter, I can get books to read from the prison library, and I can write down the stories that I dream up. The only thing I lack now is a cassette/radio. I'd like to be able to listen to music when the electricity goes off here or when I'm trying to go to sleep. And something that I don't think anyone can help me get: A lady-friend that I can say "I Love You" to and have it returned in kind. A lady who would care for me the way I would care about her. I hear about someone falling in love with Richard Rameriz and marrying him, and I ache beyond belief. I'm the type of person who **needs** love in my life. Without someone to care for, I feel incomplete.

The medical people came through the building giving TB tests to everyone. No choice. You get one or you get written up. Now I have a needle hole in my left forearm (I hate getting needles in my left arm) and a dime-sized red spot where the TB test serum was injected. No, it's not a positive reaction. I don't have TB. It's just the normal reaction of my body fighting off a foreign substance that was administered to it. My body doesn't like stuff put in it that doesn't belong there. That's just one of the reasons I never took drugs of any kind. I've never even smoked marijuana. It never bothered me that other people I knew chose that course of enjoyment (?) in their lives. I've always let people live the life-path they chose. I've always believed in the live and let credo. I'm not one to judge others for what they do. Just as long as they don't try to push their choices unto me. After all, I've never attempted to push my beliefs on others.

Regarding that book by Brian Lane. Did you get that one or the one that was co-written by Christine Keers (the one who was fired from the police force)? Both of them presented erroneous views of me. The author has either misplaced the facts or I have a split personality. If I had a split personality, it would have exhibited itself in my letters and my daily life here. Such is not the case. So it leaves only one answer: The books are wrong!

Sorry, I can't tell you anything regarding my appeal(s). It still hasn't started. It won't until I finally get an appellate attorney. And if I can't find one for myself, one that will take on my case for free, I'll get appointed one by the courts that may or may not do the job right. Brian Lane told me that he was going to look for a good appellate attorney that would volunteer to take on my case free of charge (for the fame that may come from it). But I guess that's just one more lie on top of all of the others he told me. Anyway, as I said, there's nothing new I can tell you about that.

My best to all of you.

Love and more
Bill S

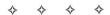

Friday – 8 August 1997
2:00 am

Dear Jenny,

I received your letter today. It was great hearing from you so quickly. Every day, I stand at the door to my cell when I know it's mail call. I rest my head against the bars, just praying that I'll get <u>something</u> in the mail. Something that will remind me that <u>someone</u> out there cares enough about me to take a little time out of their day to write a few lines to me and spend a little money on me (the material and stamp). Usually, though, it's a letter from someone who wants something from me. My civil attorney wants more information that he can use to make more money on. He just let me know that my mother and a sister are trying to contact someone back east that wants to buy memorabilia of mine because I'm supposed to be this infamous serial killer. They are promoting my guilt! One of my brothers wants to sell my van to the highest bidder, touting it as the infamous vehicle of the killer. Again, promoting my guilt! The investigative team that worked on my defense has suddenly turned on me, not wanting anything further to do with me. I've heard that they read something that I was supposed to have written wherein I supposedly blasted and belittled their efforts to defend me. The problem is, I never wrote anything of the sort! They didn't even pay me the courtesy of confronting <u>me</u> with their accusations. They refuse my phone calls, send my letters back unopened. One of those people was a lady that I really began to care a lot for. I guess you could say I was beginning to actually fall in love with her. And now she won't have anything to do with me. That really hurts. So, from all of this, I hope you can see how much I treasure a letter from someone who isn't really trying to exploit me. However, when the officer handing out the mail passes me by, the let-down is almost heart-breaking. And you know, even getting the next issue of the magazines I used to get eased that let-down from getting to me. (I used to subscribe to TV Guide, Dell Crossword Puzzle Magazine, People Magazine, Arizona Highway, and Omni Magazine. All of those subscriptions have expired, though.) Anyway, like I said, it was great getting your letter.

As to your proposal — I agree, with one proviso: That no photographs of me or from my case be used without my prior approval. The use of my letters is okay with me. By the way, which publisher did you approach? I like the point that it will focus on the <u>Person</u>, rather than the supposed crimes. Very few people look at that side of the equation.

A page from one of Bill Suff's letters.

The Anonymous Letters

The following letters are from people who did not want to be included in the book. Their letters were so interesting, I really didn't want to leave them out, so as a compromise, I decided to include them, but I omitted their names and in some places I have changed or omitted other identifying information.

"Mr. X"

April 29, 97

Hi,

How's thing's?

Your letter arrived yesterday and I've been trying to decide <u>how</u> to respond to it ... and even <u>if</u> I should.

Over the past — almost — 10 years, I've heard from a lot of people, all over the world ... some, sincere in their efforts, others, merely looking to make a name or money, off the suffering of me, my family and others.

You seem like a bright, well-written/spoken young woman, so I'm sure you can comprehend my need to be very cautious, as to who I write to or communicate with. Yes?

Due to my situation, I have developed my own way in which to communicate with someone, and — I've found — quickly discover if they are someone worth devoting a portion of my writing time — or not.

You say you're not a cop or reporter (AKA shiteaters) and well ... talk is cheap. You can <u>say</u> anything, but that doesn't make it true.

I give you the benefit of the doubt though, Jenny. And I give you the opportunity to <u>show</u> me I can trust you. <u>Show</u> me you are one of the very few I really communicate with, and get to know.

Because I'll tell you from the start, that's the "<u>only</u>" kind of writing I do. My time is too valuable, to waste writing anything else but <u>serious</u> efforts to "communicate."

Do you understand what I'm saying?

It's okay though.

This is <u>entirely</u> up to y - o - u!

If you're up to it ... willing ... and want to .... we can start working towards making you the 6th of this very select group.

Believe me, the great letters these girls write to me, the length and depth of them ——————— keep me <u>very</u> busy.

But I am willing to consider adding you to that group ... if you wish (?)

All you need to do, is show me!

Yes, the dynamics between male + female, interest me, as they do you.

Maybe it surprises you , but I am fascinated by the female perspectives on thing's ... and that's a <u>primary</u> subject of my communications with females.

That <u>is</u> a primary area of interest I have in <u>you</u>!

And I've found it's best and fastest, to find out from the Get/Go, if the person I'm writing, is willing or not, to allow me to get to know + understand them as I need and want to.

Would it surprise you to know I don't deal with frustration, very well? (Because I don't.)

I ask thing's, and go "places" in my letters, that I realize — probably — nobody has asked or gone before ... and quite possibly <u>never</u> will.

Much of it involves what's between your ears .... much of it involves what's between your legs ... <u>all</u> of it has a reason, and a meaning, that sometimes you will be able to guess; but other times, you will <u>think</u> you understood, but don't. (Can't?)

Are you still reading ... or have you thrown my letter into the air, and run out of the room — screaming!!

I want you to know + understand<u> from the start</u>, how this is going to be between us ... <u>if</u> you decide to pursue it.

It's just how it's <u>going</u> to be.

There is no compromize ... no slacking up ... if I want to know something about you, about your perspectives, or about your body ... the only acceptable response, is that you tell me. No holding back, no bullshit — I'll know if you do either — I need to <u>know</u> from the start, you're willing to spread yourself open for me ... completely.

Well...are you?

These are words on paper — the <u>only</u> way I can communicate with you — —— but they <u>can</u> mean a lot.

You initiated this with me; so as far as I'm concerned, the "<u>burden of proof</u>" so to speak, is on <u>you</u>.

Show me I can trust you ... and you really <u>do</u> want to pursue this in a serious + open way. Once I see <u>that</u> in you, I'll feel much more comfortable in following you where <u>you</u> wish to go. (As long as it <u>doesn't</u> involve any of my cases, charges, convictions ... all of which are under appeal.)

You mention "honesty" ... "reasoning" ... Baby, I don't give a fuck what ANYBODY outside of my family + a very small group of friends — think. Couldn't care less, in fact.

Trying to explain thing's, or get the TRUTH out, is something I gave up on, long, long ago.

The TRUTH means <u>nothing</u> ... the shiteaters + vultures twist, add and delete, in order to further sensationalize and freak-ify me and my family. Fuck em <u>All</u>!

<u>Where</u> did you learn of my situation?

<u>What</u> did you read, see, hear about it?

<u>What</u> caught your attention, and prompted you to write to me?

You have an interest in the "Bizarre"?

Me <u>too</u>!!

<u>How</u> "Bizarre" do you like to get?

...maybe a little bondage? ... S&M? ... do you know about Pony-Boys and Pony-Girls?

I get some interesting materials in here from time to time. If you'd like I can share some of it with you (?) ... as long as I know you're up to it! That is. Are you, Jenny? Are you 'up' to it? ☺

S-H-O-W M-E!!!

I have no idea what you may consider "Bizarre". Your idea of "Bizarre", and mine, <u>may</u> be much different. Fair statement?

Have you had any experiences you'd call "Bizarre"? If so, maybe you'd tell me about it/them (?). I'd like that ... seeing that you're willing to let me get to <u>know</u> you.

I have some older, pre-arrest photos I could send you, as we go along. Would you like that?

Letters & photos are about all you can send me here.

But I <u>do</u> like seeing photos ... especially if <u>you're</u> in them!!!

Would you send me some?

Hey ... Jen-Jen ... I'll show you mine, if you'll show me yours!! ☺

You mention "kids" ... where's Dad?

I'd rather <u>not</u> get off on this about your kids and all, until I get a <u>much</u> better understanding of you. Maybe you'll run the "<u>Basics</u>" by me?

Something I <u>would</u> like to know concerning your kids... Did you nurse them, when they were little ... or were they Bottle-Babies?

Nursing fascinates the hell out of me.

If you nursed them, tell me about it (?).

<u>Where</u> did you <u>usually</u> nurse them?

How old were you with the <u>first</u> one?

What did you usually think about, as you nursed them? ... as they sucked milk from your nipples?

How did it <u>feel</u>?

Did you see any physical differences, in your nipples from <u>before</u> you nursed ... <u>while</u> you nursed ... <u>now</u>?

Did nursing permanantly change/alter the physical appearance of your nipples?

Talk to me Jenny ... tell me...

... did you ever let <u>someone else</u> taste your milk?

Did <u>you</u> taste it? What did it taste like, to you? I'll leave it at that, for now. Let's see how you do with that!! ☺

Do you have a good imagination, Jen?

That is a quality I very much treasure ... a <u>good</u> imagination.

How about we find out, just how good a one you have?

Let's say ... you can snap your fingers, and poof, there I am, right now, in front of you.

Snap!!! ... there I am, seeing you through my 46 year old eyes ... from my almost a decade in a cage perspective...

... Now <u>what</u>?

Try it first, from <u>my</u> perspective ... see you, through <u>my</u> eyes ... tell me what I see as I look at you, <u>right now</u>. Tell me true ... <u>what</u> do you think happens.

Then, see the same scenario through <u>your</u> eyes, and your perspectives. Tell me what <u>you</u> see, think, expect to happen. And tell me, <u>what</u> happens next.

Would you Jenny ... right now, the mood you're in ... would you? Would you be the "curious" little thing you claim to be? What would you be <u>most</u> curious about, concerning me?

Let your "unconventional" mind go ... turn it loose ... let me see the <u>real</u> you!

C'mon Baby ... open-up ... let me have a little taste of "Bizarre", according to Jenny. ☺ I'd like that!

First, I'd like you to describe yourself to me, in extreme detail ... from head to toe. Skip nothing. **N-O-T-H-I-N-G**...okay?

Be sure to include the following ... Height; weight; measurements (including cup size); how long your hair is; what's your natural and current hair color; color of your eyes; Are your ears pierced, and if so, how many holes in each; Any other piercings or tattoos; and I'd also like to know what you think is your best feature ... as well as what I would think is your best feature, if I saw you stripped down.

(You like Bizarre, Kitten ... we can do Bizarre!! ☺)

Something else you may like to know about me ... I am completely fascinated with "FIRSTS" in your life ... sexually speaking.

I will, no doubt, get around to asking you about them ... or, you can start to tell me about them now, on your own.

Don't wimp-out on me Jen ... I mean, tell me **IN DETAIL** ... what happened, where it happened, who it was with, what you thought & felt, as it was happening.

I know you remember your "FIRSTS" ... and I'd very much like to start to hear about them ... in as much detail as you're able to use.

(Have you tasted your own sex juices? Don't lie to me, Jenny ☺
Did you like the way you taste? Are you as SWEET as I think you are?)

There are so many things I'd like to ask, and get to know about you.

If you're still interested, when you write back, start to **SHOW ME** you're interested. **SHOW ME** your taste for — The Bizarre! ☺

I hope you've enjoyed my letter ... and it has had the desired affect on you (?). If so, you can tell me about it (the affect, I mean) in your next letter.

Keep I mind, I say and ask what I do, because I truly <u>would</u> like to get to know you and I want to hear the responses.

The quickest way to put a stop to any communications between us, is to skip-over something I ask or say ... that clearly requires a response from you.

I absolutely **HATE** to repeat myself.

So please, keep that in mind next time you write ... and skip nothing.

DON'T GET SCARED ... NOW ! ☺

See what you can do with my letter ... and let's get this started ... "if" you're serious about doing it with with me ... I mean (?).

Write when you can ... no big hurry. I know how busy little ones can keep you.

Sincerely,

"X"

PS: One last question for you, before I go ... Do <u>you</u> have any interesting "Toys"? If so, tell me about them/it . If I was to peak into the drawer you keep your bra's & panty's in, **what** would surprise me — **most**? Do you like the color Blue? ... Sapphire Blue, in particular? That's my favorite color. What's yours? Do you own anything, in Sapphire Blue?

❖   ❖   ❖   ❖

May 20, 97

Jenny,

Your very short 2nd letter arrived about a week ago. I was sorry to see you don't write long letters, or respond to <u>all</u> that needed responding to — in mine to you.

I tend to write very long letters, and unless I get the same in return, it tends not to work-out very well.

May I suggest you go back to my first letter, and respond to **ALL** that requires a response?

It also concerns me, that you don't seem to understand, I cannot & will not go anywhere near my legal situation, cases, charges, etc ...

Having explained this once, I won't do so again.

Listen Baby ...

... you <u>sound</u> like one I would be willing to make time for in my writing.

This time of year, due to heat & humidity, my writing is pretty much limited to the cooler, morning hours. If you wish to be one of the very few I write to — in any <u>meaningful fashion</u> ... show me!

Get caught-up on your letter-debt, and we'll see what happens.

Please ... don't make me repeat myself, and respond to what I ask you about. Fair enough?

I like it that you have a "Toy" (vibrator).

Next time you write, Draw/Outline it for me on one of the pages of your letter ... and tell me more/all about exactly how you use it, and how it feels <u>best</u>. Do you like **PENETRATION**, or does the **clitoral stimulation** get it done for you ... Jen-Jen?

Does your "Toy" have a name?

If not, I'd like you to call it "------EEEE", if you would (?). Think you could do that? ... name it after me like "------EEEE", when it makes you cum? I'd <u>like</u> that.

Go back to my first letter, and respond to everything in it. Fix this Jenny, and let's move <u>forward</u> ... yes? ☺

Have you seen me before?

Enclosing a photo so you can put a face to the name. Hope you <u>like</u> it. Almost 10 years ago ... and I guess all that time in this hell-hole has taken a toll.

Nothing about a month of good food, good sleep, lots of Sun & exercise ... and plenty of Jenny-Pussy wouldn't fix, anyway. ☺

If you don't want the photo, send it back to me, and I'll not send more.

Naturally, I'd like very much to see you, as well. You have **long** legs, don't you Mooky!

Even if you need them returned ... send them so I can <u>see</u> you. If you tell me to return them, I will. You have my word on that. I'd just like to see you so I can put a face & form to you.

Do you have a camera? If so, what kind?

That's it for now, till I see your response to this letter. I'm already so far ahead in pages written ... I don't wish to <u>add</u> to my lead.

Let me know what you want to do ...

"X"

PS...How long is your hair?

✦ ✦ ✦ ✦

June 10, 97

Hey Kitten

... Just a short note ...

Hoping to <u>see</u> some photos of you ... when you can find the time to send em! ☺ I bet you have some great legs on you, don't ya Sweety!! Looking forward to seeing them, and all the Sweetness they lead to ! "X"

I hope you took my last long letter as it was intended, and are either working on a response covering **ALL** I had in my first letter to you ... Or, that such a letter is en route, as I write this!! Can't think of **ANYTHING** about you, that I wouldn't love to know, and hear about. N-U-T-T-I-N, Honey! ☺

... Here's hoping you're up to it.

For now, that's really about it, till I hear from you on thing's. (What are you wearing, right now? ... underneath? ... I mean, actually **touching** you in your sweetest, most secret places??? Hmmmmmm....)

Later,
"X"

Jenny,

So ... what happened ? ☺

... CHICKEN ??? ☺

July 14, 97

✦ ✦ ✦ ✦

July 15, 97

Jenny,

Your letter arrived yesterday. I've been thinking about it a lot. Wanted to let you know a couple of thing's.

To start ... I'm really sorry to see our communicating and my getting to know you as I'd like to ... is linked to my supplying you with material to "print" (?) my letters. Not surprised ... but yeah ...sorry.

Listen Jen-Jen ... and maybe you'll understand ... <u>if</u> I wanted to put something out there, I'd write it myself. The offers to "print" have been coming in since the 4th day after I was arrested.

I have — for many reasons — <u>no</u> inclination to do that. **NONE**.

At least you're honest and up front about your intentions. And I appreciate that. However, I wouldn't feel comfortable knowing thing's of a personal nature I write — TO <u>YOU</u>, may end up in the public domain, somehow.

Maybe I'm wrong, but I see the potential and possibility of much FRUSTRATION in trying to get to know you. After 10 years of <u>this</u>, I don't tend to react very well to <u>more</u> FRUSTRATION in my life. I certainly get enough of that in day to day existence in this nut-house.

So ... I guess this is <u>it</u>. Hey ... I gave it a shot ... and missed.

It goes like that, sometimes...........I guess.

I'm probably not a lot different — most of the time — from most of the men you know ... "IF" they could throw off their shackles, and be 'REAL'.

I'll go ahead and scratch you out of my book. That way, I won't see your name in the future and write to you in a <u>moment of weakness.</u>

Take care of yourself Jenny. No hard feelings,

"X"

  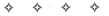

July 29, 97

Jennifer,

I've been thinking about your last note ..... thought I'd try <u>one more time</u>, to see how serious you are about communicating, by suggesting — once again — that you go back to my letters and <u>RESPOND</u> to <u>ALL</u> in them, that needs to be responded to.

This "back and forth banter" is a waste of time and energy, leading <u>nowhere</u>. I have niether the time to waste, nor the inclination to waste it, in that manner!

It's too <u>HOT</u> for this!!!

Listen to me Jen-Jen ...

...<u>if</u> we're going to communicate and get to know each other, this is going to go how I know it must.

You also owe me a photo!!!

Ya know Kitten, you contacted me ... I didn't contact you.

You're going to do it my way; or, we just aren't going to do it ... period. Do you understand?

This will be the last time I **TRY** to communicate this with you, unless you SHOW me you're going to do it RIGHT.

I want at least one photo of you wearing something minimal ... preferably more than one ... **front and back** views.

And, you need to go back and respond to all that was in my first coupla letters, that needs to be responded to.

I don't mean to get shitty ... really, I don't.

But my writing time is very valuable to me, and believe it or not, I have a LOT of people to write to ... who don't want to publish my letters.

No ... I don't want my letters in a book.

And NO ... **I'm** not "chicken"!

I am however, tired of wasting my time and energy, writing this kind of letter. You sound like a little pussy-cat I'd be interested in getting to know ... but you best make up your mind now, if you're going to do it ... and do it RIGHT.

Comprende Chiquita? ☺

"X"

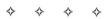

You wrote to me under false pretenses.

Ignore the letter enclosed [above] that I had written and was sending out tonight ... when our letter (also enclosed) arrived.

Keep your photo.

Keep your letters, and **don't** write to me again.

I'm not interested in my name **EVER** coming up in **ANYTHING** connected to you. Not the Internet (And I **do** know a lot of true friends who use the Net.) ... and certainly **not** in any fucking book!!!

I'm telling you in a "friendly" way here .... do **NOT** play fast & loose with my name.

Don't make me have to have people I know in Seattle look you up and explain the error of your ways to you ... Do you understand?

I want my photo RETURNED to me ... something else you obtained under false pretenses.

I'm sure you have plenty of morons more than willing to let you High-Light them ... I'm **NOT** one of them. And you need to realize I'm **not**.

"Mr. Y"

Dear Jenny,

In a place like this, one can only dwell on the Christmases I used to know. Such heartfelt memories never fail to put a lump in my throat and a smile on my face. But one thing I still can do, is pass on a wish for others to experience the unity of love, peace, & happiness, both now & into the new year.

Yes it's true, I don't know you, but I do wish all this for you & your 2 precious children.

Thank you for taking time out of your comfort zone to reach into my world.

With Respect,

"Y"

✧   ✧   ✧   ✧

2-19-97

Dear Jenny,

I was surprised to hear from you again. I truly thought you had changed your mind about having contact + communication.

Yes I see you found out how strict our prison mailroom is with such things as addresses, etc.

OK, now to get down to business with a response to your letters. Jenny it would really give me some comfort and peace of mind if we could get to know more about each other before we cover some of the heavy areas you desire to discuss. Whether you believe it or not, you are hearing from the true me. There are no split personalities etc. But you are correct, when I was out there in society, I was living 2 different lives in my behavior. It was a very sad situation.

Now Jenny the first thing that needs to occur here, is for you to put aside that book you read on me, any bias + personally passed judgment towards me, and give me a chance. Please get to know me from our communications. That book is not even close to being accurate as an account of my life of criminal behavior, or life over-all. It was written soley from State witnesses (mainly cops + prostitutes). Myself, + those from my camp, such as Attorneys, Private

302

Investigators, or Defense Witnesses, had no contact or involvement with that author or his book.

Keep in mind something here, too this very day I have never talked too, or been interviewed by police or media about the case period. I never will. I don't believe in doing so. One would have to be a fool to do so. Neither are my friend, and neither would have my best interest in mind. Plus, I have never taken the witness stand in the W------- case. Nobody <u>but</u> <u>myself</u> knows what I actually did, didn't do, or why. But I will say this, I in no way condone my criminal behavior either. I stand in utter shame and deserve to be in prison for the rest of my life. I can not, nor will I even attempt to justify, excuse, or ignore how I have come to be in this serious situation. One truly has to give an accounting for their actions. Whenever society is harmed the injury needs to be repaired. When the rights of others are violated, they need to be restored and protected for the future. I'm a firm believer that punishment serves to restore the common good as long as it reformation type punishment. In other words, restorative justice or legalized vengeance by the way of the Death Penalty. Whether viewed by others as right or wrong, state sanctioned killing is not reformation type punishment. I realize this may seem out of character coming from a convicted killer, but yes, I personally oppose the Death Penalty of today. And no, not because I'm one facing possible execution. I do not fear death nor the method used to snuff me out. However, being here in this sad situation, I've had the blessed freedom to spend countless hours studying into this entire issue Biblically, Philosophically, Politically, + otherwise. As for whatever my fate will be, I am ready to face it. I have long since made my peace with both my God + myself. I know what + who I am + not, and that's what counts for me.

Jenny I'm trusting blindly that you truly desire to be in contact as a type of friend out of genuine concern, with no hidden agenda, etc. Is this accurate? Due to the gravity of what I'm facing + my over-all situation, it is a must that you share honestly, openly + up-front with me at all times — as I will with you. Putting trust in people is one of my weak areas, so please be patient with me ok. I've received mail from numerous information + curiosity seekers over the coarse of time, to be everything , but a friend. I'm open to friendship and helping others, but I'm not open to work with anyone to be studied, analyzed, or cited for a report, article, book, etc., for their own personal gain $$ wise. I'm trusting you are not one of these kinds of people.

Anyway do I understand right that you are married, have 2 children, enjoy life, but have it in your heart to do certain things? What kind of things? Tell it to me as it really is. You say in your letter — "Ask me anything about myself", well Jenny I'm sure I'll have plenty of questions as we continue to share. One thing that would help for both of us is if we could put a face together with our communications. I recently had some photos taken of myself. Are you willing to send me a photo of yourself, etc.?

By the way, in your letter you said thank-you for not sending vile letters. Help me understand something here, in your thoughts before any contact with me, did you 1/2 expect to receive such a letter? Jenny I'm a fairly intelligent individual + very caring. Even in my current sad situation I find enough quality to my life to keep hanging in there and try to be helpful to others around me. Yes I've done vile things in my life to get here, but that's as far as it goes. I've received plenty of hate mail, but I never respond back with such. I hurt to much inside myself to be hateful back.

Well I best rap this up and get it sent. So until I hear from you again, thanks for answering my mail.

With Respect,

"Y"

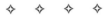

4-8-97

Hi Jenny

Actually I was hoping I'd hear from you before I wrote this letter. I mean so I at least know you still desire to communicate. Anyway this letter is in further response of your (3-15-97) letter.

That letter started out with — "You so much as admitted your guilt in the murders of all those women." Jenny whether I had taken life or not never was a question. You see, here's something the D.A. didn't want the public to know. Before trial, I met with my attorney and relayed to him what occured, what didn't occur, and why. I've always been a person who was willing to own up to and accept responsibility for my own actions. So I asked my attorney to tell me what I was legally guilty of by Law. He told me it was either Intentional Murder or Felony Murder. But not Aggravated Murder. I told him ok, would you please take all this and meet with both the Judge + the D.A. Tell them what you told me. And tell them I'm not asking for any deals, just that I want to plead guilty to what you told me I was responsible for. Nothing more, nothing less. This all occured in the Judge's Chambers. The Judge told the D.A. he should accept this and that it would be the best way to resolve things. But since the D.A. is not bound by what the Judge recommends, the D.A. said "no", I'm out for Mr. Y's blood, + I'm going to get it. So we went to trial in the M-------- case. The D.A. went for the Death Penalty, but the jury said no. I was give a life sentence. So the D.A. went for the Death Penalty again in the M case. That time the jury chose the Death Penalty. So no Jenny, I'm not trying to impress you. It's called being open + honest. Their's numerous things the D.A. never wanted the public nor my jury to know. That's why I now wish that I could have taken the witness stand.

By the way, the only reason I can live with myself, is because I have forgiven myself. But it was a long + hard process for me. Life is so precious.

Another thing you said in your letter that I want to respond too — "I don't know why some men hate certain women, especially prostitutes, but maybe it isn't just that they are prostitutes...just easily accessible targets..." None of this was the basis for my actions. And if we do in fact visit, it would be the proper forum for such intense sharing. So far, you only write about once a month. And each time I hear from you I wonder if I'll hear from you again. I guess it's because I've never been able to grasp whether you truly desire to befriend me and understand things, my life, + who I am, or whether you simply wanted to see what I'd have to say in contrast to that book, + then fade away.

I'd love to talk on the phone if you're willing. In your letter you said — "Meanwhile, ask me about anything you may be curious about". Well yes I have many questions + curiosities, but as you may have noticed, I haven't felt free to do so. Your letters are not very long or revealing so I figured for now if you wanted me to know or understand something about you, you'd share it as you desired. This thing about trust goes both ways you know.

I was saddened to hear about that case in your area of that 7 yr. old. Also the Port Angeles case of the father taking the lives of his 2 children. Have you ever tried to understand such cases where the parent take's the live of their own offspring? Heavy stuff!

Before I close, I thought I'd share a little something. On (3-31-97) I was standing up to my cell bars watching both rain + hail pound down outside. It was fascinating to watch old Mother nature do her thing. When it subsided, I went back to my radio + put my headphones on. A news broadcast broke in + announced that I-5 south of Wilsonville (which is near here) had a 30-car pile-up due to this same rain + hail storm. I thought it was rather amazing to think about in contrast how the storm was such a neat thing to gaze upon for me, yet it was misery and a harmful mess for others. Life is so eventful + impacting isn't it?

Well Jenny I best close + hit my sack so I can check out the backside of my eyelids. Write soon ok?

With Respect,
"Y"

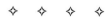

4-13-97

Dear Jenny,

Maybe you had a change of heart about writing. If so, I will certainly honor it. I thought I'd at least write this letter, + if I did hear from you then I would proceed from there.

By the way, if I shouldn't have sent that holiday card, then I apologize. I merely wanted to express some seasonal greetings regardless of the fact that we didn't know each other.

Yes I would like very much to correspond with you if you're willing. I'm sure we could learn from each other if given the chance, and keep an open mind. Your letter sounded sincere, are you? There's plenty I wanted to respond to from your letter. But I didn't want to share on such personal + sensitive issues unless we really were going to correspond for real. Over the coarse of time I've encountered a few information + curiosity seekers for their own hidden agenda + gain. By a few things you stated in your letter it didn't seem like you were that kind of person so I chose to trust you with a reply. I'm sure you can understand, due to the gravity of what I'm facing and my over-all situation, why I'd be cautious.

Thank-you again for your letter + I hope to hear from you soon.

Take Care,
"Y"

(P.S.) I've never been in your area (the Puget Sound) but it certainly sounds wonderful by your letter.

7-27-97

Dear Jenny,

You haven't heard from me because it seems you haven't been honest with me, starting with your very first letter. In my very first letter to you, I related to you that I don't cater to cops, media, analyst's, <u>+ writers</u>. Curiosity seekers + those with hidden agenda's have nothing coming from me. Either you want to become a true friend or you don't. Your letters don't reflect friendship, they have been mainly business + non-personal. You told me in your 1st letter that your weren't a judge or a journalist, which was not being up-front + honest. A journalist is one who is a writer — whether for book's, articles in periodicals, etc. Employed or unemployed as such, is immaterial. Your letters were always short + unrevealing from your end, yet you sought to gain information from me. You told me "they" wouldn't let you send me a photo. I don't know who "they" is, but why would you let a false statement like that fall out. I can receive photos from any person. Jenny I am only interested in open + honest communication. If you can't be such, then don't expect further communication with me. Even for you to visit me requires you to supply your full name, address, phone number, Soc. Sec. No., Birth date, + much more. So if you were trying to play me for information, yet keep the real you unknown, then you should simply write to others — not me. I have been nothing but open + honest with you. I don't play people anymore. My life, your life, etc., are too precious, + time too short to play such games. I'm a very serious + mature thinking individual.

Your most recent letter asked permission to copy or publish my letters previously written to you. The answer is <u>absolutely not</u>!! I wrote to you, not the world.

Jenny you received the kind of letters you did from me because I'm one who serves God now, not man, my former lusts + sinful thinking etc. I am a brother in Christ to those who are genuine believers. Anyway you take what I said here + think on it awhile. If you are being genuine with me, then why no photo, why not have a chat on the phone just for starters. I found it very peculiar that you'd tell me in your letters to ask you anything, yet when I did, you never answered back on it.

It's Your Call,

Sincerely,
"Y"...

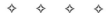

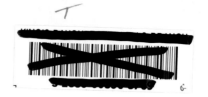